Gene Polymorphism and Nutrition: Relationships with Chronic Disease

Gene Polymorphism and Nutrition: Relationships with Chronic Disease

Editors

Daniel-Antonio de Luis Roman
Ana B. Crujeiras

MDPI • Basel • Beijing • Wuhan • Barcelona • Belgrade • Manchester • Tokyo • Cluj • Tianjin

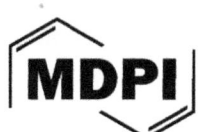

Editors
Daniel-Antonio
de Luis Roman
Hospital Clínico
Universitario de Valladolid,
Valladolid, Spain

Ana B. Crujeiras
Instituto de Investigación
Sanitaria de Santiago (IDIS),
Complejo Hospitalario
Universitario de Santiago
(CHUS/SERGAS)
and CIBERobn,
A Coruña, Spain

Editorial Office
MDPI
St. Alban-Anlage 66
4052 Basel, Switzerland

This is a reprint of articles from the Special Issue published online in the open access journal *Nutrients* (ISSN 2072-6643) (available at: https://www.mdpi.com/journal/nutrients/special_issues/gene_polymorphism_nutrition).

For citation purposes, cite each article independently as indicated on the article page online and as indicated below:

LastName, A.A.; LastName, B.B.; LastName, C.C. Article Title. *Journal Name* **Year**, *Volume Number*, Page Range.

ISBN 978-3-0365-7770-8 (Hbk)
ISBN 978-3-0365-7771-5 (PDF)

© 2023 by the authors. Articles in this book are Open Access and distributed under the Creative Commons Attribution (CC BY) license, which allows users to download, copy and build upon published articles, as long as the author and publisher are properly credited, which ensures maximum dissemination and a wider impact of our publications.

The book as a whole is distributed by MDPI under the terms and conditions of the Creative Commons license CC BY-NC-ND.

Contents

Daniel Antonio de Luis Roman, David Primo, Olatz IZaola, Emilia Gómez and Juan Jose López
Adiponectin Gene Variant rs3774261, Effects on Lipid Profile and Adiponectin Levels after a High Polyunsaturated Fat Hypocaloric Diet with Mediterranean Pattern
Reprinted from: *Nutrients* **2021**, *13*, 1811, doi:10.3390/nu13061811 1

Germán Alberto Nolasco-Rosales, José Jaime Martínez-Magaña, Isela Esther Juárez-Rojop, Thelma Beatriz González-Castro, Carlos Alfonso Tovilla-Zarate, Ana Rosa García, et al.
Association Study among Comethylation Modules, Genetic Polymorphisms and Clinical Features in Mexican Teenagers with Eating Disorders: Preliminary Results
Reprinted from: *Nutrients* **2021**, *13*, 3210, doi:10.3390/nu13093210 13

Zhen Zhang, Xuena Yang, Yumeng Jia, Yan Wen, Shiqiang Cheng, Peilin Meng, et al.
Vitamin D and the Risks of Depression and Anxiety: An Observational Analysis and Genome-Wide Environment Interaction Study
Reprinted from: *Nutrients* **2021**, *13*, 3343, doi:10.3390/nu13103343 27

José Ignacio Martínez-Montoro, Isabel Cornejo-Pareja, Ana María Gómez-Pérez and Francisco J. Tinahones
Impact of Genetic Polymorphism on Response to Therapy in Non-Alcoholic Fatty Liver Disease
Reprinted from: *Nutrients* **2021**, *13*, 4077, doi:10.3390/nu13114077 43

Liana Najjar, Joshua Sutherland, Ang Zhou and Elina Hyppönen
Vitamin D and Type 1 Diabetes Risk: A Systematic Review and Meta-Analysis of Genetic Evidence
Reprinted from: *Nutrients* **2021**, *13*, 4260, doi:10.3390/nu13124260 59

Ricardo Usategui-Martín, Daniel-Antonio De Luis-Román, José María Fernández-Gómez, Marta Ruiz-Mambrilla and José-Luis Pérez-Castrillón
Vitamin D Receptor (*VDR*) Gene Polymorphisms Modify the Response to Vitamin D Supplementation: A Systematic Review and Meta-Analysis
Reprinted from: *Nutrients* **2022**, *14*, 360, doi:10.3390/nu14020360 75

Jinyoung Shon, Yerim Han and Yoonjung Park
Effects of Dietary Fat to Carbohydrate Ratio on Obesity Risk Depending on Genotypes of Circadian Genes
Reprinted from: *Nutrients* **2022**, *14*, 478, doi:10.3390/nu14030478 85

Karina dos Santos, Eliane Lopes Rosado, Ana Carolina Proença da Fonseca, Gabriella Pinto Belfort, Letícia Barbosa Gabriel da Silva, Marcelo Ribeiro-Alves, et al.
FTO and ADRB2 Genetic Polymorphisms Are Risk Factors for Earlier Excessive Gestational Weight Gain in Pregnant Women with Pregestational Diabetes Mellitus: Results of a Randomized Nutrigenetic Trial
Reprinted from: *Nutrients* **2022**, *14*, 1050, doi:10.3390/nu14051050 105

Gemma Rodriguez-Carnero, Paula M. Lorenzo, Ana Canton-Blanco, Leire Mendizabal, Maddi Arregi, Mirella Zulueta, et al.
Genetic Variants in Folate and Cobalamin Metabolism-Related Genes in Pregnant Women of a Homogeneous Spanish Population: The Need for Revisiting the Current Vitamin Supplementation Strategies
Reprinted from: *Nutrients* **2022**, *14*, 2702, doi:10.3390/nu14132702 123

Claudia Vales-Villamarín, Jairo Lumpuy-Castillo, Teresa Gavela-Pérez, Olaya de Dios, Iris Pérez-Nadador, Leandro Soriano-Guillén and Carmen Garcés
Sex-Dependent Mediation of Leptin in the Association of Perilipin Polymorphisms with BMI and Plasma Lipid Levels in Children
Reprinted from: *Nutrients* **2022**, *14*, 3072, doi:10.3390/nu14153072 . . . . **135**

Article

Adiponectin Gene Variant rs3774261, Effects on Lipid Profile and Adiponectin Levels after a High Polyunsaturated Fat Hypocaloric Diet with Mediterranean Pattern

Daniel Antonio de Luis Roman *, David Primo, Olatz IZaola, Emilia Gómez and Juan Jose López

Center of Investigation of Endocrinology and Nutrition, Department of Endocrinology and Investigation, Medicine School, Hospital Clinico Universitario, University of Valladolid, 47005 Valladolid, Spain; dprimoma@saludcastillayleon.es (D.P.); oizaolaj@saludcastillayleon.es (O.I.); egomezho@saludcastillayleon.es (E.G.); jlopezgo@saludcastillayleon.es (J.J.L.)
* Correspondence: dluisro@saludcastillayleon.es; Tel.: +34-9-8342-0000

Abstract: The role of *ADIPOQ* gene variants on metabolic improvements after weight change secondary to different hypocaloric diets remained unclear. We evaluate the effect of rs3774261 of *ADIPOQ gene* polymorphism on biochemical improvements and weight change after high polyunsaturated fat hypocaloric diet with a Mediterranean dietary pattern for 12 weeks. A population of 361 obese subjects was enrolled in an intervention trial with a calorie restriction of 500 calories over the usual intake and 45.7% of carbohydrates, 34.4% of fats, and 19.9% of proteins. The percentages of different fats was; 21.8% of monounsaturated fats, 55.5% of saturated fats, and 22.7% of polyunsaturated fats. Before and after intervention, an anthropometric study, an evaluation of nutritional intake and a biochemical evaluation were realized. All patients lost weight regardless of genotype and diet used. After 12 weeks with a similar improvement in weight loss (AA vs. AG vs. GG); total cholesterol (delta: −28.1 ± 2.1 mg/dL vs. −14.2 ± 4.1 mg/dL vs. −11.0 ± 3.9 mg/dL; $p = 0.02$), LDL cholesterol (delta: −17.1 ± 2.1 mg/dL vs. −6.1 ± 1.9 mg/dL vs. −6.0 ± 2.3 mg/dL; $p = 0.01$), triglyceride levels (delta: −35.0 ± 3.6 mg/dL vs. 10.1 ± 3.2 mg/dL vs. −9.7 ± 3.1 mg/dL; $p = 0.02$), C reactive protein (CRP) (delta: −2.3 ± 0.1 mg/dL vs. −0.2 ± 0.1 mg/dL vs. −0.2 ± 0.1 mg/dL; $p = 0.02$), serum adiponectin (delta: 11.6 ± 2.9 ng/dL vs. 2.1 ± 1.3 ng/dL vs. 3.3 ± 1.1 ng/dL; $p = 0.02$) and adiponectin/leptin ratio (delta: 1.5 ± 0.1 ng/dL vs. 0.3 ± 0.2 ng/dL vs. 0.4 ± 0.3 ng/dL; $p = 0.03$), improved only in AA group. AA genotype of *ADIPOQ variant* (rs3774261) is related with a significant increase in serum levels of adiponectin and ratio adiponectin/leptin and decrease on lipid profile and C-reactive protein (CRP).

Keywords: adiponectin; dietary intervention; insulin resistance; obesity; rs3774261

1. Introduction

The pandemic of obesity has been termed "globesity" to remark the global nature of the problem. Lifestyle modifications with a low-calorie diet produce weight loss and the secondary improvement of many of the components of associated comorbidities, including hyperlipidemia, diabetes mellitus type 2, hypertension, and inflammatory markers [1]. Now, adipose tissue has been considered an important cornerstone endocrine organ secreting several adipokines implied in the regulation of metabolism and energy status. Some adipokines have a proinflammatory role as leptin and resistin and other groups such as adiponectin has an anti inflammatory function [2]. Adiponectin is the most important adipokine secreted by this tissue [3]. Adiponectin has an anti-inflammatory role and its levels are reduced in obese subjects and are enhanced after weight reduction [4]. Low adiponectin levels have been related with a high risk of obesity, diabetes mellitus, and hyperlipidemia [5], with a potential therapeutic effect with agonists of adiponectin [6].

The adiponectin levels are highly heritable, and the *ADIPOQ* gene is the principal locus promoting variations in serum levels [7]. Single nucleotide polymorphisms (SNPs)

are genetic variants that can sometimes have functional implications in the *ADIPOQ* gene, which is situated on chromosome 3q27. One of these SNPs, 712 G/A rs3774261 in the *ADIPOQ* has been related to diabetes mellitus in obese subjects [7] and with coronary heart disease [8,9]. Interestingly, this genetic variant has been associated with eating behavior [10], and there are nutritional intervention studies [11,12], too. These interventional designs [11,12] reported significant results on serum lipid profile and inflammatory markers. Our previous study with a Mediterranean diet [11] had a lower percentage of fat in the diet than the current intervention and low sample size; with this new study, we will evaluate more precisely the effect of the quantity and quality of fat in a larger sample of patients. Perhaps the metabolic effects found in these studies and their relationship with this genetic variation are due to both factors; weight loss and the Mediterranean diet pattern used. The beneficial effects of a diet with a Mediterranean style can be due to the presence of different foods and nutrients such as type of dietary unsaturated fatty acids [13]. Unsaturated fatty acids are ligands for the transcription factor PPAR gamma [14], which increases *ADIPOQ* gene expression and improves adiponectin concentration [15]. Perhaps increasing the amount of unsaturated fat in a hypocaloric diet would have greater benefits than a conventional hypocaloric diet and rs3774261 would modulate these changes. In previous studies [11,12], the beneficial effects found with the Mediterranean diet were related to the high consumption of olive oil, and therefore, of monounsaturated fatty acids. Notwithstanding that the polyunsaturated fatty acids may also play a relevant role and interact with this genetic variant of the ADIPOQ gene, this hypothesis has not yet been evaluated.

Given this lack of information, we conducted a study to evaluate the effects of a high polyunsaturated fat hypocaloric diet with a Mediterranean style during 12 weeks on metabolic changes considering the rs3774261 of *ADIPOQ*.

2. Subjects and Methods

2.1. Subjects and Clinical Investigation

Obese subjects were enrolled by the primary care physicians of our health area to treat obesity. These subjects were evaluated in a single-arm clinical trial with a high fat polyunsaturated hypocaloric diet with a dietary Mediterranean pattern. The local ethics committee (Hospital Clinico Universitario Valladolid committee 7/2017, code: GRS588/A/11) approved the protocol; it was in accordance with the guidelines laid down in the Declaration of Helsinki and all subjects gave written informed consent. Clinical and biochemical variables were recorded at the beginning and after 12 weeks of dietary interventions. All the enrolled obese subjects met the following inclusion criteria; age between 30 and 60 years old and an obesity category as a body mass index (BMI) $\geq$ 30 kg/m^2. The exclusion criteria were any of the following data: previous cardiovascular event, chronic renal failure, chronic liver failure, alcoholism, malignant tumor, and within the 24 weeks before the study were taking any medications or nutrient-supplements or have been on a low-calorie diet.

The main objective of our study was serum adiponectin change after 12 weeks versus baseline. The secondary objectives were improvements in lipid profile and glucose metabolism after dietary intervention. Lipid profile (LDL-cholesterol, HDL-cholesterol, triglycerides, and total cholesterol), C-reactive protein (CRP), insulin, and adipokines (resistin leptin and total adiponectin) levels were analyzed. Homeostasis model assessment (HOMA-IR) and adiponectin/leptin ratio were calculated, too. The anthropometric evaluation was realized with body weight, height, waist circumference, fat mass by bioimpedance, and calculated body mass index (BMI). Systolic and diastolic blood pressure was recorded. All clinical and biochemical parameters were determined at the basal time and after 3 months of dietary intervention. The genetic variant rs3774261 of the *ADIPOQ* gene was assessed.

2.2. Dietary Intervention

A total of 361 obese patients met the above-mentioned criteria, and they were included to observe a hypocaloric diet for 12 weeks. The diet (high-polyunsaturated fatty acid hypocaloric diet Mediterranean diet) was based on a calorie restriction of 500 calories over the usual intake, 45.7% of carbohydrates, 34.4% of fats, and 19.9% of proteins. The percentages of different fats were: 21.8% of monounsaturated fats, 55.5% of saturated fats, and 22.7% of polyunsaturated fats (13 g per day of w-6 fatty acids, 3 g per day of w-3 fatty acids, and a ratio w6/w3 of 4.3).

Food tables were used with a Mediterranean dietary style, including (legumes, vegetables, and fresh fruit 5 servings per day, poultry, whole grains, fish 3 times per week, using 20 g olive oil per day, 40 g of walnuts daily, and limit unhealthy fats such as margarine, fatty meats, snacks, industrial pastries) [16]. To improve compliance with dietary intervention, the completion of diet recommendations was evaluated every 10 days with a phone call. Records of daily dietary intake for 4 days were parameterized with software (Dietosource®, Geneva, Switzerland), and this software is based on national composition food tables [15]. The recommendations for physical activity were aerobic physical activities at least 3 times each week (60 min each). The physical activity allowed by protocol were (cycling, running, walking, and swimming). Each patient with a self-reported questionnaire recorded the physical activity.

2.3. Biochemical Parameters

Blood samples were drawn after a minimum of 10 h overnight and these samples were stored at $-80\ °C$ until analyzed. Lipid profile (low-density lipoprotein (LDL)-cholesterol, high-density lipoprotein (HDL)-cholesterol, triglycerides, and total cholesterol), C reactive protein (CRP), fasting glucose, and insulin levels were determined on the same day using the clinical chemistry automated analyzer COBAS INTEGRA 400 analyzer (Roche Diagnostic, Montreal, Canada). LDL cholesterol was calculated using the Friedewald formula (LDL cholesterol = total cholesterol-HDL cholesterol-triglycerides/5) [17]. Insulin resistance was calculated using the homeostasis model assessment (HOMA-IR) with the following equation (glucosexinsulin/22.5) [18].

Serum adipokines were measured by enzyme-linked immunosorbent assays (ELISA). Resistin kit had with a normal range of 4–12 ng/mL [19] (Biovendor Laboratory, Inc., Brno, Czech Republic). The leptin kit had a normal range of 10–100 ng/mL (Diagnostic Systems Laboratories, Inc., Webster, TX, USA) [20]. Finally, the adiponectin kit had a normal range of 8.65–21.43 ng/mL (R&D Systems, Inc., Minneapolis, MN, USA) [21]. Adiponectin/leptin ratio was calculated in all samples.

2.4. Genotyping ADIPOQ Gene

The genotype of SNP rs3774261 of *ADIPOQ* was determined with a polymerase chain reaction in real-time from peripheral blood leucocytes. Genomic DNA was obtained from a 150 uL buffy coat using a blood genomic kit (Bio-Rad®, Hercules, CA, USA) in accordance with the manufacturer's instructions. Probes and oligonucleotide primers and were designed with the Beacon Designer 5.0 (Premier Biosoft International®, LA, CA, USA). The polymorphic region of adiponectin was amplified using the polymerase chain reaction (PCR) with 50 ng of this genomic DNA, with allele-specific sense primers (primer forward: 5'-ACGTTGGATGCTCCTCCTTGAAGCCTTCAT-3' and reverse 5'-ACGTTGGATGCAAGTATTCAAAGTATGGAGC-3' in a 2 µL final volume (Termocicler Life Technologies, LA, CA, USA). Cycling parameters were as follows: after DNA denaturation at $95\ °C$ for 1 min and annealing at $65\ °C$ for 30 s. The PCR was run in a 25 µL final volume containing 10.5 µL of IQTM Supermix (Bio-Rad®, Hercules, CA, USA) with hot start Taq DNA polymerase. Duplicates in the arrays were the methodology to internal controls and the accuracy. Hardy Weinberg equilibrium was determined with a statistical test (Chi-square) to compare our expected and observed counts. The variant was in Hardy Weinberg equilibrium ($p = 0.31$).

2.5. Anthropometric Parameters and Blood Pressure

Bodyweight, height, and waist circumference (WC) were determined in the morning before breakfast at baseline and after 3 months. Body mass index was determined by the equation (weight in kg divided by the height in meters squared). Bodyweight was determined with a scale (Omron, LA, CA, USA), and the obese subjects were minimally unclothed to the nearest 0.1 kg and not wearing shoes (Omron, LA, CA, USA). Fat mass was estimated by bioimpedance (Akern, EFG, Pisa, Italy) with an accuracy of 50 g [22]. WC was measured with a measuring tape in the narrowest diameter between the xiphoid process and iliac crest. Systolic and diastolic blood pressures were measured three times and averaged after a 5 min rest with a random zero mercury sphygmomanometer, (Omron, LA, CA, USA).

2.6. Statistical Analysis

We used the software SPSS for Windows, version 23.0 software package (SPSS Inc. Chicago, IL, USA) to analyze the data. The sample size was determined to assess changes over 5 ng/mL of adiponectin levels with 90% power and 5% significance ($n = 300$). Results were expressed as average ± standard deviation. Each variable was evaluated for normality with the Kolmogorov–Smirnov test. The parametric test was investigated with the ANOVA test and Bonferroni post hoc test. Non-parametric parameters were evaluated with the Mann-Whitney U-test. Categorical variables were revised with the chi-square test, with Yates correction as necessary, and Fisher's test. The gene–diet interaction was assessed with a univariate ANCOVA adjusted by gender, and baseline weight. Correction for multiple hypotheses testing for single SNP analyses was performed. A Chi-square test was used to determine the Hardy–Weinberg equilibrium. A p-value < 0.05 was considered significant.

2.7. Ethical Approval

All methodology of our study were in accordance with the ethical standards of the institutional and/or national research committee (Hospital Clinico Universitario Valladolid committee 7/2017, code: GRS588/A/11) and with the 1964 Helsinki declaration and its later amendments or comparable ethical standards. Informed consent was signed from all individual participants included in the study.

3. Results

3.1. Characteristics of Participants and Dietary Intakes

We evaluated the role of SNP rs3774261 on the modification of adiposity markers and biochemical variables in 361 obese outpatients. The average age of the sample was 47.1 ± 3.1 years (range: 29–63) and the average body mass index (BMI) was 37.3 ± 4.9 kg/m^2 (range: 33.5–49.9). Sex distribution was 259 females (71.7%) and 102 males (28.3%). The genotype distribution of this sample was as follows: 117 patients (32.4%) AA, 164 patients AG (45.4%), and 80 patients GG (22.2%). Allelic frequency was 0.62 A and 0.38 G. Sex distribution and the average age was similar in all genotype groups (Table 1).

Following the sessions of the dietitian, the dietary recommendations were reached at 12 weeks in all genotype groups with a significant decrease of total caloric amount, carbohydrates, fats and proteins (Table 1). A significant increase was observed in the percentage of monounsaturated and polyunsaturated fats (Table 1).

At basal time, the physical activity was similar in the three groups (Table 1). In addition, after the intervention, the physical activity improved, but this improvement did not show differences in total quantity deltas (AA vs. AG vs. GG) (28.2 ± 1.2 min/week vs. 29.8 ± 2.1 min/week vs. 29.1 ± 1.1 min/week; $p = 0.52$).

Table 1. Changes in anthropometric parameters, dietary intakes, and physical activity rs3774261 (mean ± S.D).

	AA (n = 117)		AG (n = 164)		AG (n = 80)		p Time AA Time AG Time GG Basal Genotype 12 weeks Genotype
	0 time	At 12 weeks	0 time	At 12 weeks	0 time	At 12 weeks	
Age	46.3 ± 4.1	-	47.3 ± 4.0	-	46.9 ± 2.3	-	$p = 0.46$ Basal genotype
Gender/male/female%	76.1/23.9%	-	73.2/26.8%	-	71.7/28.3%	-	$p = 0.43$ Basal genotype
BMI	37.9 ± 4.1	35.9 ± 3.8 *	37.8 ± 4.0	36.1 ± 3.4 *	38.0 ± 2.0	36.3 ± 2.9 *	$p = 0.01$ $p = 0.02$ $p = 0.01$ $p = 0.46$ $p = 0.43$
Weight (kg)	96.4 ± 2.1	92.4 ± 3.0 *	97.5 ± 2.1	93.1 ± 1.4 *	97.3 ± 2.1 *	93.4 ± 2.2 *	$p = 0.01$ $p = 0.01$ $p = 0.02$ $p = 0.45$ $p = 0.11$
Fat mass (kg)	39.8 ± 2.1	36.4 ± 2.0 *	39.7 ± 2.0	36.0 ± 2.1 *	39.8 ± 2.0 *	36.2 ± 1.1 *	$p = 0.02$ $p = 0.03$ $p = 0.03$ $p = 0.39$ $p = 0.31$
WC (cm)	113.1 ± 7.0	109.2 ± 5.2 *	113.4 ± 6.1	109.1 ± 4.1 *	116.2 ± 4.0 *	111.7 ± 3.9 *	$p = 0.03$ $p = 0.04$ $p = 0.02$ $p = 0.35$ $p = 0.59$
SB (mmHg)	127.1 ± 5.1	123.2 ± 6.0 *	127.8 ± 5.0	122.3 ± 4.1 *	126.2 ± 4.0 *	123.1 ± 3.1 *	$p = 0.02$ $p = 0.03$ $p = 0.02$ $p = 0.33$ $p = 0.41$
DB (mmHg)	81.5 ± 4.1	79.3 ± 3.1	81.7 ± 5.1	79.1 ± 6.0	78.7 ± 4.1	78.7 ± 3.1	$p = 0.41$ $p = 0.42$ $p = 0.51$ $p = 0.49$ $p = 0.61$
Energy intake (cal day)	1739.2 ± 129.2	1439.1 ± 119.2	1801.7 ± 113.1	1503.1 ± 112.2	1718.9 ± 112.1	1489.1 ± 123.1	$p = 0.01$ $p = 0.02$ $p = 0.01$ $p = 0.48$ $p = 0.46$
Carbohydrates (g/day)	181.9 ± 14.1	159.1 ± 19.1	192.7 ± 13.2	148.1 ± 13.2	179.7 ± 11.1	149.1 ± 10.1	$p = 0.02$ $p = 0.03$ $p = 0.02$ $p = 0.41$ $p = 0.39$
Fat (g/day)	61.5 ± 4.1	53.3 ± 3.2	79.7 ± 4.1	50.1 ± 7.2	76.9 ± 3.9	49.9 ± 4.1	$p = 0.01$ $p = 0.01$ $p = 0.02$ $p = 0.33$ $p = 0.37$
Protein (g/day)	84.5 ± 5.1	75.1 ± 9.2	86.7 ± 2.1	76.2 ± 7.2	88.0 ± 2.1	77.1 ± 8.1	$p = 0.02$ $p = 0.02$ $p = 0.03$ $p = 0.60$ $p = 0.49$
Monounsaturated fat (%)	34.5%	55.5%	34.9%	55.0%	35.1%	55.1%	$p = 0.02$ $p = 0.03$ $p = 0.01$ $p = 0.37$ $p = 0.48$

Table 1. Count.

	AA (n = 117)		AG (n = 164)		AG (n = 80)		
Polyunsaturated fat (%)	13.4%	22.7%	13.8%	22.0%	14.0%	23.0%	p = 0.02 p = 0.03 p = 0.04 p = 0.41 p = 0.42
Saturated fat (%)	52.1%	21.8%	53.5%	23.0%	50.9%	21.9%	p = 0.01 p = 0.02 p = 0.03 p = 0.38 p = 0.43
Physical activity (min/week)	121.1 ± 12.3	149.3 ± 21.1	123.1 ± 9.9	152.0 ± 23.2	122.1 ± 7.2	151.9 ± 18.1	p = 0.11 p = 0.22 p = 0.34 p = 0.30 p = 0.33

BMI: body mass index. SB: Systolic blood pressure. DB: Diastolic blood pressure WC: Waist circumference. (*) $p < 0.05$, in each genotype group. No differences between genotype groups.

3.2. Anthropometric Results

For rs3774261, there were no statistical differences in anthropometric parameters and systolic/diastolic blood pressure in basal and post-intervention values (AA vs. AG vs. GG) (Table 1). After a high polyunsaturated fat hypocaloric diet with a Mediterranean style, we observed a significant improvement of body mass index, weight, waist circumference, fat mass, and systolic blood pressure. These statistically significant changes were similar in all genotype groups. Diastolic blood pressure remained unchanged.

3.2.1. Biochemical Parameters

In the second analysis of our design, we evaluated the actions of this dietary intervention on glucose metabolism, C Reactive protein and lipid profile (Table 2). After a significant body weight loss (AA vs. AG vs. GG); insulin levels (delta: -3.7 ± 0.2 UI/L vs. -3.8 ± 0.3 UI/L vs. -3.6 ± 0.2 UI/L; $p = 0.33$) and HOMA-IR (delta: -1.3 ± 0.2 units vs. -1.2 ± 0.3 units vs. -1.1 ± 0.4 units; $p = 0.36$) improved in all genotypes without intergroup differences. Finally, after 12 weeks (AA vs. AG vs. GG); total cholesterol (delta: -28.1 ± 2.1 mg/dL vs. -14.2 ± 4.1 mg/dL vs. -11.0 ± 3.9 mg/dL; $p = 0.01$), LDL cholesterol (delta: -17.1 ± 2.1 mg/dL vs. -6.1 ± 1.9 mg/dL vs. -6.0 ± 2.3 mg/dL; $p = 0.01$), triglyceride levels (delta: -35.0 ± 3.6 mg/dL vs. 10.1 ± 3.2 mg/dL vs. -9.7 ± 3.1 mg/dL; $p = 0.03$) and C reactive protein (CRP) (delta: -2.3 ± 0.1 mg/dL vs. -0.2 ± 0.1 mg/dL vs. -0.2 ± 0.1 mg/dL; $p = 0.01$) improved only in the AA group.

3.2.2. Adipokine Levels

Table 3 reports changes on serum adipokines and ratio adiponectin/leptin. After dietary intervention, in the AA genotype group (AA vs. AG vs. GG), serum adiponectin (delta: 11.6 ± 2.9 ng/dL vs. 2.1 ± 1.3 ng/dL vs. 3.3 ± 1.1 ng/dL; $p = 0.01$) improved. Adiponectin/leptin ratio improved in the AA genotype group (delta: 1.5 ± 0.1 ng/dL vs. 0.3 ± 0.2 ng/dL vs. 0.4 ± 0.3 ng/dL; $p = 0.02$). In all genotype groups, leptin decreased in a significant way. Serum resistin levels did not change after the dietary intervention.

Table 2. Biochemical parameters rs3774261 (mean ± S.D).

	AA (n = 117)		AG (n = 164)		AG (n = 80)		p Time AA Time AG Time GG Basal Genotype 12 weeks Genotype
	0 time	At 12 weeks	0 time	At 12 weeks	0 time	At 12 weeks	
Glucose (mg/dL)	102.1 ± 7.0	99.3 ± 7.1	101.5 ± 7.1	99.9 ± 5.1	101.1 ± 5.1	98.9 ± 4.1	$p = 0.16$ $p = 0.19$ $p = 0.30$ $p = 0.45$ $p = 0.34$
Total ch. (mg/dL)	204.1 ± 7.2	186.3 ± 4.2 *	208.7 ± 3.5	196.7 ± 6.0	205.1 ± 3.1	194.3 ± 7.2	$p = 0.01$ $p = 0.22$ $p = 0.30$ $p = 0.41$ $p = 0.31$
LDLch. (mg/dL)	127.3 ± 6.1	110.3 ± 7.2 *	129.1 ± 4.3	123.1 ± 8.2	127.1 ± 4.1	121.1 ± 9.1	$p = 0.01$ $p = 0.32$ $p = 0.31$ $p = 0.35$ $p = 0.51$
HDL-ch. (mg/dL)	52.8 ± 3.1	50.6 ± 4.0	51.9 ± 3.0	50.1 ± 2.1	52.3 ± 3.0	51.1 ± 3.1	$p = 0.21$ $p = 0.32$ $p = 0.39$ $p = 0.25$ $p = 0.41$
TG (mg/dL)	128.9 ± 11.1	93.1 ± 10.4 *	131.1 ± 6.2	121.1 ± 10.8	129.8 ± 4.2	123.9 ± 9.3	$p = 0.03$ $p = 0.32$ $p = 0.30$ $p = 0.29$ $p = 0.31$
Insulin (mUI/L)	13.1 ± 2.0	9.4 ± 1.9 *	13.3 ± 2.1	9.5 ± 1.1 *	12.7 ± 3.0	9.1 ± 3.0 *	$p = 0.01$ $p = 0.02$ $p = 0.01$ $p = 0.45$ $p = 0.39$
HOMA-IR	3.3 ± 0.6	2.0 ± 0.3 *	3.4 ± 0.5	2.1 ± 0.4 *	3.1 ± 0.2	1.8 ± 0.9 *	$p = 0.01$ $p = 0.02$ $p = 0.02$ $p = 0.35$ $p = 0.41$
CRP (mg/dL)	5.1 ± 1.0	3.8 ± 0.8 *	5.0 ± 2.9	4.9 ± 2.1	5.1 ± 3.1	5.0 ± 3.2	$p = 0.01$ $p = 0.42$ $p = 0.41$ $p = 0.55$ $p = 0.19$

Total Ch: Cholesterol. TG: Triglycerides LDL-ch: Low density lipoprotein cholesterol, HDL-ch: High density lipoprotein cholesterol. CRP: c reactive protein. HOMA-IR: Homeostasis model assessment. LDL: low density lipoprotein, HDL: High density lipoprotein. (*) $p < 0.05$, in each group. No statistical differences among genotypes in basal time or after 12 weeks. See significant deltas in the text.

Table 3. Serum levels of adipocytokines (mean ± S.D).

	AA (n = 117)		AG (n = 164)		AG (n = 80)		p
	0 time	At 12 weeks	0 time	At 12 weeks	0 time	At 12 weeks	Time AA Time AG Time GG Basal Genotype 12 weeks genotype
Adiponectin (ng/mL)	10.0 ± 3.1	21.6 ± 3.2 *	12.3 ± 3.3	14.4 ± 4.7	12.0 ± 2.8	15.5 ± 4.2	$p = 0.01$ $p = 0.12$ $p = 0.31$ $p = 0.45$ $p = 0.11$
Resistin (ng/mL)	5.1 ± 2.0	5.0 ± 1.6	5.2 ± 2.1	5.1 ± 1.1	5.3 ± 3.9	5.1 ± 3.2	$p = 0.31$ $p = 0.32$ $p = 0.41$ $p = 0.45$ $p = 0.33$
Leptin (ng/mL)	49.1 ± 9.1	12.9 ± 7.3 *	42.0 ± 7.1	22.1 ± 6.1 *	46.8 ± 4.2	19.4 ± 4.1 *	$p = 0.01$ $p = 0.02$ $p = 0.03$ $p = 0.41$ $p = 0.31$
Ratio Adiponectin/leptin	0.2 ± 0.1	1.7 ± 0.3 *	0.3 ± 0.2	0.6 ± 0.3	0.3 ± 0.2	0.7 ± 0.3	$p = 0.02$ $p = 0.33$ $p = 0.34$ $p = 0.41$ $p = 0.51$

(*) $p < 0.05$, in each group with basal values. No statistical differences among genotypes in basal time or after 12 weeks. See significant deltas in the text.

4. Discussion

We revealed, in this study on a high-polyunsaturated fat hypocaloric diet with a Mediterranean dietary pattern, a decline in LDL-cholesterol, triglycerides, and C reactive protein (CRP) and a rise in serum adiponectin levels and adiponectin/leptin ratio that were statistically significant in obese subjects with the AA genotype of rs3774261. In addition, all subjects in all genotype groups showed a significant decline of adiposity parameters and systolic blood pressure after dietary intervention.

In the literature, some investigations have shown the relationship between this genetic variant (rs3774261) on *ADIPOQ* gene and obesity, metabolic syndrome, diabetes mellitus, and serum adiponectin levels [23,24], with an increased risk to present type 2 diabetes, obesity, and hypoadiponectinemia in a non-Caucasian population [24,25]. In addition to this association with high cardiovascular risk pathology, the G allele of rs3774261 *ADIPOQ* has also been related to coronary heart disease [8]. The exact pathways by which genetic variants in the *ADIPOQ* gene produce coronary heart disease is not well known. Moreover, adiponectin, the adipokine encoded by this gene, has been reported to have anti-inflammatory properties that have important effects in fighting against atherosclerosis [26].

There is little information in the literature about the effect of nutritional treatment and this genetic variant. A recent study with a normal hypocaloric Mediterranean diet reported [11] better changes in lipid profile, CRP, and adiponectin levels in subjects with AA genotype compared in a dominant model with (AG + GG). This previous study [11] had a small sample size (n = 135) and a separate analysis of the three genotypes could not be performed. In another design with 284 Caucasian obese subjects [12] reported that after a high-fat hypocaloric diet, the response of lipid levels, CRP, and adiponectin was better on AA genotype than GA or GG genotypes, as our present results. The amount of lipid profile improvement was similar in both studies [11,12] and our present study; however, the rise in adiponectin levels and the decline in CRP was two times greater in the study with a high-fat diet [12] than in the other one [11]. In addition, these changes in lipids and CRP are of a similar magnitude to those found in the current study with a high-polyunsaturated fat hypocaloric diet. The caloric restriction was similar in these three studies, about 500 calories to the previous intake. Although both strategies were carried out with a Mediterranean diet pattern, it is important to remark that in the last study [12] and the present study, the percentage of fat in the diet was higher than the old one; 38% [12] and 34% (current) vs. 25% [11]. In our investigation, patients reached a daily intake of almost 30 g of monounsaturated fat and 16 of polyunsaturated fat, compared to 14 g and 3.6 g [11], and 25 g and 13 g [12], respectively.

This relationship of the quality of dietary fats with the biochemical changes due to weight loss and its interaction with this genetic variate of the ADIPOQ gene could be explained with some findings in the literature with other SNPs in this gene. For example, Alsahel et al. [27] showed that the genetic variant (-1006G/A) increased serum adiponectin after a high-monounsaturated diet, whereas in A-allele carriers it is decreased. This differential response was not detected with a low-fat hypocaloric diet. Moreover, the molecular mechanism could be related to the potential action of dietary unsaturated fat as ligands of PPAR gamma. The role of polyunsaturated fatty acids is being evaluated in the literature, and more intervention studies are recommended with known doses of fatty acids to evaluate their effect on adipokines [28]. In addition, this metabolic way could explain our findings on inflammatory status with CRP levels. The NF-kB pathway in the endothelium, which would produce CRP; was inhibited by adiponectin [29], for example, adiponectin contributes more powerfully to CRP elevation than for example smoking habit, age, and other metabolic parameters [29].

It seems clear in the literature that this genetic variance is related to a pro-inflammatory status, not only related to ischemic heart disease [8] but also with ischemic stroke patients [30]. In our interventional design, the response of insulin resistance was similar in all genotypes. Moreover, some studies have reported that patients carrying the A allele have better insulin sensitivity demonstrated by the euglycemic clamp [31]. The response of triglycerides found in our trial may also be important since the association between rs3774261 and coronary heart disease [8] was influenced by interactions with serum triglycerides [8]. We must not forget the differentiated response of adiponectin levels as a function of genotype found in our study to explain our metabolic findings. A novelty finding in our study was the association of this genetic variant with the adiponectin/leptin ratio and its secondary modifications to the diet. The adiponectin/leptin ratio is a biomarker of adipose tissue dysfunction and inflammation [32], which related leptin as an adipokine related to the degree of adiposity [33]. Moreover, an adiponectin/leptin quotient higher than the unit is considered as normal whereas a ratio below or near to 0.5 units may show an increase in the metabolic risk [34], as reported by the three genotypes in our study before weight loss and near to 0.5 in GA and GG genotypes after dietary intervention.

In addition to the relationship between inflammatory pathways and adiponectin response to explain our findings, unknown genetic mechanisms may also be implicated. The rs3774261 variant is in an intron located, a non-coding region. Moreover, the genetic variant in non-coding regions may alter gene splicing, transcription product binding, mRNA deterioration, and gene expression. Thus, any of these above-mentioned mechanisms can be possible pathways to explain our findings. For example, with different levels of adiponectin circulating in a case-control study, a relationship of the G allele of this genetic variant with the prevalence of metabolic syndrome was found [35]. All these relationships are complicated by the existence of a relevant role of adiponectin at the level of the central nervous system in the pathways of hunger and satiety. Recently it has been observed that the rs3774261 variant is related to disinhibition in eating behaviors [10] influencing daily total food uptake.

There are some limitations of this study. First, we only evaluated one SNP of ADIPOQ, so other variants could be related to metabolic parameters. Moreover, some synthetic associations of specific unusual variants may be in partial linkage disequilibrium with usual variants as rs3774261. Second, the lack of a control group without diet might be a bias. It might provide more valuable information on the relationship of ADIPOQ *variants* (rs3774261) with metabolic parameters if the comparative study was conducted on an unrelated control population. Third, the self-reported dietary intake of energy and macronutrients is not reliable and it might include bias of under-or over-reporting. Finally, we studied a Caucasian population, and extrapolation to other populations is not possible.

5. Conclusions

In conclusion, the AA genotype of the *ADIPOQ variant* (rs3774261) is related to a significant increase in serum levels of adiponectin and ratio adiponectin/leptin and decrease in the lipid profile and C-reactive protein (CRP) after a hypocaloric high polyunsaturated fat Mediterranean diet.

Author Contributions: D.A.d.L.R. and J.J.L. designed the study and realized statistical analysis; O.I. and E.G., anthropometric status and monitoring of dietary intake; D.P. performed biochemical evaluation and genotype studies. All authors have read and agreed to the published version of the manuscript.

Funding: This research did not receive any specific grant from funding agencies in the public, commercial, or not-for-profit sectors.

Institutional Review Board Statement: The study was conducted according to the guidelines of the Declaration of Helsinki, and approved by the Institutional Review Board (or Ethics Committee) of Hospital Clinico Universitario Valladolid committee 7/2017, code: GRS588/A/11).

Informed Consent Statement: Informed consent was obtained from all subjects involved in the study.

Conflicts of Interest: All authors have no conflict of interest.

References

1. Klein, S. Outcome Success in Obesity. *Obes. Res.* **2001**, *9*, 354S–358S. [CrossRef] [PubMed]
2. Yang, W.-S.; Chuang, L.-M. Human genetics of adiponectin in the metabolic syndrome. *J. Mol. Med.* **2005**, *84*, 112–121. [CrossRef] [PubMed]
3. Weyer, C.; Funahashi, T.; Tanaka, S.; Hotta, K.; Matsuzawa, Y.; Pratley, R.E.; Tataranni, P.A. Hypoadiponectinemia in obesity and type 2 diabetes: Close association with insulin resistance and hyperinsulinemia. *J. Clin. Endocrinol. Metab.* **2001**, *86*, 1930–1935. [CrossRef] [PubMed]
4. Ouchi, N.; Kihara, S.; Arita, Y.; Maeda, K.; Kuriyama, H.; Okamoto, Y.; Hotta, K.; Nishida, M.; Takahashi, M.; Nakamura, T.; et al. Novel modulator for endotelial adhesion molecules: Adipocyte-derived plasma protein adiponectin. *Circulation* **1999**, *100*, 2473–2476. [CrossRef]
5. Vasseur, F.; Meyre, D.; Froguel, P. Adiponectin, type 2 diabetes and the metabolic syndrome: Lessons from human genetic studies. *Expert Rev. Mol. Med.* **2006**, *8*, 1–12. [CrossRef]
6. Berg, A.H.; Scherer, P.E. Adipose Tissue, Inflammation, and Cardiovascular Disease. *Circ. Res.* **2005**, *96*, 939–949. [CrossRef]
7. Cesari, M.; Narkiewicz, K.; De Toni, R.; Aldighieri, E.; Williams, C.; Rossi, G.P. Heritability of Plasma Adiponectin Levels and Body Mass Index in Twins. *J. Clin. Endocrinol. Metab.* **2007**, *92*, 3082–3088. [CrossRef] [PubMed]
8. Kanu, J.S.; Gu, Y.; Zhi, S.; Yu, M.; Lu, Y.; Cong, Y.; Liu, Y.; Li, Y.; Yu, Y.; Cheng, Y.; et al. Single nucleotide polymorphism rs3774261 in the AdipoQ gene is associated with the risk of coronary heart disease (CHD) in Northeast Han Chinese population: A case-control study. *Lipids Health Dis.* **2016**, *15*, 1–11. [CrossRef]
9. Apalasamy, Y.D.; Rampal, S.; Salim, A.; Moy, F.M.; Bulgiba, A.; Mohamed, Z. Association of ADIPOQ gene with obesity and adiponectin levels in Malaysian Malays. *Mol. Biol. Rep.* **2014**, *41*, 2917–2921. [CrossRef]
10. Rohde, K.; Keller, M.; Horstmann, A.; Liu, X.; Eichelmann, F.; Stumvoll, M.; Villringer, A.; Kovacs, P.; Tönjes, A.; Böttcher, Y. Role of genetic variants in ADIPOQ in human eating behavior. *Genes Nutr.* **2014**, *10*, 1. [CrossRef] [PubMed]
11. De Luis, D.A.; Primo, D.; Izaola, O.; Gómez, E.; Bachiller, R. Serum Lipid and Adiponectin Improvements after a Mediterranean Dietary Pattern in Non-G-Allele Carriers of the Variant rs3774261. *Lifestyle Genom.* **2020**, *13*, 164–171. [CrossRef]
12. De Luis, D.A.; Primo, D.; Izaola, O.; Bachiller, R. Role of the variant rs37774261 of ADIPOq gene on cardiovascular risk factors and adipoencton levels after a high fat hypocaloric diet with Mediterranean Pattern. *Cardiol. Cardiovasc. Med.* **2021**, *5*, 1–16.
13. Mancini, J.G.; Filion, K.B.; Atallah, R.; Eisenberg MJMancini, J.G.; Filion, K.B.; Atallah, R.; Eisenberg, M.J. Systematic Review of the Mediterranean Diet for Long-Term Weight Loss. *Am. J. Med.* **2016**, *129*, 407–415. [CrossRef]
14. Maeda, N.; Takahashi, M.; Fiunahashi, T.; Kihara, S. PPArgamma ligands increase expression and plasma concentrations of adiponectin, and adipose derived protein. *Diabetes* **2001**, *50*, 2094–2096. [CrossRef] [PubMed]
15. Iwaki, M.; Matsuda, M.; Maeda, N.; Funahashi, T.; Matsuzawa, Y.; Makishima, M.; Shimomura, I. Induction of Adiponectin, a Fat-Derived Antidiabetic and Antiatherogenic Factor, by Nuclear Receptors. *Diabetes* **2003**, *52*, 1655–1663. [CrossRef] [PubMed]
16. Mataix, J.; Mañas, M. *Tablas de Composición de Alimentos Españoles*; University of Granada: Granada, Spain, 2003.

17. Friedewald, W.T.; Levy, R.I.; Fredrickson, D.S. Estimation of the Concentration of Low-Density Lipoprotein Cholesterol in Plasma, without Use of the Preparative Ultracentrifuge. *Clin. Chem.* **1972**, *18*, 499–502. [CrossRef]
18. Mathews, D.R.; Hosker, J.P.; Rudenski, A.S.; Naylor, B.A.; Treacher, D.F. Homeostasis model assessment: Insulin resistance and beta cell function from fasting plasma glucose and insulin concentrations in man. *Diabetologia* **1985**, *28*, 412–414. [CrossRef]
19. Pfützner, A.; Langenfeld, M.; Kunt, T.; Löbig, M.; Forst, T. Evaluation of human resistin assays with serum from patients with type 2 diabetes and different degrees of insulin resistance. *Clin. Lab.* **2003**, *49*, 571–576.
20. Suominen, P. Evaluation of an Enzyme Immunometric Assay to Measure Serum Adiponectin Concentrations. *Clin. Chem.* **2004**, *50*, 219–221. [CrossRef]
21. Khan, S.S.; Smith, M.S.; Reda, D.; Suffredini, A.F.; McCoy, J.P. Multiplex bead array assays for detection of soluble cytokines: Comparisons of sensitivity and quantitative values among kits from multiple manufacturers. *Cytom. B Clin. Cytom.* **2004**, *61*, 35–39. [CrossRef]
22. Lukaski, H.C.; Johnson, P.E.; Bolonchuk, W.W.; Lykken, G.I. Assessment of fat-free mass using bioelectrical impedance measurements of the human body. *Am. J. Clin. Nutr.* **1985**, *41*, 810–817. [CrossRef]
23. Wassel, C.L.; Pankow, J.S.; Jacobs, D.R., Jr.; Steffes, M.W.; Li, N.; Schreiner, P.J. Variants in the Adiponectin Gene and Serum Adiponectin: The Coronary Artery Development in Young Adults (CARDIA) Study. *Obesity* **2010**, *18*, 2333–2338. [CrossRef]
24. Ramya, K.; Ashok Ayyappa, K.; Ghosh, S.; Mohan, V. Radha Genetic Association of ADIPOQ Gene Variants with Type 2 Diabetes, Obesity and Serum Adiponectin Levels in South Indian Population. *Gene* **2013**, *32*, 253–262. [CrossRef] [PubMed]
25. Ezzidi, I.; Mtiraoui, N.; Ali, M.E.M.; Al Masoudi, A.; Abu Duhier, F. Adiponectin (ADIPOQ) gene variants and haplotypes in Saudi Arabian women with polycystic ovary syndrome (PCOS): A case—Control study. *Gynecol. Endocrinol.* **2019**, *36*, 66–71. [CrossRef] [PubMed]
26. Ouchi, N.; Kihara, S.; Arita, Y. Adiponectin and adipocyte-derived plasma protein, inhibits endothelial NFkappa B signaling through a C AMP dependent pathway. *Circulation* **2000**, *102*, 1296–1301. [CrossRef]
27. Alsaleh, A.; O´Dell, S.D.; Frost, G.S.; Griffin, B.A.; Lovegrove, J.A.; Jebb, S.A.; Sanders, T.A. RISK Study Group SNP at the DIPOQ gene locus interact with age and dietary intake of fat to determine serum adiponectin in subjects at risk of the metabolic syndrome. *Am. J. Clin. Nutr.* **2011**, *94*, 262–269.
28. Matsushita, K.; Yatsuya, H.; Tamakoshi, K.; Wada, K.; Otsuka, R.; Zhang, H.; Sugiura, K.; Kondo, T.; Murohara, T.; Toyoshima, H. Inverse association between adiponectin and C-reactive protein in substantially healthy Japanese men. *Atherosclerosis* **2006**, *188*, 184–189. [CrossRef]
29. Rausch, J.; Gillespie, S.; Orchard, T.; Tan, A.; McDaniel, J.C. Systematic review of marine-derived omega-3 fatty acid supplementation effects on leptin, adiponectin, and the leptin-to-adiponectin ratio. *Nutr. Res.* **2021**, *85*, 135–152. [CrossRef]
30. Li, S.; Lu, N.; Li, Z.; Jiao, B.; Wang, H.; Yang, J.; Yu, T. Adiponectin Gene Polymorphism and Ischemic Stroke Subtypes in a Chinese Population. *J. Stroke Cerebrovasc. Dis.* **2017**, *26*, 944–951. [CrossRef]
31. Specchia, C.; Scott, K.; Fortina, P.; Devoto, M.; Falkner, B. Association of a Polymorphic Variant of the Adiponectin Gene with Insulin Resistance in African Americans. *Clin. Transl. Sci.* **2008**, *1*, 194–199. [CrossRef] [PubMed]
32. Frühbeck, G.; Catalán, V.; Rodríguez, A.; Ramírez, B.; Becerril, S.; Salvador, J.; Colina, I.; Gómez-Ambrosi, J. Adiponectin-leptin Ratio is a Functional Biomarker of Adipose Tissue Inflammation. *Nutrients* **2019**, *11*, 454. [CrossRef] [PubMed]
33. Frühbeck, G.; Gómez-Ambrosi, J. Control of body weight: A physiologic and transgenic perspective. *Diabetologia* **2003**, *46*, 143–172. [CrossRef] [PubMed]
34. Frühbeck, G.; Catalán, V.; Rodríguez, A.; Gómez-Ambrosi, J. Adiponectin-leptin ratio: A promising index to estimate adipose tissue dysfunction. Relation with obesity-associated cardiometabolic risk. *Adipocyte* **2018**, *7*, 57–62. [CrossRef] [PubMed]
35. Wang, Q.; Ren, D.; Bi, Y.; Yuan, R.; Li, D.; Wang, J.; Wang, R.; Zhang, L.; He, G.; Liu, B. Association and functional study between ADIPOQ and metabolic syndrome in elderly Chinese Han population. *Aging* **2020**, *12*, 25819–25827. [CrossRef] [PubMed]

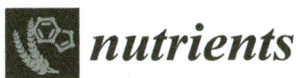

Article

Association Study among Comethylation Modules, Genetic Polymorphisms and Clinical Features in Mexican Teenagers with Eating Disorders: Preliminary Results

Germán Alberto Nolasco-Rosales [1], José Jaime Martínez-Magaña [2], Isela Esther Juárez-Rojop [1], Thelma Beatriz González-Castro [3], Carlos Alfonso Tovilla-Zarate [4], Ana Rosa García [5], Emmanuel Sarmiento [5], David Ruiz-Ramos [1], Alma Delia Genis-Mendoza [2,*] and Humberto Nicolini [2,*]

1. Biomedical Postgraduate Program, Academic Division of Health Sciences, Juárez Autonomous University of Tabasco, Villahermosa 86000, Mexico; ganr_1277@live.com.mx (G.A.N.-R.); iselajuarezrojop@hotmail.com (I.E.J.-R.); daruiz_914@hotmail.com (D.R.-R.)
2. Genomics of Psychiatric and Neurodegenerative Diseases Laboratory, National Institute of Genomic Medicine (INMEGEN), Mexico City 01090, Mexico; martinezmaganajjaime@gmail.com
3. Genomics Laboratory, Academic Division Jalpa de Mendez, Juárez Autonomous University of Tabasco, Jalpa de Mendez 86200, Mexico; thelma.glez.castro@gmail.com
4. Genomics Laboratory, Comalcalco Multidisciplinary Academic Division, Juárez Autonomous University of Tabasco, Villahermosa 86000, Mexico; alfonso_tovillaz@yahoo.com.mx
5. Children's Psychiatric Hospital "Dr. Juan N. Navarro", Mexico City 01090, Mexico; anarosagarciab@gmail.com (A.R.G.); emmanuelsarmientoh@hotmail.com (E.S.)
* Correspondence: adgenis@inmegen.gob.mx (A.D.G.-M.); hnicolini@inmegen.gob.mx (H.N.); Tel: +52-(53)-501900 (ext. 1196/1197) (A.D.G.-M. & H.N.)

Citation: Nolasco-Rosales, G.A.; Martínez-Magaña, J.J.; Juárez-Rojop, I.E.; González-Castro, T.B.; Tovilla-Zarate, C.A.; García, A.R.; Sarmiento, E.; Ruiz-Ramos, D.; Genis-Mendoza, A.D.; Nicolini, H. Association Study among Comethylation Modules, Genetic Polymorphisms and Clinical Features in Mexican Teenagers with Eating Disorders: Preliminary Results. *Nutrients* **2021**, *13*, 3210. https://doi.org/10.3390/nu13093210

Academic Editors: Daniel-Antonio de Luis Roman and Ana B. Crujeiras

Received: 9 July 2021
Accepted: 7 September 2021
Published: 15 September 2021

Publisher's Note: MDPI stays neutral with regard to jurisdictional claims in published maps and institutional affiliations.

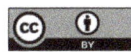

Copyright: © 2021 by the authors. Licensee MDPI, Basel, Switzerland. This article is an open access article distributed under the terms and conditions of the Creative Commons Attribution (CC BY) license (https://creativecommons.org/licenses/by/4.0/).

Abstract: Eating disorders are psychiatric disorders characterized by disturbed eating behaviors. They have a complex etiology in which genetic and environmental factors interact. Analyzing gene-environment interactions could help us to identify the mechanisms involved in the etiology of such conditions. For example, comethylation module analysis could detect the small effects of epigenetic interactions, reflecting the influence of environmental factors. We used MethylationEPIC and Psycharray microarrays to determine DNA methylation levels and genotype from 63 teenagers with eating disorders. We identified 11 comethylation modules in WGCNA (Weighted Gene Correlation Network Analysis) and correlated them with single nucleotide polymorphisms (SNP) and clinical features in our subjects. Two comethylation modules correlated with clinical features (BMI and height) in our sample and with SNPs associated with these phenotypes. One of these comethylation modules (yellow) correlated with BMI and rs10494217 polymorphism (associated with waist-hip ratio). Another module (black) was correlated with height, rs9349206, rs11761528, and rs17726787 SNPs; these polymorphisms were associated with height in previous GWAS. Our data suggest that genetic variations could alter epigenetics, and that these perturbations could be reflected as variations in clinical features.

Keywords: comethylation modules; genetic polymorphisms; eating disorders; WGCNA

1. Introduction

Eating disorders (EDs) are severe psychiatric disorders characterized by disturbances of eating behavior, affecting the health and quality of life of individuals. These disorders have an early teenage onset and a hereditary component [1]. EDs have a complex etiology in which genetic and environmental factors interact [2]. Genome-wide association studies (GWAS) and other genetic studies have revealed loci and single nucleotide polymorphisms (SNP) associated with ED [1,3,4]. The clinical characteristics of EDs have been associated in genetic studies. In this sense, significant genetic correlations have been reported in anorexia nervosa with psychiatric disorders, physical activity and metabolic, lipid and anthropometric traits [5]. In addition, genetic associations between ED and substance use have been described [6]. Additionally, the genetic-environment relationship in ED has been studied through DNA methylation, reporting perturbations in the methylation levels of some genes (*DRD2, SLC6A3, POMC, OXTR,* among others) [2,7,8]. However, genes do not function alone: on average, each gene is estimated to interact with another four or eight genes, and to be involved with 10 biological functions. Furthermore, recent studies suggest that gene networks provide the potential to identify hundreds of disease-related genes [9]. Analyzing gene-environment interactions in EDs could help us to identify the mechanisms involved in their etiology. Nowadays, new technologies evaluating thousands of genes apply statistic approaches that integrate different information sources from gene interactions (e.g., comethylation module construction) [10]. Comethylation modules are clusters of highly interconnected CpG sites. These modules are detected through the construction of a correlation network. Correlation networks are used to analyze large, high-dimensional data sets. These correlation networks are constructed on the basis of correlations among quantitative measurements (e.g., gene expression profiles, methylation levels) [11]. Comethylation modules are formed by using methylation data as quantitative measurements of gene-environment interactions [10]. Additionally, comethylation modules alleviate various testing problems which are inherent to microarray data analyses, and have been found to be useful for describing pairwise relationships among methylated genes [9–11]. In brief, comethylation modules (1) consider all genes as interconnected, (2) identify groups of CpG sites with similar methylation levels, (3) increase statistical power, and (4) detect small effects of epigenetic interactions [9–11]. Thus, evaluating correlations among genetic factors, comethylation modules, and clinical features in EDs could be a means by which to identify biological markers in such disorders. The objective of the present study was to detect comethylation modules from DNA methylation samples from children and teenagers with an ED, and to correlate these modules with clinical features and genetic variability.

2. Materials and Methods

2.1. Study Population

We included 63 subjects diagnosed with anorexia nervosa (AN), bulimia nervosa, (BN) or binge eating disorder (BED) using DSM 5 criteria [12]. Individuals were recruited in the outpatient center of the Children's Psychiatric Hospital "Dr. Juan N. Navarro" from May 2014 to August 2016. Inclusion criteria were subjects with at least three generations of Mexican lineage, 12–18 years of age, and individuals not using psychotropic or psychoactive drugs. The clinical features of the sample are described in Table 1.

Table 1. Clinical features of study population.

Features	Sample ($n = 50$)
Age (years)	13.98 ± 1.74
Gender	
Male	13 (26)
Female	37 (74)
Body Mass Index (BMI) zscore	1.03 ± 0.97
BMI classification	
Underweight	1 (2)
Normal weight	20 (40)
Overweight	11 (22)
Obesity	18 (36)
Diagnosis	
Binge eating disorder	17 (34)
Bulimia nervosa	22 (44)
Anorexia nervosa	11 (22)
Comorbidities	
Any	46 (92)

Table 1. *Cont.*

Features	Sample (*n* = 50)
Major depressive disorder	21 (42)
Suicide behavior	16 (32)
Dysthymia disorder	18 (36)
Attention-Deficit/Hyperactivity Disorder	15 (30)
Generalized Anxiety Disorder	10 (20)
Oppositional Defiant Disorder	6 (12)
Conduct Disorder	5 (10)
Psychotic Disorder	5 (10)
Eating Attitudes	
Fear of gain weight	35 (70)
Binge	34 (68)
Restriction	24 (48)
Vomit	21 (42)
Other behaviors	10 (20)

Features of subjects who satisfied inclusion criteria. Continuous variables are expressed as mean ± standard deviation. Categorical variables are expressed as *n* (%).

This study followed the principles of the Declaration of Helsinki. Sample recollection and processing were approved by the Ethics Committee of the Children's Psychiatric Hospital "Dr. Juan N. Navarro" with approval No. II3/01/0913 (11 October 2017), and by the Ethics Committee of the National Institute of Genomic Medicine (INMEGEN) with approval No. 06/2018/I.

2.2. Evaluation Instruments

BED was screened with the QEWP-R (Questionnaire on Eating and Weight Pattern-Revised) [13]. AN was screened with EAT-26 (Eating Attitudes Test) [14]. We evaluated the presence of psychiatric comorbidity with the Spanish version of MINI Kid (Mini International Neuropsychiatric Interview for Children and Adolescent) [15]. A pedopsychiatrist performed all ED diagnoses.

2.3. DNA Extraction and Microarray Analysis

After diagnostic evaluation of each individual, a blood sample was collected using an EDTA tube; DNA was subsequently extracted from this sample. We used the salting-out method from the Gentra Puregene Blood (Qiagen, Germantown, MD, USA) commercial kit. DNA extraction quality and integrity were evaluated by analysis with a NanoDrop spectrophotometer (Thermofisher, Waltham, MA, USA) and 2% agarose gel. DNA samples met the following quality criteria: visible genomic DNA band, 230/260 and 260/230 ratios >1.8, concentration >50 ng/µL, and no signs of DNA degradation. For genotypification, we hybridized DNA with commercial microarray Infinium Psycharray Beadchip (Illumina, San Diego, CA, USA). For methylation analysis, DNA was bisulfite converted using an EZ DNA Methylation Kit (Zymo Research, Irvine, CA, USA). Converted DNA was hybridized with the Infinium MethylationEPIC BeadChip (Illumina, San Diego, CA, USA). Each microarray was processed in the Microarray and Expression Unit of the National Institute of Genomic Medicine.

2.4. Quality Control of Genotypification Data

We transformed fluorescence intensities from the Psycharray into genotypes using the GenomeStudio (v. 2.0) software, and quality control was done with the PLINK (v. 1.9) toolset [16]. We eliminated: (1) SNPs with less than 95% genotype calls, (2) individuals with less than 95% genotype calls, (3) individuals with sex discrepancy, (4) SNPs located in chromosomes X and Y, (5) SNPs with less than 0.05 minor allele frequency (MAF), (6) SNPs deviating from Hardy-Weinberger equilibrium ($p < 1 \times 10^{-6}$), and (7) SNPs with A/T and C/G alleles. Subsequently, filtrated data were exported to the R (v. 4.0) software [17], and we removed SNPs with missing data and SNPs without homozygous individuals to minor alleles. Only 193,314 SNPs passed the quality control.

2.5. Quality Control of DNA Methylation Data

The fluorescence intensities of the MethylationEPIC microarray were transformed into *idat* files, which were filtered with ChAMP pipeline (v.2.18) [18] for R (v. 4.0) software. Quality control removed: (1) probes with detection *p*-value > 0.01, (2) probes with <3 beads in at least 5% of samples per probe, (3) non-CpG probes, (4) multihit probes, (5) probes located in chromosome X and Y, and (6) individuals with sex discrepancy in their genotypification data. We converted filtered methylation data into β-values, which were normalized using the BMIQ (Beta-Mixture Quantile Normalization) method [19]. Afterwards, we evaluated the presence of the batch effect with a singular value decomposition (SVD) method. We preserved CpG sites with standard deviation (SD) > 0.05, keeping 105,393 sites. Likewise, we made many cut points in SD (0.05, 0.06, 0.07, 0.08, 0.09, 0.10, 0.15, 0.20) to find an optimal point for the construction of comethylation modules.

2.6. Comethylation Modules Construction

In order to identify comethylation modules, we processed methylation values with the WGCNA (Weighted correlation network analysis) package [11,20] (R software). Later, we applied the means method to achieve hierarchical clustering, and eliminated individuals with atypical samples. For the final analysis, we only considered 50 subjects. Furthermore, an analysis of network topology was used to determine a soft-thresholding power less than 20 with suitable independence (>0.8) and mean connectivity (<1000). The CpG sites with SD > 0.06 in their methylation values had the best network topology. We applied *blockwiseModules* function (WGCNA package [11,20]) to detect comethylation modules, using a minimum module size of 175 and a threshold of 20. In a subsequent analysis, we discarded the CpG sites clustered in the grey module, and identified a new set of modules. The 11 constructed comethylation modules included 11,418 CpG sites. Each module was automatically assigned a color by WGCNA, indicating its size. The grey module was discarded from further analysis as it groups unassigned CpG sites to other modules; thus, these sites are unrelated.

2.7. Enrichment Analysis of Modules

The CpG sites inside modules were annotated using IlluminaHumanMethylationEPI-Canno.ilm10b4.hg19 package [21]. Genes of CpG sites were extracted and enriched using the WebGestalt online tool [22]. We accomplished the enrichments with Over-Representation Analysis of KEGG Database (Kyoto Encyclopedia of Genes and Genomes) [23]; this was considered to be significant with an adjusted *p*-value by FDR ≤ 0.05.

2.8. Correlation of Comethylation Modules with Clinical Features and SNPs

The eigengene of each comethylation module was correlated with clinical data and SNPs using Pearson's correlations. We calculated the R^2 and *p* values with *cor* and *corPvalueStudent* functions and set the significant value $p < 5 \times 10^{-3}$ for clinical data and $p < 5 \times 10^{-8}$ for SNPs. In order to find associations between SNPs and phenotypes, we used the PheWAS tool on the GWAS Atlas website [24]. Associations were considered to be significant for any phenotype with a $p < 1 \times 10^{-10}$.

3. Results

3.1. Description of Comethylation Modules

There were 11 modules in our study. Modules were turquoise (5073 sties), blue (2928 sites), brown (193 sites), yellow (166 sites), green (151 sites), red (150 sites), black (148 sites), pink (145 sites), magenta (135 sites), purple (111 sites), and grey (2218 sites). The CpG sites of these modules were located in 4005 genes. According to relative position to gene, the gene body was the most common annotated location, ranging from 40 sites

(56.34%) in the purple module to 2430 sites (69.27%) in the turquoise module. Table 2 shows the details of functional annotation of CpG sites from comethylation modules regarding gene location.

Table 2. Comethylation module CpG sites classification.

Module		TSS1500	TSS200	5′UTR	Body	1stExon	ExonBnd	3′UTR
Turquoise		359 (10.23)	97 (2.77)	436 (12.43)	2430 (69.27)	33 (0.94)	37 (1.05)	116 (3.31)
Blue		158 (7.85)	75 (3.72)	309 (15.34)	1366 (67.83)	23 (1.14)	16 (0.79)	67 (3.33)
Brown		14 (10.77)	4 (3.08)	23 (17.69)	78 (60.00)	2 (1.54)	3 (2.31)	6 (4.62)
Yellow		13 (12.15)	6 (5.61)	13 (12.15)	69 (64.49)	2 (1.87)	0 (0)	4 (3.74)
Green		11 (11.22)	3 (3.06)	13 (13.27)	68 (69.39)	1 (1.02)	1 (1.02)	1 (1.02)
Red		20 (18.52)	1 (0.93)	15 (13.89)	66 (61.11)	2 (1.85)	1 (0.93)	3 (2.78)
Black		11 (11.22)	2 (2.04)	9 (9.18)	66 (67.35)	2 (2.04)	2 (2.04)	6 (6.12)
Pink		13 (13.00)	2 (2.00)	9 (9.00)	71 (71.00)	2 (2.00)	1 (1.00)	2 (2.00)
Magenta		10 (11.36)	4 (4.55)	12 (13.64)	56 (63.64)	1 (1.14)	0 (0)	5 (5.68)
Purple		8 (11.27)	5 (7.04)	8 (11.27)	40 (56.34)	1 (1.41)	2 (2.82)	7 (9.86)

CpG sites were annotated with the IlluminaHumanMethylationEPICanno.ilm10b4.hg19 [21] package. Data expressed as n of sites, (%) by rows. TSS: Transcription Start Site. UTR: Untranslated Region. ExonBnd: Exon Boundaries.

Concerning the distribution of CpG sites with respect to CpG islands, a majority of comethylation modules corresponded to Open Sea (71.11–84.56%, 85–4207 sites); on the other hand, the purple comethylation module had a high percentage of CpG sites annotated on islands (15.32%, 17 sites) (Table 3). CpG sites in comethylation modules were heterogeneously distributed among chromosomes (Table S1). Additionally, we observed two groups of comethylation modules given the methylation levels from beta values. One group had partially methylated values (0.2 < β value < 0.8) (turquoise, blue and purple), while the other group had hypermethylated values (β value ≥ 0.8) (brown, yellow, green, red, black, pink and magenta) (Table S2).

Table 3. CpG site position with respect to CpG islands.

Module		OpenSea	Island	N Shore	S Shore	N Shelf	S Shelf
Turquoise		4207 (82.93)	13 (0.26)	247 (4.87)	212 (4.18)	202 (3.98)	192 (3.78)
Blue		2476 (84.56)	15 (0.51)	128 (4.37)	83 (2.83)	104 (3.55)	122 (4.17)
Brown		153 (79.27)	6 (3.11)	9 (4.66)	17 (8.81)	4 (2.07)	4 (2.07)
Yellow		125 (75.30)	1 (0.60)	14 (8.43)	10 (6.02)	12 (7.23)	4 (2.41)
Green		114 (75.50)	5 (3.31)	10 (6.62)	8 (5.30)	9 (5.96)	5 (3.31)
Red		121 (80.67)	1 (0.67)	6 (4.00)	2 (1.33)	8 (5.33)	12 (8.00)
Black		115 (77.70)	1 (0.68)	7 (4.73)	6 (4.05)	11 (7.43)	8 (5.41)
Pink		114 (78.62)	6 (4.14)	7 (4.83)	7 (4.83)	8 (5.52)	3 (2.07)
Magenta		96 (71.11)	6 (4.44)	9 (6.67)	9 (6.67)	8 (5.93)	7 (5.19)
Purple		85 (76.58)	17 (15.32)	4 (3.60)	3 (2.70)	1 (0.90)	1 (0.90)
Total		7606 (82.67)	71 (0.77)	441 (4.79)	357 (3.88)	367 (3.99)	358 (3.89)

CpG sites were annotated with the IlluminaHumanMethylationEPICanno.ilm10b4.hg19 [21] package. Data expressed in n of sites, (%) by rows.

3.2. Enriched Pathways on Each Module

We found significant enriched pathways of genes annotated on the CpG sites from turquoise and blue modules (Table S3). Genes in the turquoise module were enriched for the longevity regulating pathway (adjusted p value = 0.0047), GnRH (Gonadotropin-releasing hormone) signaling pathway (adjusted p value = 0.0042), glioma (adjusted p value = 0.0126), cholinergic synapse (adjusted p value = 0.0091), human cytomegalovirus infection (adjusted p value = 0.0126), and endocytosis (adjusted p value = 0.0126). Genes from blue comethylation module were enriched in pathways for Th1 and Th2 cell differentiation (adjusted p value = 6.8672 × 10^{-7}), allograft rejection (adjusted p value = 0.0185), endometrial cancer (adjusted p value = 0.0111), and TNF signaling pathway (adjusted p value = 0.0007). Another enrichment pathways within the same module included the AGE-RAGE signaling pathway in diabetic complications (adjusted p value = 0.0033), phosphatidylinositol signaling system (adjusted p value = 0.0074), glioma (adjusted p value = 0.0365), longevity regulating pathway (adjusted p value = 0.0325), human cytomegalovirus infection (adjusted p value = 0.0008), and focal adhesion (adjusted p value = 0.0039).

3.3. Correlations of Modules with Clinical Features in Our Population

In our results, seven clinical features and comorbidities correlated with different comethylation modules (Figure 1). The yellow comethylation module correlated with body mass index (BMI) zscore ($R^2 = 0.47$, $p = 0.0006$), conduct disorder ($R^2 = -0.41$, $p = 0.0030$), and psychotic disorder ($R^2 = -0.45$, $p = 0.0010$). Meanwhile, the purple comethylation module correlated with gender ($R^2 = -1$, $p < 1 \times 10^{-50}$), suicidal behavior ($R^2 = 0.41$, $p = 0.0030$), and attention-deficit/hyperactivity disorder ($R^2 = -0.59$, $p = 6 \times 10^{-6}$). Finally, the black module correlated with height ($R^2 = 0.4$, $p = 0.0040$). Notably, clinical features did not correlate with more than one module at a time.

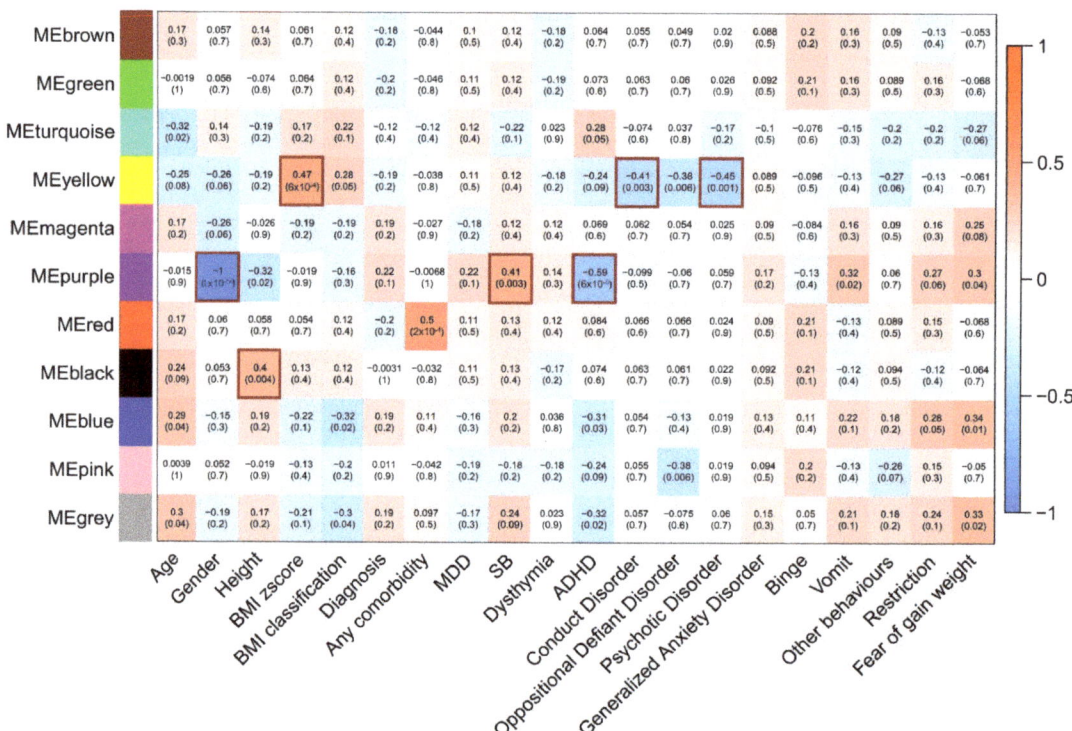

Figure 1. Correlations between modules and clinical features. MDD: major depressive disorder. SB: suicidal behavior. ADHD: attention deficit hyperactivity disorder. Red borders indicate significant correlations. Significance indicates p-values $< 5 \times 10^{-3}$.

3.4. Correlations of SNPs with Modules

Seven comethylation modules had correlations with any SNP (brown, green, yellow, magenta, red, black and pink) (Table S4). SNPs were located mostly in intronic regions, ranging from 33.96% in the red module (18 SNPs) to 55.56% in the yellow module (15 SNPs). Another frequent location was intergenic regions, ranging from 14.81% in the yellow module (4 SNPs) to 31.71% in the black module (13 SNPs). The most frequent location in the green module was intergenic regions (28.13%, 9 SNPs), followed by intronic regions (21.88%, 7 SNPs).

The most correlated SNPs (89.95%, 206 SNPs) were in nonprotein-coding transcript regions, while 10.05% (23 SNPs) were in protein-coding regions (synonymous and missense). Seventeen SNPs (7.42%) were annotated as missense variants; the red and black modules had four missense SNPs each. Meanwhile, six correlated SNPs (2.62%) were annotated as synonymous variants, with two SNPs per module (brown, yellow, and red). We observed 10 correlated SNPs (4.37%) in regulatory regions, although no SNPs were found in the yellow comethylation module. The magenta comethylation module had no SNPs annotated in the upstream and downstream regions. Finally, correlated SNPs annotated in 3′ untranslated regions (UTR) were the least frequent (2 SNPs, 0.87%), found within the magenta and red modules (Table 4).

Table 4. Annotations of SNPs correlated with modules.

	Brown	Green	Yellow	Magenta	Red	Black	Pink	Total
3′UTR	0 (0.00)	0 (0.00)	0 (0.00)	1 (5.88)	1 (1.89)	0 (0.00)	0 (0.00)	2 (0.89)
Downstream	0 (0.00)	2 (6.25)	1 (3.70)	0 (0.00)	4 (7.55)	1 (2.44)	1 (5.00)	9 (4)
Intergenic	7 (17.95)	9 (28.13)	4 (14.81)	5 (29.41)	13 (24.53)	13 (31.71)	4 (20.00)	55 (24.4)
Intron	19 (48.72)	7 (21.88)	15 (55.56)	7 (41.18)	18 (33.96)	14 (34.15)	7 (35.00)	87 (38.67)
Missense	3 (7.69)	1 (3.13)	2 (7.41)	1 (5.88)	4 (7.55)	4 (9.76)	2 (10.00)	17 (7.56)
Non coding transcript	3 (7.69)	8 (28.13)	2 (7.41)	1 (5.88)	6 (13.21)	5 (14.64)	3 (20.00)	28 (12.44)
Regulatory	1 (2.56)	3 (9.38)	0 (0.00)	2 (11.76)	2 (3.77)	1 (2.44)	1 (5.00)	10 (4.44)
Synonymous	2 (5.13)	0 (0.00)	2 (7.41)	0 (0.00)	2 (3.77)	0 (0.00)	0 (0.00)	6 (2.67)
Upstream	4 (10.26)	1 (3.13)	1 (3.70)	0 (0.00)	2 (3.77)	2 (4.88)	1 (5.00)	11 (4.89)

dbSNP codes were annotated with InfiniumPsychArray-24v1-3_A1_b150_rsids file. Coding regions were annotated with Ensembl Variant Effect Predictor. Data expressed as n of SNPs, (%) by columns.

3.5. Correlated SNP PheWAS

Regarding clinical features, BMI, body fat, and height were the most frequent phenotypes associated with SNPs (Figure 2).

Concerning psychiatric disorders, we found several SNPs to be associated with three comethylation modules. The brown comethylation module had a SNP associated with depressive symptoms and neuroticism (rs4598994). Meanwhile, the pink comethylation module was associated with depressive affect (rs4800995); two SNPs were associated with schizophrenia (rs3129012 and rs356971) in the black comethylation module. Moreover, seven correlated SNPs with four comethylation modules were associated with autoimmune diseases. The magenta comethylation module was associated with rheumatoid arthritis and Crohn's disease (rs1893217). Likewise, the red (rs3095345) and pink (rs9267546 and rs9267547) comethylation modules were associated with rheumatoid arthritis and type 1 diabetes. The black module was associated with primary sclerosing cholangitis (rs3129012 and rs356971), autoimmune vitiligo, and systemic lupus erythematosus (rs356971). Finally, the yellow and black comethylation modules were correlated with clinical features in our population (BMI zscore, conduct disorder, psychotic disorder, and height); likewise, these comethylation modules were correlated with SNPs associated with similar phenotypes. Meanwhile, the yellow module correlated with one SNP (rs10494217) associated with the waist–hip ratio in PheWAS, and the black comethylation module correlated with three SNPs associated with height (rs9349206, rs11761528 and rs17726787).

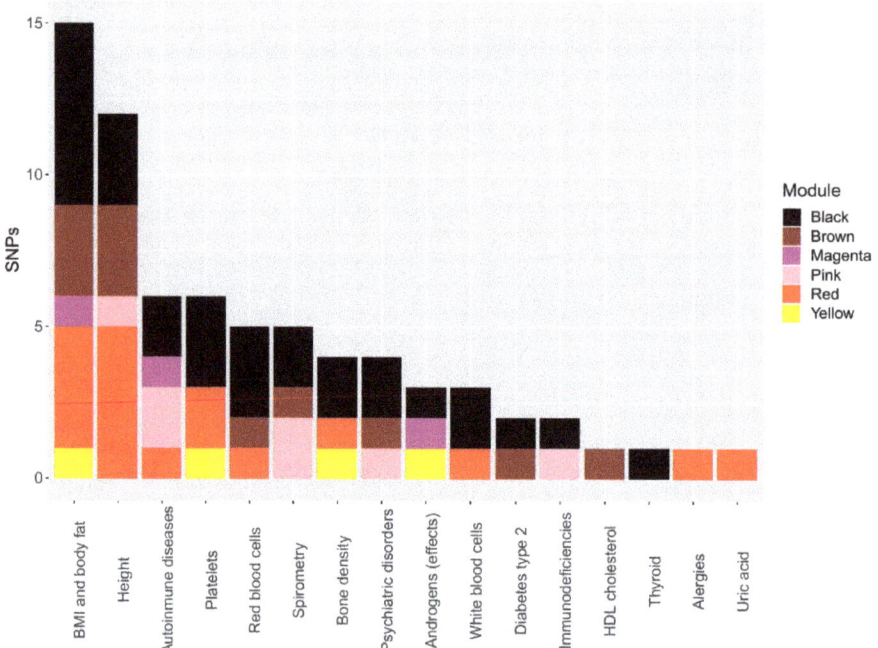

Figure 2. Phenotypes associated with correlated single nucleotide polymorphisms (SNP) in PheWAS.

4. Discussion

Several studies have evaluated the clinical features, genetic variants, and single DNA methylation sites involved in ED, but none has considered these factors together to date [1,5,7]. As such, little information is available about the integration of these different levels of biological information. As far as we know, this is the first study to integrate clinical features, genetic variants, and DNA methylation using a comethylation network analysis in teenagers with EDs.

BMI is an important clinical characteristic of the individuals diagnosed with ED, and it has a high impact on metabolic profiles [25]. Low BMI is a diagnosis criterion for anorexia nervosa [12]; on the other hand, bulimia nervosa and binge-eating disorder are related to risk of overweight/obesity [26]. In our analysis, the yellow module could be important in the changes in BMI found in individuals with EDs. The yellow module was correlated with BMI and rs10494217. This SNP is a missense genetic variant changing a histidine aminoacid for an asparagine in position 50 of *TBX15* gene (p.His50Asn). Previously, GWAS associated rs10494217 with waist-hip index, a variable related to BMI [27]. The *TBX15* gene is a member of the T-box gene family, i.e., transcriptional regulators which play an important role in the development of skeletal elements of limbs, vertebral column, and head, as well as other organs [28,29]. Likewise, this gene was reported as a regulator of metabolism of adipose tissue and muscle fibers, and shown to indirectly regulate body fat and BMI [30–32]. *TBX15* is highly expressed in adipose tissue, and it binds to the promoter of *PRDM16* gene. *PRDM16* is essential for the browning of adipose tissue; reduced expression of its protein promotes obesity with high-fat diet and increases visceral fat [33]. As a missense variant, rs10494217 could reduce the binding of *TBX15* protein to the promoter of *PRDM16*, and thus disturb adipose tissue function and alter BMI in individuals diagnosed with an ED. A possible alteration of *PRDM16* expression could induce epigenetic reprogramming, as it is found in the yellow module in this study. CpG sites of the yellow module were enriched in alpha-linolenic acid metabolism (*PLA2G4E* and *PLB1*) and VEGF signaling pathway (*AKT3*,

NFATC2, *PLA2G4E* and *SHC2*); both pathways are involved in adipose tissue function and BMI [34–37].

The black module could also be related to BMI in ED-diagnosed individuals. This module was correlated with rs11761528, a SNP associated with BMI and androsterone sulfate metabolism [27,38]. rs11761528 is an intronic polymorphism of the *ZKSCAN5* gene. There is little information about *ZKSCAN5* (zinc finger with KRAB and SCAN domains 5) and its mechanism; however, animal models suggest that this gene is correlated with adipocyte volume, systolic blood pressure, and cardiac mass [39]. Similarly, rs17726787 was previously associated with height and trunk fat-free mass in GWAS [24,40]. This SNP is an intronic variant of the *CELF1* gene. Disturbances in gene expression of *CELF1* are related with cardiopathies [41–43]. The black module was enriched in mTOR signaling pathway (*IGF1R*, *LPIN1* and *RPS6KA2*), suggesting that genetic variations like rs11761528 and rs17726787 could alter the epigenetics of this pathway. The mTOR signaling pathway is essential for cardiac development [44,45]. Heart complications are frequent in anorexia nervosa patients, reaching 80% in some studies. Severe anorexia nervosa can change cardiac structure, although most structural abnormalities are reversible [46,47]. Nevertheless, there is a lack of analyses which explore the relationships between altered genes in the module, genetic variation, and cardiopathies in ED-diagnosed individuals.

Although schizophrenia was not correlated in our sample, we found genes and SNPs associated with the disorder. Schizophrenia and other psychiatric disorders are associated with anorexia nervosa [3,5]. Also, there is reportedly a high prevalence of schizophrenia among individuals with eating disorders [48]. CpG sites conforming the black module were enriched in morphine addiction (*GABBR2*, *GABRP* and *PDE4B*), and polymorphisms of the *PDE4B* gene have been associated with susceptibility to schizophrenia [49]. rs356971 and rs3129012 SNPs were correlated with the black module; these SNPs are associated with schizophrenia [50] and waist–hip index [27]. Furthermore, rs356971 and rs3129012 are associated with phenotypes related with the immunological system, hemoglobin concentration, white blood cells, and platelet count [51]. These SNPs are also associated with primary sclerosing cholangitis [52], autoimmune vitiligo [53], IgA deficiency [54], and systemic lupus erythematosus [55]. Immune-mediated mechanisms have been suggested in the development of EDs; an increased risk for autoimmune diseases in EDs has been reported [56,57]. Likewise, a locus in chromosome 12 was associated with anorexia nervosa, diabetes type 1, and autoimmune diseases [3].

Some modules could have comethylation of CpG sites which was not altered by a genetic effect in individuals diagnosed with an ED, like the turquoise and blue modules. These modules were enriched in pathways associated with the immunological system (Th1 and Th2 cell differentiation, TNF signaling pathway, focal adhesion). The same modules were also enriched in pathways related with development status. The construction of these modules could be influenced by the developmental stage of individuals in the sample, i.e., mainly teenagers [58]. One pathway is the GnRH (Gonadotropin Release Hormone) signaling pathway, which is activated at the beginning of pubertal development, and it depends on neuroendocrine signaling [59–61]. Another enriched pathway was associated with adiponectin (adiponectin/CaMKK/AMPK) [62,63]. Many authors suggest that adiponectin levels change with pubertal development [64,65]. Also, partial methylation of these modules suggests transcriptional activation of these pathways. The detection of these modules is more likely to be an effect of background epigenetic alterations and the cell development stage in the tissue (white blood cells) used for the analysis.

Our study has some limitations. Firstly, we note the absence of a control group. However, in this exploratory study, our primary aim was to detect comethylation modules in ED patients and assess the relationship between such modules and clinical phenotypes in ED. Second, we had a small sample with many variables evaluated. Although these conditions could affect the statistic power of our analysis, comethylation modules aggregate covarying CpGs and evaluate grouped CpGs, reducing the number of tests needed. Besides, WGCNA requires at least 20 samples to construct biologically meaningful modules [66].

Third, our data was from a sample made up of Mexican teenagers; therefore, our results should not be applied to all populations with EDs.

5. Conclusions

This is the first study integrating clinical features, genetic variants, and DNA methylation using comethylation network analysis in teenagers with ED. Our findings showed that two comethylation modules correlated with physical features as well as with SNPs previously associated with metabolic and psychiatric phenotypes. These data suggest that genetic variations could alter epigenetics, and that these perturbations could be reflected as variations in clinical features.

Supplementary Materials: The following are available online at https://www.mdpi.com/2072-6643/13/9/3210/s1, Table S1: CpG sites per chromosome and normalized value per chromosomic size, Table S2: Descriptive statistics of comethylation modules' beta values, Table S3: Functional enrichments of comethylation modules, Table S4: Characteristics of SNPs correlated with comethylation modules.

Author Contributions: Conceptualization, H.N. and A.D.G.-M.; methodology, G.A.N.-R. and I.E.J.-R.; software, G.A.N.-R. and J.J.M.-M.; validation, I.E.J.-R. and C.A.T.-Z.; formal analysis, G.A.N.-R. and J.J.M.-M.; investigation, A.R.G., E.S., G.A.N.-R. and T.B.G.-C.; resources, H.N.; data curation, G.A.N.-R.; writing—original draft preparation, G.A.N.-R.; writing—review and editing, G.A.N.-R., J.J.M.-M., I.E.J.-R., T.B.G.-C., C.A.T.-Z., A.R.G., E.S., D.R.-R., A.D.G.-M. and H.N.; visualization, G.A.N.-R.; supervision, J.J.M.-M. and I.E.J.-R.; project administration, A.D.G.-M.; funding acquisition, H.N. All authors have read and agreed to the published version of the manuscript.

Funding: This research was funded by Fundación Gonzalo Río Arronte, grant number S591, and Instituto Nacional de Medicina Genómica (INMEGEN), grant number 06/2018/I.

Institutional Review Board Statement: This study was conducted according to the guidelines of the Declaration of Helsinki and approved by the Ethics Committees of the Psychiatric Hospital "Dr. Juan N. Navarro" (protocol code No. II3/01/0913; 11 October 2017), and National Institute of Genomic Medicine (INMEGEN) (protocol code No. 06/2018/I; June 2018).

Informed Consent Statement: Informed consent was obtained from all subjects involved in the study.

Data Availability Statement: The data presented in this study are available on request from the corresponding author, which were omitted due to privacy and ethical issues.

Acknowledgments: We want to acknowledge Microarray and Expression Unit of National Institute of Genomic Medicine for their technical support. Germán Alberto Nolasco-Rosales and David Ruiz-Ramos are students of Master of Biomedical Sciences degree in Juárez Autonomous University of Tabasco and were supported by CONACYT.

Conflicts of Interest: The authors declare no conflict of interest.

References

1. Bulik, C.M.; Blake, L.; Austin, J. Genetics of Eating Disorders: What the Clinician Needs to Know. *Psychiatr. Clin. N. Am.* **2019**, *42*, 59–73. [CrossRef]
2. Steiger, H.; Booij, L. Eating Disorders, Heredity and Environmental Activation: Getting Epigenetic Concepts into Practice. *J. Clin. Med.* **2020**, *9*, 1332. [CrossRef] [PubMed]
3. Duncan, L.; Yilmaz, Z.; Gaspar, H.; Walters, R.; Goldstein, J.; Anttila, V.; Bulik-Sullivan, B.; Ripke, S.; Thornton, L.; Hinney, A.; et al. Significant Locus and Metabolic Genetic Correlations Revealed in Genome-Wide Association Study of Anorexia Nervosa. *Am. J. Psychiatry* **2017**, *174*, 850–858. [CrossRef]
4. Yilmaz, Z.; Hardaway, J.A.; Bulik, C.M. Genetics and Epigenetics of Eating Disorders. *Adv. Genom. Genet.* **2015**, *5*, 131–150. [CrossRef]
5. Watson, H.J.; Yilmaz, Z.; Thornton, L.M.; Hübel, C.; Coleman, J.R.I.; Gaspar, H.A.; Bryois, J.; Hinney, A.; Leppä, V.M.; Mattheisen, M.; et al. Genome-wide association study identifies eight risk loci and implicates metabo-psychiatric origins for anorexia nervosa. *Nat. Genet.* **2019**, *51*, 1207–1214. [CrossRef]

6. Munn-Chernoff, M.A.; Johnson, E.C.; Chou, Y.-L.; Coleman, J.R.I.; Thornton, L.M.; Walters, R.K.; Yilmaz, Z.; Baker, J.H.; Hübel, C.; Gordon, S.; et al. Shared genetic risk between eating disorder- and substance-use-related phenotypes: Evidence from genome-wide association studies. *Addict. Biol.* **2021**, *26*, e12880. [CrossRef]
7. Hübel, C.; Marzi, S.J.; Breen, G.; Bulik, C.M. Epigenetics in eating disorders: A systematic review. *Mol. Psychiatry* **2019**, *24*, 901–915. [CrossRef] [PubMed]
8. Rodríguez-López, M.L.; Martínez-Magaña, J.J.; Ruiz-Ramos, D.; García, A.R.; Gonzalez, L.; Tovilla-Zarate, C.A.; Sarmiento, E.; Juárez-Rojop, I.E.; Nicolini, H.; Gonzalez-Castro, T.B.; et al. Individuals Diagnosed with Binge-Eating Disorder Have DNA Hypomethylated Sites in Genes of the Metabolic System: A Pilot Study. *Nutrients* **2021**, *13*, 1413. [CrossRef]
9. Zhao, W.; Langfelder, P.; Fuller, T.; Dong, J.; Li, A.; Hovarth, S. Weighted Gene Coexpression Network Analysis: State of the Art. *J. Biopharm. Stat.* **2010**, *20*, 281–300. [CrossRef] [PubMed]
10. Lin, X.; Barton, S.; Holbrook, J.D. How to make DNA methylome wide association studies more powerful. *Epigenomics* **2016**, *8*, 1117–1129. [CrossRef]
11. Langfelder, P.; Horvath, S. WGCNA: An R package for weighted correlation network analysis. *BMC Bioinform.* **2008**, *9*, 559. [CrossRef]
12. APA. *Diagnostic and Statistical Manual of Mental Disorders*, 5th ed.; American Psychiatric Association: Arlington, VA, USA, 2013.
13. Yanovski, S.Z.; Marcus, M.D.; Wadden, T.A.; Walsh, B.T. The Questionnaire on Eating and Weight Patterns-5: An updated screening instrument for binge eating disorder. *Int. J. Eat. Disord.* **2015**, *48*, 259–261. [CrossRef]
14. Garner, D.M.; Olmsted, M.P.; Bohr, Y.; Garfinkel, P.E. The Eating Attitudes Test: Psychometric features and clinical correlates. *Psychol. Med.* **1982**, *12*, 871–878. [CrossRef]
15. Sheehan, D.V.; Sheehan, K.H.; Shytle, R.D.; Janavs, J.; Bannon, Y.; Rogers, J.E.; Milo, K.M.; Stock, S.L.; Wilkinson, B. Reliability and validity of the Mini International Neuropsychiatric Interview for Children and Adolescents (MINI-KID). *J. Clin. Psychiatry* **2010**, *71*, 313–326. [CrossRef]
16. Chang, C.C.; Chow, C.C.; Tellier, L.C.A.M.; Vattikuti, S.; Purcell, S.M.; Lee, J.J. Second-generation PLINK: Rising to the challenge of larger and richer datasets. *GigaScience* **2015**, *4*, s13742-015-0047-8. [CrossRef]
17. R Core Team. *R: A Language and Environment for Statistical Computing*; R Foundation for Statistical Computing: Vienna, Austria, 2020.
18. Morris, T.J.; Butcher, L.M.; Feber, A.; Teschendorff, A.E.; Chakravarthy, A.R.; Wojdacz, T.K.; Beck, S. ChAMP: 450k Chip Analysis Methylation Pipeline. *Bioinformatics* **2014**, *30*, 428–430. [CrossRef]
19. Teschendorff, A.E.; Marabita, F.; Lechner, M.; Bartlett, T.; Tegner, J.; Gomez-Cabrero, D.; Beck, S. A beta-mixture quantile normalization method for correcting probe design bias in Illumina Infinium 450 k DNA methylation data. *Bioinformatics* **2013**, *29*, 189–196. [CrossRef] [PubMed]
20. Zhang, B.; Horvath, S. A General Framework for Weighted Gene Co-Expression Network Analysis. *Stat. Appl. Genet. Mol. Biol.* **2005**, *4*. [CrossRef] [PubMed]
21. Hansen, K.D. *IlluminaHumanMethylationEPICanno.ilm10b4.hg19: Annotation for Illumina's EPIC Methylation Arrays*, R Package Version 0.6.0. 2017.
22. Liao, Y.; Wang, J.; Jaehnig, E.J.; Shi, Z.; Zhang, B. WebGestalt 2019: Gene set analysis toolkit with revamped UIs and APIs. *Nucleic Acids Res.* **2019**, *47*, W199–W205. [CrossRef] [PubMed]
23. Kanehisa, M.; Goto, S. KEGG: Kyoto Encyclopedia of Genes and Genomes. *Nucleic Acids Res.* **2000**, *28*, 27–30. [CrossRef]
24. Watanabe, K.; Stringer, S.; Frei, O.; Umićević Mirkov, M.; de Leeuw, C.; Polderman, T.J.C.; van der Sluis, S.; Andreassen, O.A.; Neale, B.M.; Posthuma, D. A global overview of pleiotropy and genetic architecture in complex traits. *Nat. Genet.* **2019**, *51*, 1339–1348. [CrossRef]
25. Genis-Mendoza, A.D.; Martínez-Magaña, J.J.; Ruiz-Ramos, D.; Gonzalez-Covarrubias, V.; Tovilla-Zarate, C.A.; Narvaez, M.L.L.; Castro, T.B.G.; Juárez-Rojop, I.E.; Nicolini, H. Interaction of FTO rs9939609 and the native American-origin ABCA1 p.Arg230Cys with circulating leptin levels in Mexican adolescents diagnosed with eating disorders: Preliminary results. *Psychiatry Res.* **2020**, *291*, 113270. [CrossRef] [PubMed]
26. Hay, P. Current approach to eating disorders: A clinical update. *Intern. Med. J.* **2020**, *50*, 24–29. [CrossRef]
27. Pulit, S.L.; Stoneman, C.; Morris, A.P.; Wood, A.R.; Glastonbury, C.A.; Tyrrell, J.; Yengo, L.; Ferreira, T.; Marouli, E.; Ji, Y.; et al. Meta-analysis of genome-wide association studies for body fat distribution in 694 649 individuals of European ancestry. *Hum. Mol. Genet.* **2019**, *28*, 166–174. [CrossRef] [PubMed]
28. Papaioannou, V.E. T-box genes in development: From hydra to humans. In *International Review of Cytology*; Academic Press: Cambridge, MA, USA, 2001; Volume 207, pp. 1–70.
29. Singh, M.K.; Petry, M.; Haenig, B.; Lescher, B.; Leitges, M.; Kispert, A. The T-box transcription factor Tbx15 is required for skeletal development. *Mech. Dev.* **2005**, *122*, 131–144. [CrossRef]
30. Lee, K.Y.; Singh, M.K.; Ussar, S.; Wetzel, P.; Hirshman, M.F.; Goodyear, L.J.; Kispert, A.; Kahn, C.R. Tbx15 controls skeletal muscle fibre-type determination and muscle metabolism. *Nat. Commun.* **2015**, *6*, 8054. [CrossRef]
31. Lee, K.Y.; Sharma, R.; Gase, G.; Ussar, S.; Li, Y.; Welch, L.; Berryman, D.E.; Kispert, A.; Bluher, M.; Kahn, C.R. Tbx15 Defines a Glycolytic Subpopulation and White Adipocyte Heterogeneity. *Diabetes* **2017**, *66*, 2822. [CrossRef] [PubMed]
32. Sun, P.; Zhang, D.; Huang, H.; Yu, Y.; Yang, Z.; Niu, Y.; Liu, J. MicroRNA-1225-5p acts as a tumor-suppressor in laryngeal cancer via targeting CDC14B. *Biol. Chem.* **2019**, *400*, 237–246. [CrossRef] [PubMed]

33. Cohen, P.; Levy, J.D.; Zhang, Y.; Frontini, A.; Kolodin, D.P.; Svensson, K.J.; Lo, J.C.; Zeng, X.; Ye, L.; Khandekar, M.J.; et al. Ablation of PRDM16 and Beige Adipose Causes Metabolic Dysfunction and a Subcutaneous to Visceral Fat Switch. *Cell* **2014**, *156*, 304–316. [CrossRef]
34. Arensdorf, A.M.; Dillard, M.E.; Menke, J.M.; Frank, M.W.; Rock, C.O.; Ogden, S.K. Sonic Hedgehog Activates Phospholipase A2 to Enhance Smoothened Ciliary Translocation. *Cell Rep.* **2017**, *19*, 2074–2087. [CrossRef]
35. Iyer, A.; Lim, J.; Poudyal, H.; Reid, R.C.; Suen, J.Y.; Webster, J.; Prins, J.B.; Whitehead, J.P.; Fairlie, D.P.; Brown, L. An Inhibitor of Phospholipase A^2; Group IIA Modulates Adipocyte Signaling and Protects Against Diet-Induced Metabolic Syndrome in Rats. *Diabetes* **2012**, *61*, 2320. [CrossRef] [PubMed]
36. Kuefner, M.S.; Deng, X.; Stephenson, E.J.; Pham, K.; Park, E.A. Secretory phospholipase A2 group IIA enhances the metabolic rate and increases glucose utilization in response to thyroid hormone. *FASEB J.* **2019**, *33*, 738–749. [CrossRef] [PubMed]
37. Sato, H.; Taketomi, Y.; Ushida, A.; Isogai, Y.; Kojima, T.; Hirabayashi, T.; Miki, Y.; Yamamoto, K.; Nishito, Y.; Kobayashi, T.; et al. The Adipocyte-Inducible Secreted Phospholipases PLA2G5 and PLA2G2E Play Distinct Roles in Obesity. *Cell Metab.* **2014**, *20*, 119–132. [CrossRef]
38. Shin, S.-Y.; Fauman, E.B.; Petersen, A.-K.; Krumsiek, J.; Santos, R.; Huang, J.; Arnold, M.; Erte, I.; Forgetta, V.; Yang, T.-P.; et al. An atlas of genetic influences on human blood metabolites. *Nat. Genet.* **2014**, *46*, 543–550. [CrossRef]
39. Coan, P.M.; Hummel, O.; Garcia Diaz, A.; Barrier, M.; Alfazema, N.; Norsworthy, P.J.; Pravenec, M.; Petretto, E.; Hübner, N.; Aitman, T.J. Genetic, physiological and comparative genomic studies of hypertension and insulin resistance in the spontaneously hypertensive rat. *Dis. Models Mech.* **2017**, *10*, 297–306. [CrossRef] [PubMed]
40. Yengo, L.; Sidorenko, J.; Kemper, K.E.; Zheng, Z.; Wood, A.R.; Weedon, M.N.; Frayling, T.M.; Hirschhorn, J.; Yang, J.; Visscher, P.M.; et al. Meta-analysis of genome-wide association studies for height and body mass index in ~700000 individuals of European ancestry. *Hum. Mol. Genet.* **2018**, *27*, 3641–3649. [CrossRef]
41. Belanger, K.; Nutter, C.A.; Li, J.; Tasnim, S.; Liu, P.; Yu, P.; Kuyumcu-Martinez, M.N. CELF1 contributes to aberrant alternative splicing patterns in the type 1 diabetic heart. *Biochem. Biophys. Res. Commun.* **2018**, *503*, 3205–3211. [CrossRef]
42. Chang, K.-T.; Cheng, C.-F.; King, P.-C.; Liu, S.-Y.; Wang, G.-S. CELF1 Mediates Connexin 43 mRNA Degradation in Dilated Cardiomyopathy. *Circ. Res.* **2017**, *121*, 1140–1152. [CrossRef]
43. Fang, Y.; Tao, Y.; Zhou, H.; Lai, H. Promoting role of circ-Jarid2/miR-129-5p/Celf1 axis in cardiac hypertrophy. *Gene Ther.* **2020**, *27*, 1–11. [CrossRef]
44. Sciarretta, S.; Forte, M.; Frati, G.; Sadoshima, J. New Insights into the Role of mTOR Signaling in the Cardiovascular System. *Circ. Res.* **2018**, *122*, 489–505. [CrossRef]
45. Sciarretta, S.; Volpe, M.; Sadoshima, J. Mammalian Target of Rapamycin Signaling in Cardiac Physiology and Disease. *Circ. Res.* **2014**, *114*, 549–564. [CrossRef]
46. Fayssoil, A.; Melchior, J.C.; Hanachi, M. Heart and anorexia nervosa. *Heart Fail. Rev.* **2021**, *26*, 65–70. [CrossRef]
47. Westmoreland, P.; Krantz, M.J.; Mehler, P.S. Medical Complications of Anorexia Nervosa and Bulimia. *Am. J. Med.* **2016**, *129*, 30–37. [CrossRef] [PubMed]
48. Kouidrat, Y.; Amad, A.; Lalau, J.-D.; Loas, G. Eating Disorders in Schizophrenia: Implications for Research and Management. *Schizophr. Res. Treat.* **2014**, *2014*, 791573. [CrossRef] [PubMed]
49. Feng, Y.; Cheng, D.; Zhang, C.; Li, Y.; Zhang, Z.; Wang, J.; Shi, Y. Association of PDE4B Polymorphisms with Susceptibility to Schizophrenia: A Meta-Analysis of Case-Control Studies. *PLoS ONE* **2016**, *11*, e0147092. [CrossRef] [PubMed]
50. Pardiñas, A.F.; Holmans, P.; Pocklington, A.J.; Escott-Price, V.; Ripke, S.; Carrera, N.; Legge, S.E.; Bishop, S.; Cameron, D.; Hamshere, M.L.; et al. Common schizophrenia alleles are enriched in mutation-intolerant genes and in regions under strong background selection. *Nat. Genet.* **2018**, *50*, 381–389. [CrossRef]
51. Astle, W.J.; Elding, H.; Jiang, T.; Allen, D.; Ruklisa, D.; Mann, A.L.; Mead, D.; Bouman, H.; Riveros-Mckay, F.; Kostadima, M.A.; et al. The Allelic Landscape of Human Blood Cell Trait Variation and Links to Common Complex Disease. *Cell* **2016**, *167*, 1415–1429.e1419. [CrossRef] [PubMed]
52. Ji, S.-G.; Juran, B.D.; Mucha, S.; Folseraas, T.; Jostins, L.; Melum, E.; Kumasaka, N.; Atkinson, E.J.; Schlicht, E.M.; Liu, J.Z.; et al. Genome-wide association study of primary sclerosing cholangitis identifies new risk loci and quantifies the genetic relationship with inflammatory bowel disease. *Nat. Genet.* **2017**, *49*, 269–273. [CrossRef] [PubMed]
53. Jin, Y.; Andersen, G.; Yorgov, D.; Ferrara, T.M.; Ben, S.; Brownson, K.M.; Holland, P.J.; Birlea, S.A.; Siebert, J.; Hartmann, A.; et al. Genome-wide association studies of autoimmune vitiligo identify 23 new risk loci and highlight key pathways and regulatory variants. *Nat. Genet.* **2016**, *48*, 1418–1424. [CrossRef] [PubMed]
54. Bronson, P.G.; Chang, D.; Bhangale, T.; Seldin, M.F.; Ortmann, W.; Ferreira, R.C.; Urcelay, E.; Pereira, L.F.; Martin, J.; Plebani, A.; et al. Common variants at PVT1, ATG13–AMBRA1, AHI1 and CLEC16A are associated with selective IgA deficiency. *Nat. Genet.* **2016**, *48*, 1425–1429. [CrossRef]
55. Julià, A.; López-Longo, F.J.; Pérez Venegas, J.J.; Bonàs-Guarch, S.; Olivé, À.; Andreu, J.L.; Aguirre-Zamorano, M.Á.; Vela, P.; Nolla, J.M.; de la Fuente, J.L.M.; et al. Genome-wide association study meta-analysis identifies five new loci for systemic lupus erythematosus. *Arthritis Res. Ther.* **2018**, *20*, 100. [CrossRef] [PubMed]
56. Raevuori, A.; Haukka, J.; Vaarala, O.; Suvisaari, J.M.; Gissler, M.; Grainger, M.; Linna, M.S.; Suokas, J.T. The Increased Risk for Autoimmune Diseases in Patients with Eating Disorders. *PLoS ONE* **2014**, *9*, e104845. [CrossRef]

57. Zerwas, S.; Larsen, J.T.; Petersen, L.; Thornton, L.M.; Quaranta, M.; Koch, S.V.; Pisetsky, D.; Mortensen, P.B.; Bulik, C.M. Eating Disorders, Autoimmune, and Autoinflammatory Disease. *Pediatrics* **2017**, *140*, e20162089. [CrossRef] [PubMed]
58. Almstrup, K.; Lindhardt Johansen, M.; Busch, A.S.; Hagen, C.P.; Nielsen, J.E.; Petersen, J.H.; Juul, A. Pubertal development in healthy children is mirrored by DNA methylation patterns in peripheral blood. *Sci. Rep.* **2016**, *6*, 28657. [CrossRef]
59. Abreu, A.P.; Kaiser, U.B. Pubertal development and regulation. *Lancet Diabetes Endocrinol.* **2016**, *4*, 254–264. [CrossRef]
60. Herbison, A.E. Control of puberty onset and fertility by gonadotropin-releasing hormone neurons. *Nat. Rev. Endocrinol.* **2016**, *12*, 452–466. [CrossRef]
61. Livadas, S.; Chrousos, G.P. Control of the onset of puberty. *Curr. Opin. Pediatrics* **2016**, *28*, 551–558. [CrossRef]
62. Fang, H.; Judd, R.L. Adiponectin Regulation and Function. *Compr. Physiol.* **2018**, *8*, 1031–1063. [CrossRef]
63. Wang, Z.V.; Scherer, P.E. Adiponectin, the past two decades. *J. Mol. Cell Biol.* **2016**, *8*, 93–100. [CrossRef] [PubMed]
64. Sitticharoon, C.; Sukharomana, M.; Likitmaskul, S.; Churintaraphan, M.; Maikaew, P. Increased high molecular weight adiponectin, but decreased total adiponectin and kisspeptin, in central precocious puberty compared with aged-matched prepubertal girls. *Reprod. Fertil. Dev.* **2017**, *29*, 2466–2478. [CrossRef]
65. Woo, J.G.; Dolan, L.M.; Daniels, S.R.; Goodman, E.; Martin, L.J. Adolescent Sex Differences in Adiponectin Are Conditional on Pubertal Development and Adiposity. *Obes. Res.* **2005**, *13*, 2095–2101. [CrossRef] [PubMed]
66. Langfelder, P.; Horvath, S. WGCNA Package FAQ. Available online: https://horvath.genetics.ucla.edu/html/CoexpressionNetwork/Rpackages/WGCNA/faq.html (accessed on 24 August 2021).

Article

Vitamin D and the Risks of Depression and Anxiety: An Observational Analysis and Genome-Wide Environment Interaction Study

Zhen Zhang [†], Xuena Yang [†], Yumeng Jia, Yan Wen, Shiqiang Cheng, Peilin Meng, Chun'e Li, Huijie Zhang, Chuyu Pan, Jingxi Zhang, Yujing Chen and Feng Zhang *

Key Laboratory of Trace Elements and Endemic Diseases of National Health and Family Planning Commission, School of Public Health, Health Science Center, Xi'an Jiaotong University, Xi'an 710000, China; zhang785334865@yeah.net (Z.Z.); smile940323@stu.xjtu.edu.cn (X.Y.); jia.yu.meng@163.com (Y.J.); wenyan@mail.xjtu.edu.cn (Y.W.); chengsq0701@stu.xjtu.edu.cn (S.C.); mengpeilin@stu.xjtu.edu.cn (P.M.); lichune@stu.xjtu.edu.cn (C.L.); zhj2020@stu.xjtu.edu.cn (H.Z.); panchuyu_dsa@163.com (C.P.); 3120315071@stu.xjtu.edu.cn (J.Z.); c18003409402@163.com (Y.C.)
* Correspondence: fzhxjtu@mail.xjtu.edu.cn
† The two authors contributed equally to this work.

Abstract: Previous studies have suggested that vitamin D (VD) was associated with psychiatric diseases, but efforts to elucidate the functional relevance of VD with depression and anxiety from genetic perspective have been limited. Based on the UK Biobank cohort, we first calculated polygenic risk score (PRS) for VD from genome-wide association study (GWAS) data of VD. Linear and logistic regression analysis were conducted to evaluate the associations of VD traits with depression and anxiety traits, respectively. Then, using individual genotype and phenotype data from the UK Biobank, genome-wide environment interaction studies (GWEIS) were performed to identify the potential effects of gene × VD interactions on the risks of depression and anxiety traits. In the UK Biobank cohort, we observed significant associations of blood VD level with depression and anxiety traits, as well as significant associations of VD PRS and depression and anxiety traits. GWEIS identified multiple candidate loci, such as rs114086183 ($p = 4.11 \times 10^{-8}$, LRRTM4) for self-reported depression status and rs149760119 ($p = 3.88 \times 10^{-8}$, GNB5) for self-reported anxiety status. Our study results suggested that VD was negatively associated with depression and anxiety. GWEIS identified multiple candidate genes interacting with VD, providing novel clues for understanding the biological mechanism potential associations between VD and psychiatric disorders.

Keywords: vitamin D; depression; anxiety; genome-wide association study; polygenic risk score; genome-wide environment interaction study

1. Introduction

Psychiatric disorders are a group of complex diseases, which are mainly characterized by varying degrees of obstacles in mental activities such as cognition, emotion, willpower, and behavior [?]. A meta-analysis showed that overall global prevalence of psychiatric disorders was increased with odds ratio of 1.179 (95% CI: 1.065–1.305) [?]. Additionally, another study has found that the prevalence of the common mental illnesses is continuously rising, particularly in low- and middle-income countries, with many people suffering from depression and anxiety disorders simultaneously [?]. Depression and anxiety disorders are the most common mental disorders in the general population [?]. According to the latest report of World Health Organization, it is estimated that there are 322 million people (4.4% of the world's population) living with depression and more than 260 million people (3.6% of the global population) affected by anxiety disorders [?]. Furthermore, Wang et al. observed that depression and anxiety were significantly associated with higher cancer incidence, cancer-specific mortality and all-cause mortality [?]. Traditional treatment of depression and anxiety can only relieve rather than cure the condition, causing a tremendous economic burden on individual families and high suicide rate. Therefore, it is urgent to find new ways to treat and prevent depression and anxiety disorders.

Vitamin D (VD) is a member of the steroid hormone family. As a necessary vitamin to human body, it is not only cheap, but also widely available. Besides being ingested from daily diet and VD supplements, it can also be synthesized from 7-dehydrocholesterol in the skin through ultraviolet radiation-b (UVB) [?]. Previous studies on VD have found that genetic and environmental factors can affect the status and metabolism of VD. The data from twin and family studies have suggested that circulating VD concentrations are partly determined by genetics, with heritability ranging from 23% to 80% [?]. Furthermore, genetic studies of VD have found that genetic variations and alterations (e.g., deletions, amplifications, inversions) in genes involved in VD metabolism, catabolism, transport, or binding to its receptors may affect VD levels [?]. Moreover, a study of gene-environment interactions with VD has showed that specific genetic variants associated with VD metabolism may be correlated with prostate cancer risk in VD-deficient patients [?]. As for the biological function of VD, previous studies have demonstrated that VD plays an important role in bone health, reproduction and fertility, and immune function [?]. Growing evidence shows that VD also exerts a great influence on the development and adult brain, such as maintaining calcium balance and signaling, regulating neurotrophic factors, providing neuroprotection, modulating neurotransmission, and promoting synaptic plasticity [?]. In addition, a recent systematic review has shown that VD deficiency in adulthood may also be associated with adverse brain-related outcomes [?]. The discovery of the functions of VD in the brain and the continuous confirmation of the effects of VD on disease provides a new research direction for the study of psychiatric disorders in recent years.

Although a lot of research has been devoted to exploring the relationship between VD and depression and anxiety, it is still controversial whether VD was associated with the two mental disorders [?]. Some studies have observed an association between VD and depression symptoms [? ? ?], while other studies have not found this association [? ?]. Additionally, previous studies on the association between VD and anxiety symptoms observed inconsistent association [? ?]. The discrepant results may be not only related to potential confounding factors, but also to complex etiology of psychiatric disorders. Previous studies on the pathogenesis of psychiatric disorders have found that they are associated with a variety of factors. For example, numerous studies have proved that inflammation is related to the pathogenesis of psychiatric disorders, and that the increase in inflammation will affect the occurrence and development of some psychiatric disorders [? ?]. Other studies have found that both diet and the gut microbiome have a strong influence on emotional behavior and neural processes [?]. Dietary patterns and changes in the microbiome can affect symptoms of depression and anxiety disorder and increase the risk of both disease through the microbiome gut–brain axis (MGBA) [?]. Moreover, some studies have shown that psychiatric disorders are caused by the interplay between genetic susceptibility and environmental risk factors [? ?]. It has been reported that the heritability of major depression [?] and current anxiety symptoms [?] was estimated to be 38% and 31%, respectively. However, previous studies on exploring the associations between VD and depression and anxiety only focused on the influence of environmental or genetic factors, usually not considering the interactions between them, which may underestimate the effects of VD on the risks of depression and anxiety.

Polygenic risk score (PRS) is proposed by running a GWAS on a study sample, selecting SNPs according to the relevant phenotypes, and creating the sum of phenotype related alleles (usually weighted by the SNP-specific coefficients from the GWAS) that can be evaluated in other replication sample [?]. PRS analysis can not only explore the genetic associations between various complex diseases and traits, but also assess the influence of susceptible loci on disease risks [?]. For example, PRS-related studies conducted by Psychiatric Genomics Consortium have found significant associations between PRS of symptom scale score and the risk of schizophrenia [?] as well as the efficacy of antipsychotic medication [?]. Recently, Revez et al. [?] conducted a GWAS of 417,580 UK Biobank study participants and identified 143 genetic loci associated with VD. Using the PRS of VD traits as instrumental variables, we can further explore the associations between the PRS of VD traits and psychiatric disorders.

GWAS study has strong ability in identifying susceptibility genetic loci associated with psychiatric disorders [?]. However, previous studies have shown that most of the phenotypic variation in complex diseases and traits cannot be explained solely by genetic factors, because phenotypic variation can also occur through genetic environment (G × E) interactions, in which the genotypes of different individuals vary in response to environmental stimuli [?]. Therefore, we further adopted the genome-wide environment interaction study (GWEIS), which can not only assess the effects of G × E interactions, but also evaluate the effects of genetic interactions on a genome-wide scale, helping to identify new genetic risk variants and understand the potential biological mechanisms [?]. For example, Rivera et al. found 53 and 34 single nucleotide polymorphisms (SNP_S) in additive interactions with smoking in Lofgren's syndrome (LS) and non-LS, respectively, but the association did not persist when assessing the effect of smoking on sarcoidosis without genetic information [?].

Utilizing the individual blood VD levels and calculated VD PRS data in UK Biobank cohort, we conducted regression analysis to evaluate the associations between VD (including blood VD levels and calculated VD PRS data) and depression status and anxiety status in the UK Biobank. Then, based on the results of regression analysis, genome-wide environment interaction studies (GWEIS) were performed to clarify the potential effects of gene × Vitamin D interactions on depression and anxiety.

2. Materials and Methods

2.1. UK Biobank Cohort

The UK Biobank (UKB) is a large population-based prospective cohort study, with health-linked information, both regarding phenotype and genotype, on approximately 500,000 participants aged between 40 and 69 years from all over the United Kingdom in 2006 and 2010 [?]. All participants were asked to report a series of health status and demographic information through questionnaires and interviews, and approved to use their anonymous data for any health-related research. Informed consent was provided by UKB from all participants. This study was approved by UKB (Application 46478) and obtained participants' health-related records.

2.2. UK Biobank Phenotypes of Vitamin D

A total of 376,803 UKB participants' blood samples were collected for quantitative measurement of 25(OH)D levels via chemiluminescent immunoassay (CLIA), and 343,334 (91.12%) individuals had their vitamin D 25(OH)D levels (UK Biobank data field: 30,890) measured. The analysis was limited to the population of white British individuals (UK Biobank data field: 21,000).

2.3. UK Biobank Phenotypes of Depression and Anxiety

The phenotypes of depression and anxiety were defined according to the previous study [?]. The selection criteria of case group were defined based on self-reports (UK Biobank data fields: 20,002; 20,126; and 20,544). In order to classify participants as much as possible, patient health questionnaire-9 (PHQ-9) [?], general anxiety disorder-7 (GAD-7) [?], and composite international diagnostic interview short-form (CIDI-SF) [?] were used as strict inclusion and exclusion criterion. PHQ-9 and GAD-7 are score scales for depression and anxiety, used to screen and measure the severity of depression and anxiety, respectively. PHQ-9 is a classification scale focusing on nine depression symptoms and signs, with a total score (0–27) [?], and GAD-7 is a classification scale focusing on seven anxious symptoms and signs, with a total score (0–21) [?]. Detailed classification of depression and anxiety are presented in the Supplementary Information. The selection criteria of the control group were as follows: without symptoms of depression and anxiety defined by CIDI and self-reported, depression PHQ scores and anxiety GAD scores ≤ 5, and without core symptoms.

2.4. UK Biobank Genotyping, Imputation and Quality Control

A total of 488,377 participants of UKB cohort were genotyped by either the Affymetrix UK BiLEVE Axiom Array or the Affymetrix UKB Axiom arrays [?]. The imputation and the quality control of these genotype results were carried out based on UK10K project reference panel [?] and Haplotype Reference Consortium (HRC) [?] reference panel. Then, we removed the participants who reported inconsistencies between self-reported gender and genetic gender, without ethic consents and imputation data. Additionally, we excluded variants with the Hardy–Weinberg equilibrium test $p > 1.0 \times 10^{-5}$, a minor allele frequency (MAF) of < 0.01, and a genotype missing rate of > 0.05. Ultimately, we used KING software to exclude the genetically related individuals.

2.5. GWAS Data of Vitamin D

The latest large-scale GWAS summary statistics of VD were used here. Briefly, this GWAS dataset detected 18,864 independent SNPs that were statistically associated with VD [?]. The genotype data were quality-controlled and imputed against the HRC and UK10K by the UKB group. Then, a linear mixed model GWAS was implemented in fastGWA to identify the genetic loci associated with 25OHD concentrations. Additionally, a rank-based reverse normal transformation (RINT) was applied to the phenotype, age, and gender. The genotyping batch and the first 40 ancestry PCs were used as covariates in the mixed model. In order to determine the independent associations, a conditional and joint (COJO) analysis [?] was employed on the GWAS results to explain the correlation structure between SNPs in the 10-Mb window (COJO default parameters). Detailed information of the GWAS can be obtained in the published study [?].

2.6. PRS Analysis of Vitamin D

Using the VD associated SNPs from the GWAS ($p < 5 \times 10^{-8}$) [?], the PRS of VD of each individual was calculated as the sum of the risk allele they carried, weighted by the effect size of the risk allele [?]. The PRS of VD was computed by PLINK2.0 [?], according to the formula:

$$\text{PRS} = \sum_{i=1}^{n} \beta_i \text{SNP}_{im}$$

PRS denotes the PRS value of VD for UKB subject; n and i, respectively, denote the total number of sample size and genetic markers; β_i is the effect parameter of risk allele of the significant SNP associated with VD, which was obtained from the GWAS of VD [?]; and SNP_{im} is the dosage (0, 1, 2) of the risk allele of the SNP associated with VD [?].

2.7. Statistical Analysis

In the UK Biobank cohort, we evaluated associations between vitamin D and depression and anxiety through regression analysis. Specifically, logistic regression analysis was employed to evaluate the associations of self-reported depression and anxiety status with blood VD, VD PRS before COJO adjustment, and VD PRS after COJO adjustment. Linear regression analysis was conducted to test the associations of the PHQ-9 score and the GAD-7 score with blood VD, VD PRS before COJO adjustment, and VD PRS after COJO adjustment. In this regression analysis, blood VD, VD PRS before COJO adjustment, and VD PRS after COJO adjustment were used as independent variables. Self-reported depression, self-reported anxiety, PHQ-9 score, and GAD-7 score were used as outcome variables. Sex, age, and 10 principle components (PCs) of population structure were used as covariates in the regression analysis. A $p < 0.05$ indicated an association. All analyses were conducted by R.

2.8. Genome-Wide Environment Interaction Studies (GWEIS)

The generalized linear regression model of PLINK2.0 [?] was used to estimate the gene × VD interaction effects on the risk of depression and anxiety, using age, gender, and the first 10 PCs as covariates. According to previous research [?], we used PLINK2.0 genetic additive (ADD) models and selected high-quality SNPs through a quality control filters: SNPs with a low call rates (<0.90), low minor allele frequencies (<0.01), or low Hardy–Weinberg equilibrium exact test p-values (<0.01) were excluded. $p < 5.0 \times 10^{-8}$ and $p < 5.0 \times 10^{-7}$ were defined as significant and suggestive interactions, respectively. GWEIS results were visualized with the circular Manhattan plots generated by the "CMplot" R script. (https://github.com/YinLiLin/R-CMplot) (accessed on 15 February 2021).

3. Results

3.1. General Population Characteristics

3.1.1. Characteristics of UK Biobank Subjects with Blood Vitamin D Data

For depression traits, with self-reported depression status as the outcome variable, a total of 110,744 participants answered the depression-related questions, and 52,766 were classified into depression group. With the depression PHQ score as the outcome variable, a total of 109,543 participants completed the questionnaire. For anxiety traits, with self-reported anxiety status as the outcome variable, a total of 98,784 participants answered the anxiety-related questions, and 19,759 were classified into anxiety group. With the anxiety GAD score as the outcome variable, a total of 110,023 participants completed the questionnaire.

3.1.2. Characteristics of UK Biobank Subjects with Vitamin D PRS Data

In the self-reported depression status, a total of 121,685 participants answered depression-related questions, of which 58,349 were included in depression group; in the depression PHQ scores, a total of 120,033 participants completed the questionnaire. In the self-reported anxiety status, a total of 108,309 participants answered anxiety-related questions, of which 21,807 were classified into anxiety group. In addition, in the anxiety GAD scores, a total of 120,590 participants completed the questionnaire. Detailed information is shown in Table ??.

Table 1. General population characteristics of this study participants from UK Biobank.

Outcome Variable	Independent Variable	Number/(Case/Control)	Sex (Female)	Age ± SD
Depression status	Blood VD	52,766/57,978	61,458 (55.50%)	56.40 ±7.68
	VDPRS After COJO	58,349/63,336	68,365 (56.18%)	56.47 ± 7.65
	VDPRS Before COJO	58,349/63,336	68,365 (56.18%)	56.47 ± 7.65
Anxiety status	Blood VD	19,759/79,025	53,541 (54.20%)	56.42 ± 7.60
	VDPRS After COJO	21,807/86,502	59,453 (54.89%)	56.50 ± 7.57
	VDPRS Before COJO	21,807/86,502	59,453 (54.89%)	56.50 ± 7.57
Depression (PHQ score)	Blood VD	109,543	60,377 (55.12%)	56.16 ± 7.65
	VDPRS After COJO	120,033	66,934 (55.76%)	56.24 ± 7.62
	VDPRS Before COJO	120,033	66,934 (55.76%)	56.24 ± 7.62
Anxiety (GAD score)	Blood VD	110,023	60,629 (55.11%)	56.15 ± 7.65
	VDPRS After COJO	120,590	67,235 (55.76%)	56.23 ± 7.61
	VDPRS Before COJO	120,590	67,235 (55.76%)	56.23 ± 7.61

Abbreviations: VD, Vitamin D; VDPRS, polygenic risk score of vitamin D; COJO, conditional and joint analysis; SD, age was described as mean ± standard deviation (SD); PHQ score, patient health questionnaire (PHQ) is used to describe the depression; GAD score, general anxiety disorder (GAD) is used to describe the anxiety of the participants.

3.2. Regression Analysis Result

3.2.1. Associations between Blood Vitamin D and Depression, Anxiety Traits in UK Biobank Cohort

Significant associations of blood VD level with self-reported depression status (odds ratio (OR) = 0.89, $p = 5.92 \times 10^{-77}$) and self-reported anxiety status (OR = 0.92,

$p = 1.46 \times 10^{-22}$) were observed. Associations were also observed between the blood VD level, the depression PHQ score (Beta = -0.062, standard error (SE) = 0.003, $p = 5.95 \times 10^{-96}$), and the anxiety GAD score (Beta = -0.030, SE = 0.00, $p = 1.21 \times 10^{-21}$).

3.2.2. Associations between Vitamin D PRS and Depression, Anxiety Traits in UK Biobank Cohort

We observed significant associations of VD PRS before COJO adjustment with self-reported depression status (OR = 0.99, $p = 3.82 \times 10^{-2}$), depression PHQ score (Beta = -0.0060, SE = 0.003, $p = 3.25 \times 10^{-2}$), and anxiety GAD score (Beta = -0.010, SE = 0.00, $p = 4.36 \times 10^{-2}$). In addition, we also observed significant associations of VD PRS after COJO adjustment with a self-reported depression status (OR = 0.99, $p = 1.84 \times 10^{-2}$), a depression PHQ score (Beta = -0.0070, SE = 0.0030, $p = 9.15 \times 10^{-3}$), and an anxiety GAD score (Beta = -0.010, SE = 0.00, $p = 1.02 \times 10^{-2}$). Detailed information is shown in Table ??.

Table 2. The associations between Vitamin D traits and traits of depression and anxiety.

Outcome Variable	Independent Variable	Beta	SE	T	p–Value	OR
Depression status	Blood VD	-0.12	0.01	-18.57	5.92×10^{-77}	0.89
	VDPRS After COJO	-0.014	0.006	-2.36	1.84×10^{-2}	0.99
	VDPRS Before COJO	-0.012	0.006	-2.07	3.82×10^{-2}	0.99
Anxiety status	Blood VD	-0.080	0.01	-9.77	1.46×10^{-22}	0.92
	VDPRS After COJO	0.00	0.01	-0.29	7.71×10^{-1}	1.00
	VDPRS Before COJO	0.00	0.01	-0.32	7.47×10^{-1}	1.00
Depression (PHQ score)	Blood VD	-0.062	0.003	-20.81	5.95×10^{-96}	–
	VDPRS After COJO	-0.007	0.003	-2.61	9.15×10^{-3}	–
	VDPRS Before COJO	-0.006	0.003	-2.14	3.25×10^{-2}	–
Anxiety (GAD score)	Blood VD	-0.030	0.00	-9.56	1.21×10^{-21}	–
	VDPRS After COJO VDPRS	-0.010	0.00	-2.57	1.02×10^{-2}	–
	Before COJO	-0.010	0.00	-2.02	4.36×10^{-2}	–

Abbreviations: SE, standard error; T, t–test; OR, odd ratios; VD, vitamin D; VDPRS, polygenic risk score of vitamin D; COJO, conditional and joint analysis; PHQ score, patient health questionnaire (PHQ) is used to describe the depression; GAD score, general anxiety disorder (GAD) is used to describe the anxiety of the participants. Note. Logistic regression was used to evaluate the association between blood VD, VD PRS before COJO adjustment, VD PRS after COJO adjustment and self-reported depression and anxiety. Linear regression was used to evaluate the association between blood VD, VD PRS before COJO adjustment, VD PRS after COJO adjustment and PHQ score, GAD score.

3.3. GWEIS Analysis Results

For self-reported depression status, GWEIS identified a significant gene × VD PRS interaction ($p < 5.0 \times 10^{-8}$) at the LRRTM4 gene (rs114086183, $p = 4.11 \times 10^{-8}$). For self-reported anxiety status, significant gene × VD PRS interaction was detected at the GNB5 gene (rs149760119, $p = 3.88 \times 10^{-8}$). For the depression PHQ score, two significant gene × blood VD interactions were identified at SLC11A2 and HIGD1C (rs117102029, $p = 4.02 \times 10^{-8}$). For the anxiety GAD score, we detected multiple significant gene × VD trait interactions, such as SMYD3 (rs142593645, $p = 2.51 \times 10^{-8}$), SEMA3E (rs76440131, $p = 2.80 \times 10^{-10}$), and VTI1A (rs17266687, $p = 3.09 \times 10^{-8}$). Among them, three genes (SEMA3E, DOCK8, TMCO3) were identified by VD PRS before and after COJO adjustment. The visualization of the results is shown in ??????. Additional detailed results are shown in Table ??.

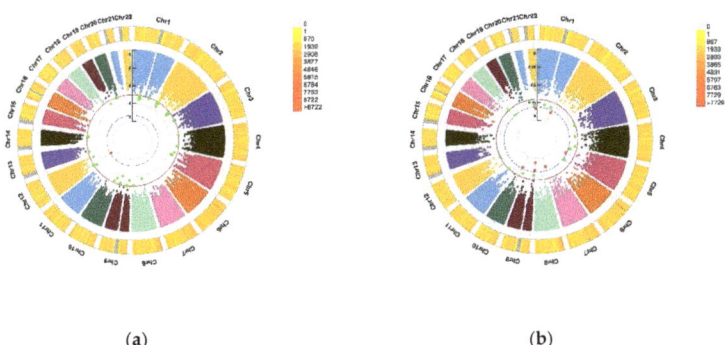

(a)   (b)

Figure 1. Genomic regions interacting with blood VD for the PHQ score and the GAD score. (**a**) Depression (PHQ score), A SNP allele was found to significantly interact with blood VD in depression (PHQ score); (**b**) Anxiety (GAD score), seven independent SNP alleles were found to significantly interact with blood VD in anxiety disorder (GAD score). From the center, the first circos depicts the $-\log 10$ p-values of each variant due to double exposure, i.e., the effect of both SNP allele and blood VD. The second circos shows chromosome density. Red dots represent the $p < 5 \times 10^{-8}$ and green dots represent $p < 1 \times 10^{-7}$. The figure was generated using the "CMplot" R script (https://github.com/YinLiLin/R-CMplot) (accessed on 15 February 2021).

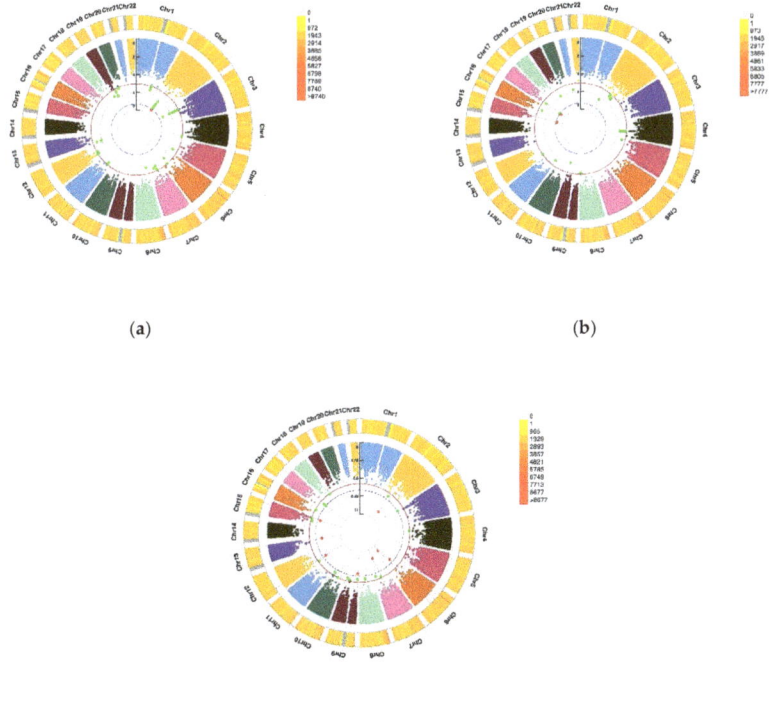

Figure 2. Genomic regions interacting with VD PRS after COJO adjustment for depression status, anxiety status, and GAD score. (**a**) Depression status, a SNP allele was found to significantly interact with blood VD in depression status; (**b**) Anxiety status, 2 independent SNP alleles were found to significantly interact with blood VD in anxiety status; (**c**) Anxiety (GAD score), 8 independent SNP alleles interacted significantly with blood VD in anxiety disorders (GAD score). From the center, the first circos depicts the $-\log 10$ p-values of each variant due to double exposure, i.e., the effect of both SNP allele and VD PRS after COJO adjustment. The second circos shows chromosome density. Red dots represent the $p < 5 \times 10^{-8}$ and green dots represent $p < 1 \times 10^{-7}$. The figure was generated using the "CMplot" R script (https://github.com/YinLiLin/R-CMplot) (accessed on 15 February 2021).

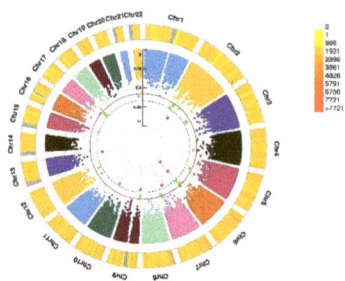

Figure 3. Genomic regions interacting with VD PRS before COJO adjustment for GAD score. This graph shows 7 independent SNP alleles interacting significantly with blood VD in anxiety disorders (GAD score). From the center, the first circos depicts the $-\log 10$ p-values of each variant due to double exposure, i.e., the effect of both SNP allele and VD PRS before COJO adjustment. The second circos shows chromosome density. Red dots represent the $p < 5 \times 10^{-8}$ and green dots represent $p < 1 \times 10^{-7}$. The figure was generated using the "CMplot" R script (https://github.com/YinLiLin/R-CMplot) (accessed on 15 February 2021).

Table 3. Summary of gene–environment interaction analysis among SNP and VD traits for depression and anxiety traits.

	CHR	SNP	Model	Beta	SE	Gene	p-Value
Depression status	2	rs114086183	ADD × VD PRS afterCOJO	0.16	0.029	LRRTM4	4.11×10^{-8}
Anxiety status	15	rs149760119	ADD × VD PRS afterCOJO	−0.22	0.04	GNB5	3.88×10^{-8}
Depression (PHQ score)	12	rs117102029	ADD × VD blood	0.01	0.002	SLC11A2, HIGD1C	4.02×10^{-8}
Anxiety (GAD score)	1	rs142593645	ADD × VD blood	1.52	0.27	SMYD3	2.51×10^{-8}
	7	rs13228257	ADD × VD blood	−1.25	0.22	DPP6	1.45×10^{-8}
	7	rs76440131	ADD × VD PRS afterCOJO	−2.64	0.42	SEMA3E	2.80×10^{-10}
	9	rs78029983	ADD × VD PRS afterCOJO	−1.08	0.19	DOCK8	2.43×10^{-10}
	13	rs76004204	ADD × VD PRS afterCOJO	2.17	0.37	TMCO3	6.38×10^{-9}
	7	rs76440131	ADD × VD PRS beforeCOJO	−2.16	0.38	SEMA3E	1.76×10^{-8}
	9	rs78029983	ADD × VD PRS beforeCOJO	−1.10	0.20	DOCK8	2.10×10^{-8}
	10	rs17266687	ADD × VD PRS beforeCOJO	−1.20	0.21	VTI1A	2.48×10^{-8}
	13	rs76004204	ADD × VD PRS beforeCOJO	1.97	0.34	TMCO3	8.89×10^{-9}

Abbreviations: CHR, chromosome; SNP, single nucleotide polymorphism; SE, standard error; ADD, additive effect; VD, vitamin D; VDPRS, polygenic risk score of vitamin D; COJO, conditional and joint analysis; PHQ score, patient health questionnaire (PHQ) is used to describe the depression; GAD score, general anxiety disorder (GAD) is used to describe the anxiety of the participants; p-value, estimates of the effect of interaction on depression and anxiety traits by using ADD × VD traits.

4. Discussion

Since many complex diseases are associated with thousands of genetic variations, GWAS study merely calculates the association between a single SNP and a phenotype, which could easily lead to a decline in the interpretation of phenotypes influenced by multiple genetic variations. In this study, using individual blood VD level and calculated VD PRS data, we systematically evaluated the associations of VD traits with depression and anxiety traits. Then, we conducted GWEIS to clarify the potential effects of gene × VD interaction on depression and anxiety traits. We observed significant associations between VD and depression and anxiety traits in the UK Biobank cohort, and GWEIS analysis identified the effects of multiple significant gene × VD interactions on depression and anxiety traits.

As mentioned before, previous studies on VD and psychiatric disorders merely focused on the effects of environmental or genetic factors on the risks of depression and anxiety, usually without considering the interaction between them. For anxiety, multiple studies have observed that VD level was associated with anxiety [?], and VD supplementation can significantly improve patients' anxiety symptoms after adjusting for covariates known to affect VD level [?]. However, there is also controversy about the association between VD and depression. For instance, Zhao et al. found that VD was not associated with an increased risk of depression after adjusting for potential confounders, such as age, gender, race, physical activity, alcohol use, and chronic diseases [?]. Some studies conducted in different regions failed to observe the association between VD and depression when controlled for potential confounding factors [? ?]. In contrast, Milaneschi et al. observed that low VD levels were associated with the presence and severity of depression, suggesting that VD represented a potential biological vulnerability for depression [?]. Additionally, a prospective association study of VD and depression using UKB cohort data found that both vitamin D deficiency and insufficiency may be risk factors for new onset depression in middle-aged adults [?]. Our results support an association between VD traits and depression and anxiety traits in the UK Biobank cohort, particularly from a genetic perspective. It is important to note that our study found an association between VD and depression and anxiety; however, further research is needed to determine whether there was a causal association and in what direction.

Currently, to the best of our knowledge, there are limited researches to explore the genetic mechanism affecting the link between VD and depression and anxiety. Therefore, we performed GWEIS and identified multiple candidate genes interacting with VD, which are implicated in the brain or neural regulation and pathology, such as LRRTM4 for depression status and GNB5 for anxiety status. The LRRTM4 is a new four-membered family of genes from human and mice. Its main function is to encode a putative leucine-rich repeat transmembrane protein, which can not only facilitate the development of glutamate synapses, but also regulate many cellular events during nervous system development and disease [? ?]. In animal experiments, it has been found that LRRTM4 is expressed in many brain regions and nervous system neurons, suggesting that LRRTM4 plays a vital role in the development and maintenance of the vertebrate nervous system [?]. In addition, the role of VD in regulating brain axon growth has been observed in previous studies [?], and prenatal VD deficiency has been shown to alter many genes involved in synaptic plasticity [?]. Whether VD deficiency alters the LRRTM4 gene remains elusive and need further studies.

For anxiety status, the identified GNB5 gene is the G protein subunit beta 5 (Gβ5) that encodes a heterotrimeric GTP binding protein. Gβ5 is enriched in the central nervous system. Its main function is to form a complex with regulatory factors of the G protein signal transduction protein family, thereby regulating and affecting the neurotransmitter signal transduction of many neurobehavioral results [?]. A previous study found that VD can affect adult brain development and function through signal transduction [?]. Furthermore, a study of the expression of genes associated with Alzheimer's disease in the presence of VD deficiency found that GNB5 expression was significantly reduced [?]. We may infer that VD can regulate G-protein-mediated signaling in the brain by influencing the GNB5 gene [?]. In addition, previous studies have indicated that GNB5 gene mutations can lead to severe speech disorders, motor delays, and attention deficit hyperactivity disorder (ADHD) as the main manifestations of recessive neurodevelopmental disorders [? ?].

For the anxiety GAD score, our GWEIS results showed that multiple genes have significant interactions with vitamin D. DPP6 is a single-channel type II transmembrane protein expressed in the brain, which mainly regulates the dendritic excitability of hippocampal neurons [?]. Cacace et al. found that DPP6 is a new genetic factor in dementia. DPP6 is involved in a variety of cellular pathways, including neurogenesis and neuronal excitability, and its deletion has been associated with low intelligence and neurodevelopmental disorders [?]. Another study in an animal model also found that DPP6 deletion affects hippocampal synaptic development and leads to behavioral impairments in recognition, learning, and memory [?]. Similar to the DPP6 gene, Tang's study found that VTI1A is mainly involved in neuronal development and neurotransmission, and mutations are likely to lead to neurological dysfunction and neurological diseases [?]. In common genes identified by VD PRS before and after COJO adjustment, SEMA3E is a member of the signaling family that binds directly to the receptor Plexin-D1 to secrete brain signals. A study found that SEMA3E-Plexin-D1 signaling is not only involved in axon growth and guidance, but also determines synaptic recognition and specificity in multiple parts of the nervous system [?]. Although these genes have been found to play a certain role in the development and conduction of the nervous system, the potential biological mechanism of the interaction between these genes and VD to affect the nervous system function and disease has not been found, which needs further research and confirmation.

In addition, we identified multiple candidate genes which interacted with vitamin D for the depression PHQ score, such as SLC11A2 and HIGD1C. The SLC11A2 gene, also called DMT1, is an iron-responsive gene mainly involved in iron absorption [?]. Mutations in this gene will affect the changes in the body's iron content. Bastian et al. [?] found that iron deficiency in the early life can damage the expression of hippocampal neuron genes, leading to long-term neurological dysfunction. Saadat et al. [?] observed that the TT genotype and the T allele of the 1254T > C polymorphism in the DMT1 gene may be a risk factor for Parkinson's disease. At present, few researches were conducted to explain the function and role of the HIGD1C gene. However, the HIGD1A gene, which came from the same family as the HIGD1C gene (HIG1 hypoxia-inducible domain family), has been found to be related to the nervous system in previous studies. Research conducted by López's et al. found that the HIGD1A gene is not only widely expressed in the rat brain, but also may play a protective role in certain areas of the central nervous system [?]. Nevertheless, no studies have shown a direct link between VD and the effects of SLC11A2 and HIGD1C genes on the nervous system and psychiatric disorders. It is worth mentioning that previous studies have found the important role of VD in the brain and nervous system, such as VD differentiates brain cells [?], which regulates axon growth [?] and can regulate calcium signaling [?]. VD can not only affect adult brain development and function through signal transduction, but also affect the nutritional support factors of developing and mature neurons and prevent the production of reactive oxygen species. These all support the importance of VD for development and function of human brain.

Molecular genetic studies have confirmed the presence of widespread pleiotropy across psychiatric disorders [?]. Previous studies have found that depression and anxiety are highly comorbid and share a common underlying basis, including symptom overlap, potential negative affectivity, shared familial risk, stress, negative cognitions, and similar neural-circuitry dysfunction related to emotion regulation [? ? ?]. According to Gray and McNaughton's theory, this comorbidity is caused by the recursive interconnection of brain regions that connect fear, anxiety, and panic, as well as hereditary personality traits such as neuroticism [?]. Twin and familial studies have shown that comorbidity of depression and anxiety disorders is largely explained by shared genetic risk factors [?]. However, a recent factor analysis and genomic structural equation modelling study on depression and anxiety found that depressive and anxiety symptoms could be affected by different factors, although the genetic correlation between the factors was high [?]. In this study, we further compared and identified genetic loci between depression and anxiety; no overlapping loci were found, suggesting that VD may have different biological mechanisms in depression and anxiety. It is considered that environmental exposure can contribute to the development of depression and anxiety through different molecular mechanisms [?]. Furthermore, based on the results of genomic structural equation modeling [?] and the differences in etiology and pathogenesis of depression and anxiety [?], it is reasonable to infer that few genetic loci interacting with VD promote the occurrence and development of depression and anxiety at the same time. Genetic research that assesses the link between VD and psychiatric disorders are limited, and further exploration is needed to confirm our findings.

It is worth noting that our study has some limitations. First, all research data in our study were derived from the UK Biobank, and the research participants were limited to people of European descent. Due to different genetic backgrounds, the results of this study should be interpreted with caution when applying the results to other populations. Secondly, in our research, we mainly used self-reports and related questionnaire scores to characterize depression and anxiety states. Since there is no systematic method to classify all the symptoms, the self-reported analysis results may not be completely consistent with the analysis results of questionnaire scores; in addition, self-reported results may increase the possibility of measurement error and recall bias. Due to the lack of temporal sequence between variables and the absence of Mendelian Randomization study, it is not possible to draw evidence for causality directly, resulting in the lack of demonstration strength of the study. Finally, there is a lack of relevant researches to investigate the influence of the identified SNPs on the biological mechanisms of depression and anxiety. More large sample prospective studies and biological studies are needed to confirm our results and elucidate the potential role of new genetic variants in the pathogenesis of psychiatric disorders.

5. Conclusions

In summary, through regression analysis and GWEIS analysis, we observed that the VD was negatively associated with depression and anxiety, and further GWEIS analysis identified multiple candidate genes related to depression and anxiety. The interaction effects observed from the results provide new direction for understanding the genetic research of psychiatric disorders. Further research is needed to clarify the underlying mechanism of gene × VD interaction effects for psychiatric disorders.

Supplementary Materials: The following are available online at https://www.mdpi.com/2072-6643/13/10/3343/s1, Table S1: Present and past depression and/or bipolar affective disorder. Table S2: Generalized anxiety disorder.

Author Contributions: Z.Z. had full access to all the data in the study and takes responsibility for the integrity of the data and the accuracy of the data analysis. X.Y. contributed equally to the work as co–senior authors. Y.W., Y.J. and F.Z. conceptualized and designed the study. Z.Z., X.Y., Y.J., Y.W., S.C., P.M., C.L., H.Z., C.P., J.Z., Y.C. and F.Z. contributed in acquisition, analysis, and interpretation of the data. Z.Z. drafted the manuscript. F.Z., X.Y. helped with critical revision of the manuscript for important intellectual content. S.C. performed statistical analysis. Y.W., Y.J. and F.Z. provided administrative, technical, or material support. F.Z. supervised the study. All authors have read and agreed to the published version of the manuscript.

Funding: This study was supported by the National Natural Scientific Foundation of China (81922059).

Institutional Review Board Statement: This study has been approved by UKB (Application 46478) and obtained participants' health-related records.

Informed Consent Statement: Informed consent was obtained from all subjects involved in the study.

Data Availability Statement: The UK Biobank data are available through the UK Biobank Access Management System https://www.ukbiobank.ac.uk/ (accessed on 20 December 2020). We will return the derived data fields following UK Biobank policy; in due course, they will be available through the UK Biobank Access Management System.

Acknowledgments: This study was conducted using the UK Biobank Resource (Application 46478).

Conflicts of Interest: All authors report no biomedical financial interests or potential conflicts of interest.

References

1. Battle, D.E. Diagnostic and Statistical Manual of Mental Disorders (DSM). *Codas* **2013**, *25*, 191–192. [CrossRef] [PubMed]
2. Richter, D.; Wall, A.; Bruen, A.; Whittington, R. Is the global prevalence rate of adult mental illness increasing? Systematic review and meta-analysis. *Acta Psychiatr. Scand.* **2019**, *140*, 393–407. [CrossRef] [PubMed]
3. Friedrich, M.J. Depression Is the Leading Cause of Disability Around the World. *JAMA* **2017**, *317*, 1517. [CrossRef] [PubMed]
4. Bekhuis, E.; Boschloo, L.; Rosmalen, J.G.; Schoevers, R.A. Differential associations of specific depressive and anxiety disorders with somatic symptoms. *J. Psychosom. Res.* **2015**, *78*, 116–122. [CrossRef]

5. Wang, Y.H.; Li, J.Q.; Shi, J.F.; Que, J.Y.; Liu, J.J.; Lappin, J.M.; Leung, J.; Ravindran, A.V.; Chen, W.Q.; Qiao, Y.L.; et al. Depression and anxiety in relation to cancer incidence and mortality: A systematic review and meta-analysis of cohort studies. *Mol. Psychiatry* **2020**, *25*, 1487–1499. [CrossRef]
6. Groves, N.J.; McGrath, J.J.; Burne, T.H. Vitamin D as a neurosteroid affecting the developing and adult brain. *Annu. Rev. Nutr.* **2014**, *34*, 117–141. [CrossRef]
7. Bahrami, A.; Sadeghnia, H.R.; Tabatabaeizadeh, S.A.; Bahrami-Taghanaki, H.; Behboodi, N.; Esmaeili, H.; Ferns, G.A.; Mobarhan, M.G.; Avan, A. Genetic and epigenetic factors influencing vitamin D status. *J. Cell Physiol.* **2018**, *233*, 4033–4043. [CrossRef] [PubMed]
8. Ahn, J.; Albanes, D.; Berndt, S.I.; Peters, U.; Chatterjee, N.; Freedman, N.D.; Abnet, C.C.; Huang, W.Y.; Kibel, A.S.; Crawford, E.D.; et al. Vitamin D-related genes, serum vitamin D concentrations and prostate cancer risk. *Carcinogenesis* **2009**, *30*, 769–776. [CrossRef]
9. Szpunar, M.J. Association of antepartum vitamin D deficiency with postpartum depression: A clinical perspective. *Public Health Nutr.* **2020**, *23*, 1173–1178. [CrossRef]
10. Bersani, F.S.; Ghezzi, F.; Maraone, A.; Vicinanza, R.; Cavaggioni, G.; Biondi, M.; Pasquini, M. The relationship between Vitamin D and depressive disorders. *Riv. Psichiatr.* **2019**, *54*, 229–234. [CrossRef] [PubMed]
11. Anglin, R.E.; Samaan, Z.; Walter, S.D.; McDonald, S.D. Vitamin D deficiency and depression in adults: Systematic review and meta-analysis. *Br. J. Psychiatry* **2013**, *202*, 100–107. [CrossRef]
12. Hoang, M.T.; Defina, L.F.; Willis, B.L.; Leonard, D.S.; Weiner, M.F.; Brown, E.S. Association between low serum 25-hydroxyvitamin D and depression in a large sample of healthy adults: The Cooper Center longitudinal study. *Mayo Clin. Proc.* **2011**, *86*, 1050–1055. [CrossRef]
13. Fond, G.; Godin, O.; Schürhoff, F.; Berna, F.; Bulzacka, E.; Andrianarisoa, M.; Brunel, L.; Aouizerate, B.; Capdevielle, D.; Chereau, I.; et al. Hypovitaminosis D is associated with depression and anxiety in schizophrenia: Results from the national FACE-SZ cohort. *Psychiatry Res.* **2018**, *270*, 104–110. [CrossRef]
14. Ikonen, H.; Palaniswamy, S.; Nordstrom, T.; Jarvelin, M.R.; Herzig, K.H.; Jaaskelainen, E.; Seppala, J.; Miettunen, J.; Sebert, S. Vitamin D status and correlates of low vitamin D in schizophrenia, other psychoses and non-psychotic depression—The Northern Finland Birth Cohort 1966 study. *Psychiatry Res.* **2019**, *279*, 186–194. [CrossRef]
15. Libuda, L.; Laabs, B.H.; Ludwig, C.; Bühlmeier, J.; Antel, J.; Hinney, A.; Naaresh, R.; Föcker, M.; Hebebrand, J.; König, I.R.; et al. Vitamin D and the Risk of Depression: A Causal Relationship? Findings from a Mendelian Randomization Study. *Nutrients* **2019**, *11*, 1085. [CrossRef]
16. Kim, S.Y.; Jeon, S.W.; Lim, W.J.; Oh, K.S.; Shin, D.W.; Cho, S.J.; Park, J.H.; Shin, Y.C. The Relationship between Serum Vitamin D Levels, C-Reactive Protein, and Anxiety Symptoms. *Psychiatry Investig.* **2020**, *17*, 312–319. [CrossRef]
17. Niles, A.N.; Smirnova, M.; Lin, J.; O'Donovan, A. Gender differences in longitudinal relationships between depression and anxiety symptoms and inflammation in the health and retirement study. *Psychoneuroendocrinology* **2018**, *95*, 149–157. [CrossRef]
18. Tanaka, M.; Tóth, F.; Polyák, H.; Szabó, Á.; Mándi, Y.; Vécsei, L. Immune Influencers in Action: Metabolites and Enzymes of the Tryptophan-Kynurenine Metabolic Pathway. *Biomedicines* **2021**, *9*, 734. [CrossRef] [PubMed]
19. Luna, R.A.; Foster, J.A. Gut brain axis: Diet microbiota interactions and implications for modulation of anxiety and depression. *Curr. Opin. Biotechnol.* **2015**, *32*, 35–41. [CrossRef] [PubMed]
20. Bear, T.L.K.; Dalziel, J.E.; Coad, J.; Roy, N.C.; Butts, C.A.; Gopal, P.K. The Role of the Gut Microbiota in Dietary Interventions for Depression and Anxiety. *Adv. Nutr.* **2020**, *11*, 890–907. [CrossRef] [PubMed]
21. Sullivan, P.F.; Neale, M.C.; Kendler, K.S. Genetic epidemiology of major depression: Review and meta-analysis. *Am. J. Psychiatry* **2000**, *157*, 1552–1562. [CrossRef]
22. Kendler, K.S.; Gatz, M.; Gardner, C.O.; Pedersen, N.L. A Swedish national twin study of lifetime major depression. *Am. J. Psychiatry* **2006**, *163*, 109–114. [CrossRef]
23. Purves, K.L.; Coleman, J.R.I.; Meier, S.M.; Rayner, C.; Davis, K.A.S.; Cheesman, R.; Bækvad-Hansen, M.; Børglum, A.D.; Wan Cho, S.; Jürgen Deckert, J.; et al. A major role for common genetic variation in anxiety disorders. *Mol. Psychiatry* **2020**, *25*, 3292–3303. [CrossRef]
24. Dudbridge, F. Power and predictive accuracy of polygenic risk scores. *PLoS Genet.* **2013**, *9*, e1003348. [CrossRef]
25. Euesden, J.; Lewis, C.M.; O'Reilly, P.F. PRSice: Polygenic Risk Score software. *Bioinformatics* **2015**, *31*, 1466–1468. [CrossRef]
26. Schizophrenia Working Group of the Psychiatric Genomics Consortium. Biological insights from 108 schizophrenia-associated genetic loci. *Nature* **2014**, *511*, 421–427. [CrossRef] [PubMed]
27. Zhang, J.P.; Robinson, D.; Yu, J.; Gallego, J.; Fleischhacker, W.W.; Kahn, R.S.; Crespo-Facorro, B.; Vazquez-Bourgon, J.; Kane, J.M.; Malhotra, A.K.; et al. Schizophrenia Polygenic Risk Score as a Predictor of Antipsychotic Efficacy in First-Episode Psychosis. *Am. J. Psychiatry* **2019**, *176*, 21–28. [CrossRef]
28. Revez, J.A.; Lin, T.; Qiao, Z.; Xue, A.; Holtz, Y.; Zhu, Z.; Zeng, J.; Wang, H.; Sidorenko, J.; Kemper, K.E.; et al. Genome-wide association study identifies 143 loci associated with 25 hydroxyvitamin D concentration. *Nat. Commun.* **2020**, *11*, 1647. [CrossRef]
29. Hou, L.; Bergen, S.E.; Akula, N.; Song, J.; Hultman, C.M.; Landén, M.; Adli, M.; Alda, M.; Ardau, R.; Arias, B.; et al. Genome-wide association study of 40,000 individuals identifies two novel loci associated with bipolar disorder. *Hum. Mol. Genet.* **2016**, *25*, 3383–3394. [CrossRef]

30. Rask-Andersen, M.; Karlsson, T.; Ek, W.E.; Johansson, Å. Gene-environment interaction study for BMI reveals interactions between genetic factors and physical activity, alcohol consumption and socioeconomic status. *PLoS Genet.* **2017**, *13*, e1006977. [CrossRef]
31. van Os, J.; Rutten, B.P. Gene-environment-wide interaction studies in psychiatry. *Am. J. Psychiatry* **2009**, *166*, 964–966. [CrossRef]
32. Rivera, N.V.; Patasova, K.; Kullberg, S.; Diaz-Gallo, L.M.; Iseda, T.; Bengtsson, C.; Alfredsson, L.; Eklund, A.; Kockum, I.; Grunewald, J.; et al. A Gene-Environment Interaction Between Smoking and Gene polymorphisms Provides a High Risk of Two Subgroups of Sarcoidosis. *Sci. Rep.* **2019**, *9*, 18633. [CrossRef]
33. Sudlow, C.; Gallacher, J.; Allen, N.; Beral, V.; Burton, P.; Danesh, J.; Downey, P.; Elliott, P.; Green, J.; Landray, M.; et al. UK biobank: An open access resource for identifying the causes of a wide range of complex diseases of middle and old age. *PLoS Med.* **2015**, *12*, e1001779. [CrossRef]
34. Davis, K.A.S.; Cullen, B.; Adams, M.; Brailean, A.; Breen, G.; Coleman, J.R.I.; Dregan, A.; Gaspar, H.A.; Hübel, C.; Lee, W.; et al. Indicators of mental disorders in UK Biobank-A comparison of approaches. *Int. J. Methods Psychiatr. Res.* **2019**, *28*, e1796. [CrossRef] [PubMed]
35. Kroenke, K.; Spitzer, R.L.; Williams, J.B. The PHQ-9: Validity of a brief depression severity measure. *J. Gen. Intern. Med.* **2001**, *16*, 606–613. [CrossRef]
36. Spitzer, R.L.; Kroenke, K.; Williams, J.B.; Löwe, B. A brief measure for assessing generalized anxiety disorder: The GAD-7. *Arch. Intern. Med.* **2006**, *166*, 1092–1097. [CrossRef]
37. Gigantesco, A.; Morosini, P. Development, reliability and factor analysis of a self-administered questionnaire which originates from the World Health Organization's Composite International Diagnostic Interview—Short Form (CIDI-SF) for assessing mental disorders. *Clin. Pract. Epidemiol. Ment. Health* **2008**, *4*, 8. [CrossRef]
38. Manea, L.; Gilbody, S.; McMillan, D. Optimal cut-off score for diagnosing depression with the Patient Health Questionnaire (PHQ-9): A meta-analysis. *CMAJ* **2012**, *184*, E191–E196. [CrossRef]
39. Kroenke, K.; Spitzer, R.L.; Williams, J.B.; Löwe, B. The Patient Health Questionnaire Somatic, Anxiety, and Depressive Symptom Scales: A systematic review. *Gen. Hosp. Psychiatry* **2010**, *32*, 345–359. [CrossRef]
40. Bycroft, C.; Freeman, C.; Petkova, D.; Band, G.; Elliott, L.T.; Sharp, K.; Motyer, A.; Vukcevic, D.; Delaneau, O.; O'Connell, J.; et al. The UK Biobank resource with deep phenotyping and genomic data. *Nature* **2018**, *562*, 203–209. [CrossRef]
41. Walter, K.; Min, J.L.; Huang, J.; Crooks, L.; Memari, Y.; McCarthy, S.; Perry, J.R.; Xu, C.; Futema, M.; Lawson, D.; et al. The UK10K project identifies rare variants in health and disease. *Nature* **2015**, *526*, 82–90. [CrossRef]
42. McCarthy, S.; Das, S.; Kretzschmar, W.; Delaneau, O.; Wood, A.R.; Teumer, A.; Kang, H.M.; Fuchsberger, C.; Danecek, P.; Sharp, K.; et al. A reference panel of 64,976 haplotypes for genotype imputation. *Nat. Genet.* **2016**, *48*, 1279–1283. [CrossRef] [PubMed]
43. Yang, J.; Ferreira, T.; Morris, A.P.; Medland, S.E.; Madden, P.A.; Heath, A.C.; Martin, N.G.; Montgomery, G.W.; Weedon, M.N.; Loos, R.J.; et al. Conditional and joint multiple-SNP analysis of GWAS summary statistics identifies additional variants influencing complex traits. *Nat. Genet.* **2012**, *44*, s361–s363. [CrossRef] [PubMed]
44. Purcell, S.; Neale, B.; Todd-Brown, K.; Thomas, L.; Ferreira, M.A.; Bender, D.; Maller, J.; Sklar, P.; de Bakker, P.I.; Daly, M.J.; et al. PLINK: A tool set for whole-genome association and population-based linkage analyses. *Am. J. Hum. Genet.* **2007**, *81*, 559–575. [CrossRef]
45. Chang, C.C.; Chow, C.C.; Tellier, L.C.; Vattikuti, S.; Purcell, S.M.; Lee, J.J. Second-generation PLINK: Rising to the challenge of larger and richer datasets. *Gigascience* **2015**, *4*, 7. [CrossRef]
46. Clarke, G.M.; Morris, A.P. A comparison of sample size and power in case-only association studies of gene-environment interaction. *Am. J. Epidemiol.* **2010**, *171*, 498–505. [CrossRef]
47. Kimball, S.M.; Mirhosseini, N.; Rucklidge, J. Database Analysis of Depression and Anxiety in a Community Sample-Response to a Micronutrient Intervention. *Nutrients* **2018**, *10*, 152. [CrossRef]
48. Zhu, C.; Zhang, Y.; Wang, T.; Lin, Y.; Yu, J.; Xia, Q.; Zhu, P.; Zhu, D.M. Vitamin D supplementation improves anxiety but not depression symptoms in patients with vitamin D deficiency. *Brain Behav.* **2020**, *10*, e01760. [CrossRef]
49. Zhao, G.; Ford, E.S.; Li, C.; Balluz, L.S. No associations between serum concentrations of 25-hydroxyvitamin D and parathyroid hormone and depression among US adults. *Br. J. Nutr.* **2010**, *104*, 1696–1702. [CrossRef]
50. Nanri, A.; Mizoue, T.; Matsushita, Y.; Poudel-Tandukar, K.; Sato, M.; Ohta, M.; Mishima, N. Association between serum 25-hydroxyvitamin D and depressive symptoms in Japanese: Analysis by survey season. *Eur. J. Clin. Nutr.* **2009**, *63*, 1444–1447. [CrossRef]
51. Pan, A.; Lu, L.; Franco, O.H.; Yu, Z.; Li, H.; Lin, X. Association between depressive symptoms and 25-hydroxyvitamin D in middle-aged and elderly Chinese. *J. Affect. Disord.* **2009**, *118*, 240–243. [CrossRef] [PubMed]
52. Milaneschi, Y.; Hoogendijk, W.; Lips, P.; Heijboer, A.C.; Schoevers, R.; van Hemert, A.M.; Beekman, A.T.; Smit, J.H.; Penninx, B.W. The association between low vitamin D and depressive disorders. *Mol. Psychiatry* **2014**, *19*, 444–451. [CrossRef] [PubMed]
53. Ronaldson, A.; Arias de la Torre, J.; Gaughran, F.; Bakolis, I.; Hatch, S.L.; Hotopf, M.; Dregan, A. Prospective associations between vitamin D and depression in middle-aged adults: Findings from the UK Biobank cohort. *Psychol. Med.* **2020**, *10*, 1–9. [CrossRef]
54. Laurén, J.; Airaksinen, M.S.; Saarma, M.; Timmusk, T. A novel gene family encoding leucine-rich repeat transmembrane proteins differentially expressed in the nervous system. *Genomics* **2003**, *81*, 411–421. [CrossRef]

55. Reichman, R.D.; Gaynor, S.C.; Monson, E.T.; Gaine, M.E.; Parsons, M.G.; Zandi, P.P.; Potash, J.B.; Willour, V.L. Targeted sequencing of the LRRTM gene family in suicide attempters with bipolar disorder. *Am. J. Med. Genet. B Neuropsychiatr. Genet.* **2020**, *183*, 128–139. [CrossRef]
56. Marini, F.; Bartoccini, E.; Cascianelli, G.; Voccoli, V.; Baviglia, M.G.; Magni, M.V.; Garcia-Gil, M.; Albi, E. Effect of 1alpha,25-dihydroxyvitamin D3 in embryonic hippocampal cells. *Hippocampus* **2010**, *20*, 696–705. [CrossRef]
57. Eyles, D.; Almeras, L.; Benech, P.; Patatian, A.; Mackay-Sim, A.; McGrath, J.; Féron, F. Developmental vitamin D deficiency alters the expression of genes encoding mitochondrial, cytoskeletal and synaptic proteins in the adult rat brain. *J. Steroid Biochem. Mol. Biol.* **2007**, *103*, 538–545. [CrossRef]
58. Shamseldin, H.E.; Masuho, I.; Alenizi, A.; Alyamani, S.; Patil, D.N.; Ibrahim, N.; Martemyanov, K.A.; Alkuraya, F.S. GNB5 mutation causes a novel neuropsychiatric disorder featuring attention deficit hyperactivity disorder, severely impaired language development and normal cognition. *Genome Biol.* **2016**, *17*, 195. [CrossRef]
59. Gezen-Ak, D.; Dursun, E.; Yilmazer, S. The effects of vitamin D receptor silencing on the expression of LVSCC-A1C and LVSCC-A1D and the release of NGF in cortical neurons. *PLoS ONE* **2011**, *6*, e17553. [CrossRef]
60. Grimm, M.O.W.; Lauer, A.A.; Grösgen, S.; Thiel, A.; Lehmann, J.; Winkler, J.; Janitschke, D.; Herr, C.; Beisswenger, C.; Bals, R.; et al. Profiling of Alzheimer's disease related genes in mild to moderate vitamin D hypovitaminosis. *J. Nutr. Biochem.* **2019**, *67*, 123–137. [CrossRef] [PubMed]
61. Mai, J.H.; Ou, Z.H.; Chen, L.; Duan, J.; Liao, J.X.; Han, C.X. Intellectual developmental disorder with cardiac arrhythmia syndrome in a family caused by GNB5 variation and literature review. *Chin. J. Pediatr.* **2020**, *58*, 833–837. [CrossRef]
62. Sun, W.; Maffie, J.K.; Lin, L.; Petralia, R.S.; Rudy, B.; Hoffman, D.A. DPP6 establishes the A-type K(+) current gradient critical for the regulation of dendritic excitability in CA1 hippocampal neurons. *Neuron* **2011**, *71*, 1102–1115. [CrossRef]
63. Cacace, R.; Heeman, B.; Van Mossevelde, S.; De Roeck, A.; Hoogmartens, J.; De Rijk, P.; Gossye, H.; De Vos, K.; De Coster, W.; Strazisar, M.; et al. Loss of DPP6 in neurodegenerative dementia: A genetic player in the dysfunction of neuronal excitability. *Acta Neuropathol.* **2019**, *137*, 901–918. [CrossRef] [PubMed]
64. Lin, L.; Murphy, J.G.; Karlsson, R.M.; Petralia, R.S.; Gutzmann, J.J.; Abebe, D.; Wang, Y.X.; Cameron, H.A.; Hoffman, D.A. DPP6 Loss Impacts Hippocampal Synaptic Development and Induces Behavioral Impairments in Recognition, Learning and Memory. *Front. Cell Neurosci.* **2018**, *12*, 84. [CrossRef]
65. Tang, B.L. Vesicle transport through interaction with t-SNAREs 1a (Vti1a)'s roles in neurons. *Heliyon* **2020**, *6*, e04600. [CrossRef]
66. Oh, W.J.; Gu, C. The role and mechanism-of-action of Sema3E and Plexin-D1 in vascular and neural development. *Semin Cell Dev. Biol.* **2013**, *24*, 156–162. [CrossRef] [PubMed]
67. Casale, M.; Borriello, A.; Scianguetta, S.; Roberti, D.; Caiazza, M.; Bencivenga, D.; Tartaglione, I.; Ladogana, S.; Maruzzi, M.; Della Ragione, F.; et al. Hereditary hypochromic microcytic anemia associated with loss-of-function DMT1 gene mutations and absence of liver iron overload. *Am. J. Hematol.* **2018**, *93*, E58–E60. [CrossRef]
68. Bastian, T.W.; von Hohenberg, W.C.; Mickelson, D.J.; Lanier, L.M.; Georgieff, M.K. Iron Deficiency Impairs Developing Hippocampal Neuron Gene Expression, Energy Metabolism, and Dendrite Complexity. *Dev. Neurosci.* **2016**, *38*, 264–276. [CrossRef] [PubMed]
69. Saadat, S.M.; Değirmenci, İ.; Özkan, S.; Saydam, F.; Özdemir Köroğlu, Z.; Çolak, E.; Güneş, H.V. Is the 1254T > C polymorphism in the DMT1 gene associated with Parkinson's disease? *Neurosci. Lett.* **2015**, *594*, 51–54. [CrossRef] [PubMed]
70. López, L.; Zuluaga, M.J.; Lagos, P.; Agrati, D.; Bedó, G. The Expression of Hypoxia-Induced Gene 1 (Higd1a) in the Central Nervous System of Male and Female Rats Differs According to Age. *J. Mol. Neurosci.* **2018**, *66*, 462–473. [CrossRef]
71. Cui, X.; McGrath, J.J.; Burne, T.H.; Mackay-Sim, A.; Eyles, D.W. Maternal vitamin D depletion alters neurogenesis in the developing rat brain. *Int. J. Dev. Neurosci.* **2007**, *25*, 227–232. [CrossRef] [PubMed]
72. Brewer, L.D.; Thibault, V.; Chen, K.C.; Langub, M.C.; Landfield, P.W.; Porter, N.M. Vitamin D hormone confers neuroprotection in parallel with downregulation of L-type calcium channel expression in hippocampal neurons. *J. Neurosci.* **2001**, *21*, 98–108. [CrossRef] [PubMed]
73. Cross-Disorder Group of the Psychiatric Genomics Consortium. Genomic Relationships, Novel Loci, and Pleiotropic Mechanisms across Eight Psychiatric Disorders. *Cell* **2019**, *179*, 1469–1482.e1411. [CrossRef]
74. Garber, J.; Brunwasser, S.M.; Zerr, A.A.; Schwartz, K.T.; Sova, K.; Weersing, V.R. Treatment and Prevention of Depression and Anxiety in Youth: Test of Cross-Over Effects. *Depress. Anxiety* **2016**, *33*, 939–959. [CrossRef]
75. Balogh, L.; Tanaka, M.; Török, N.; Vécsei, L.; Taguchi, S. Crosstalk between Existential Phenomenological Psychotherapy and Neurological Sciences in Mood and Anxiety Disorders. *Biomedicines* **2021**, *9*, 340. [CrossRef]
76. Tanaka, M.; Vécsei, L. Editorial of Special Issue "Crosstalk between Depression, Anxiety, and Dementia: Comorbidity in Behavioral Neurology and Neuropsychiatry". *Biomedicines* **2021**, *9*, 517. [CrossRef] [PubMed]
77. Middeldorp, C.M.; Cath, D.C.; Van Dyck, R.; Boomsma, D.I. The co-morbidity of anxiety and depression in the perspective of genetic epidemiology. A review of twin and family studies. *Psychol. Med.* **2005**, *35*, 611–624. [CrossRef]
78. Thorp, J.G.; Campos, A.I.; Grotzinger, A.D.; Gerring, Z.F.; An, J.; Ong, J.S.; Wang, W.; Shringarpure, S.; Byrne, E.M.; MacGregor, S.; et al. Symptom-level modelling unravels the shared genetic architecture of anxiety and depression. *Nat. Hum. Behav.* **2021**, 1–11. [CrossRef]

79. Gonda, X.; Petschner, P.; Eszlari, N.; Sutori, S.; Gal, Z.; Koncz, S.; Anderson, I.M.; Deakin, B.; Juhasz, G.; Bagdy, G. Effects of Different Stressors Are Modulated by Different Neurobiological Systems: The Role of GABA-A Versus CB1 Receptor Gene Variants in Anxiety and Depression. *Front. Cell. Neurosci.* **2019**, *13*, 138. [CrossRef] [PubMed]
80. Clark, L.A.; Cuthbert, B.; Lewis-Fernández, R.; Narrow, W.E.; Reed, G.M. Three Approaches to Understanding and Classifying Mental Disorder: ICD-11, DSM-5, and the National Institute of Mental Health's Research Domain Criteria (RDoC). *Psychol. Sci. Public Interes.* **2017**, *18*, 72–145. [CrossRef]

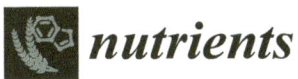

Review

Impact of Genetic Polymorphism on Response to Therapy in Non-Alcoholic Fatty Liver Disease

José Ignacio Martínez-Montoro [1,2], Isabel Cornejo-Pareja [3,4,*], Ana María Gómez-Pérez [1,*] and Francisco J. Tinahones [1,2,3,4]

[1] Department of Endocrinology and Nutrition, Virgen de la Victoria University Hospital, 29010 Málaga, Spain; joseimartinezmontoro@gmail.com (J.I.M.-M.); fjtinahones@hotmail.com (F.J.T.)
[2] Faculty of Medicine, University of Málaga, 29071 Málaga, Spain
[3] Instituto de Investigación Biomédica de Málaga (IBIMA), Virgen de la Victoria University Hospital, 29010 Málaga, Spain
[4] Spanish Biomedical Research Center in Physiopathology of Obesity and Nutrition (CIBERObn), Instituto de Salud Carlos III, 28029 Madrid, Spain
* Correspondence: isabelmaria_cornejo@hotmail.com (I.C.-P.); anamgp86@gmail.com (A.M.G.-P.); Tel.: +34-951034044 (I.C.-P.)

Abstract: In the last decades, the global prevalence of non-alcoholic fatty liver disease (NAFLD) has reached pandemic proportions with derived major health and socioeconomic consequences; this tendency is expected to be further aggravated in the coming years. Obesity, insulin resistance/type 2 diabetes mellitus, sedentary lifestyle, increased caloric intake and genetic predisposition constitute the main risk factors associated with the development and progression of the disease. Importantly, the interaction between the inherited genetic background and some unhealthy dietary patterns has been postulated to have an essential role in the pathogenesis of NAFLD. Weight loss through lifestyle modifications is considered the cornerstone of the treatment for NAFLD and the inter-individual variability in the response to some dietary approaches may be conditioned by the presence of different single nucleotide polymorphisms. In this review, we summarize the current evidence on the influence of the association between genetic susceptibility and dietary habits in NAFLD pathophysiology, as well as the role of gene polymorphism in the response to lifestyle interventions and the potential interaction between nutritional genomics and other emerging therapies for NAFLD, such as bariatric surgery and several pharmacologic agents.

Keywords: non-alcoholic fatty liver disease; gene polymorphism; dietary intervention; gene-nutrient interactions; bariatric surgery; pharmacotherapy

Citation: Martínez-Montoro, J.I.; Cornejo-Pareja, I.; Gómez-Pérez, A.M.; Tinahones, F.J. Impact of Genetic Polymorphism on Response to Therapy in Non-Alcoholic Fatty Liver Disease. *Nutrients* 2021, *13*, 4077. https://doi.org/10.3390/nu13114077

Academic Editors: Daniel-Antonio de Luis Roman and Ana B. Crujeiras

Received: 16 September 2021
Accepted: 9 November 2021
Published: 15 November 2021

Publisher's Note: MDPI stays neutral with regard to jurisdictional claims in published maps and institutional affiliations.

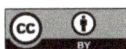

Copyright: © 2021 by the authors. Licensee MDPI, Basel, Switzerland. This article is an open access article distributed under the terms and conditions of the Creative Commons Attribution (CC BY) license (https://creativecommons.org/licenses/by/4.0/).

1. Introduction

Non-alcoholic fatty liver disease (NAFLD) has become the leading cause of chronic liver disease worldwide, with an estimated global prevalence of 25% among the adult population [1]. NAFLD comprises the full spectrum of the disease, from simple macrovesicular steatosis to non-alcoholic steatohepatitis (NASH), which is defined by the coexistence of steatosis, hepatocyte ballooning and inflammation with or without fibrosis, presenting an increased risk of progression to cirrhosis, hepatocellular carcinoma and end-stage liver disease [2]. In addition to the important clinical consequences derived from NAFLD, socioeconomic costs of this pathology have been reported to be enormous and the disease burden is expected to continue to increase in the coming years [3].

NAFLD is directly associated with the different components of the metabolic syndrome, including obesity, type 2 diabetes mellitus (T2DM), dyslipidemia and hypertension; in fact, obesity and insulin resistance/T2DM constitute the most common risk factors for NAFLD [4]. Actually, this disease is considered as the hepatic manifestation of the metabolic syndrome and bidirectional relationships between NAFLD and the rest of metabolic complications have been established [5]. Accordingly, environmental factors such as sedentary lifestyle and high-caloric intake play a major part in NAFLD development and progression [6]. However, it is important to note that NAFLD pathogenesis is complex and several factors are involved in the natural history of this pathology. In line, novel environmental modifiers, such as gut microbiota, have been proved to directly influence the course of the disease [7]. Importantly, genome-wide association studies (GWAS) and candidate gene studies have revealed, in the last few years, that NAFLD development, severity and risk of progression are strongly influenced by a number of single-nucleotide polymorphisms (SNPs), including patatin-like phospholipase domain-containing protein 3 (PNPLA3), transmembrane 6 superfamily member 2 (TM6SF2), membrane bound O-acyltransferase domain containing 7 (MBOAT7), glucokinase regulatory protein (GKRP) and hydroxysteroid 17-βdehydrogenase 13 (HSD17B13) as the main genetic determinants of NAFLD [8]. Moreover, the intricate interaction of genetic predisposition and environmental factors, such as nutrition, is considered to play a key role in the pathophysiology of NAFLD [9].

To date, the mainstay of treatment for NAFLD is weight loss [5]. Lifestyle intervention through dietary habits modifications and structured physical activity enables sustained weight loss and the subsequent hepatic fat content reduction and NASH improvement [10]. Importantly, the effect of specific training modalities, such as endurance training, may contribute to NASH improvement [11]. Furthermore, bariatric surgery (BS) has emerged as an effective therapeutic approach to NASH and fibrosis resolution [12]. However, a significant number of patients do not achieve the expected results even after adequate adherence to therapy. Thereby, among other factors, nutrient-gene interaction could explain this inter-individual variability in response to treatment and gene-based personalized therapies may constitute a useful tool in NAFLD treatment. In this article, we review the role of gene polymorphism in the variability in response to therapy in NAFLD, including the interaction between SNPs and dietary interventions, as well as the potential relationships among nutritional genomics, BS and other therapies.

2. Nutrigenetics and NAFLD Pathogenesis

In addition to the classical metabolic risk factors for NASH and fibrosis progression, several studies have identified genetic associations with NAFLD susceptibility and severity [13]. The I148M (rs738409 C > G) variant of PNPLA3 (isoleucine to methionine exchange at the amino acid position 148 due to cytosine to guanine transversion in rs738409) is the most important risk mutation related to NAFLD, and it is strongly associated with the development and progression of the disease and also with the response to treatment [14] (Figure 1). PNPLA3 exhibits triacylglycerol lipase and acylglycerol transacylase activity in the hepatocytes and the I148M variant causes loss of function, promoting triglyceride accumulation in the hepatocytes [15]. The frequency of the I148M allele is particularly high in Hispanics (0.49), with lower frequencies in European Americans and African Americans; therefore, this fact may partially explain the differences in NAFLD prevalence among different ethnic groups [16]. On the other hand, TM6SF2 regulates hepatic lipid metabolism and the E165K missense variant impairs very low-density lipoprotein (VLDL) secretion and triggers hepatic lipid accumulation [17], whereas MBOAT7 rs641738 C > T SNP increases risk of NAFLD through the imbalance of phosphatidylinositol species [18]. GKRP rs780094 C > T variant presents a reduced capacity of glucokinase inhibition and consequently enhances glycolysis and glucose uptake by the liver [19]. Conversely, HSD17B13 rs6834314 A > G variant, involved in retinol metabolism, protects against NAFLD progression [20]. Finally, other reported genetic determinants associated with NAFLD include SH2B Adaptor Protein 1 (SH2B1), superoxide dismutase 2 (SOD2), signal transducer and activator of transcription 3 (STAT3), phosphatidylethanolamine-N–methyltransferase (PEMT), apolipoprotein B (APOB) or uncoupling protein 2 (UCP2) [21]. Of note, there are some mitochondria-related SNPs among the NAFLD-associated genetic determinants, since mitochondria dysfunction increases oxidative stress which is closely related to NAFLD pathogenesis [22]. Thus, C47T variant in the mitochondrial enzyme SOD2 is linked to advanced fibrosis in NASH [23], whereas mitochondrial UCP2-866 G > A polymorphism reduces risk of NASH progression [24]. Furthermore, mitochondrial deoxyribonucleic acid (DNA) polymorphism 12361 A > G was associated with increased risk of moderate and severe NAFLD in a Chinese population [25].

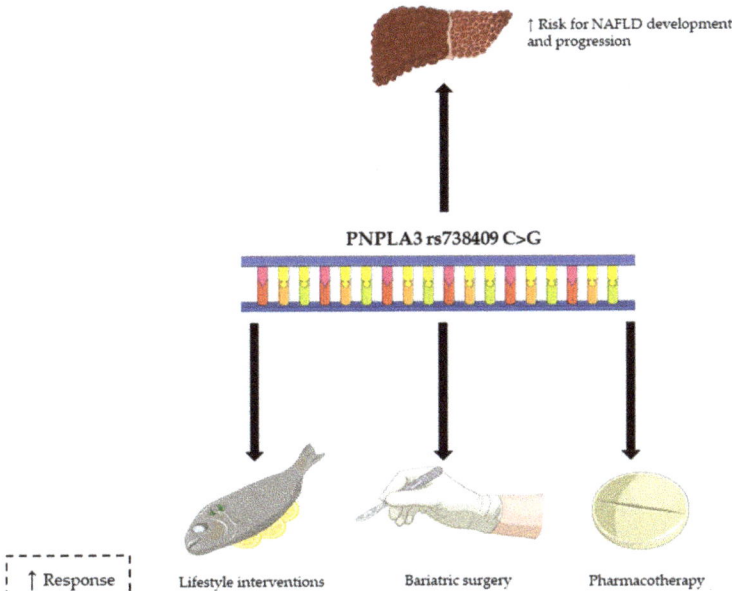

Figure 1. The role of PNPLA3 rs738409 C > G variant in NAFLD. PNPLA3 I148M is associated with NAFLD development and progression, and the interplay between this variant and environmental factors, including dietary habits, seems to be crucial in the pathophysiology of the disease. PNPLA3 I148M presence may also be related to an increased response to lifestyle interventions, bariatric surgery and certain types of therapeutic agents, such as the combination of sodium-glucose cotransporter 2 inhibitors and polyunsaturated fatty acid (PUFA). PNPL3: patatin-like phospholipase domain-containing protein 3; I148M (rs738409 C > G): isoleucine to methionine exchange at the amino acid position 148 due to cytosine to guanine transversion in rs738409); NAFLD: non-alcoholic fatty liver disease.

Notably, SNP-mediated liver damage only explains a small proportion of NAFLD pathophysiology, and synergistic interaction between these risks variants and the environment are needed to trigger significant alterations [26]. As an example, Smagris et al., showed that PNPLA3 I148M knock in mice developed sucrose diet-dependent hepatic steatosis, but no hepatic alterations were found in chow-fed animals with the mutation [27]. Moreover, a preclinical study revealed that several mitochondrial gene polymorphisms only predisposed to NASH when either a methionine and choline deficient diet or Western-style diet was administrated [28]. Thus, the interaction between nutrients and genetic factors could modulate NAFLD presence and evolution. Additionally, it is also important to bear in mind that nutrition can also give rise to modifications in gene expression through several epigenetic mechanisms, including histone modification, DNA methylation and the regulation of transcription by micro-ribonucleic acids (miRNAs) [29]. These complex pathways are encompassed within the field of nutrigenomics, which constitutes a key element in NAFLD pathogenesis [29]. However, this topic is beyond the scope of this review and we will focus on the influential effect of genetics on response to different nutrients in NAFLD.

2.1. Carbohydrates

Dietary carbohydrates, including free sugars, can promote the accumulation of liver fat by increasing intrahepatic triglyceride content [30] and the presence of some SNPs may involve an additive harmful effect. Among them, the most studied nutrient/diet-gene interactions in clinical studies include the I148M variant of PNPLA3. Thus, in a cross-sectional study, Davis et al., reported a positive association between high dietary carbohydrate/sugar consumption and hepatic fat accumulation in Hispanic children with overweight and PNPLA3 GG genotype [31]. Similarly, Nobili et al., found that carriers of this genotype with a high consumption of sweetened beverages presented higher degrees of hepatic steatosis [32]. Furthermore, in a small clinical trial including 14 adolescents, GKRP rs1260326 TT variant increased de novo lipogenesis after glucose overload [33].

Particularly, the consumption of the monosaccharide fructose has been implicated in the development and progression of NAFLD [34]. Fructose triggers hepatic de novo lipogenesis via increasing the levels of lipogenic enzymes and stimulating sterol regulatory element-binding protein (SREBP)-1, and it also inhibits fatty acid oxidation, leading to an increase of reactive oxygen species (ROS) [35]. Thus, an ongoing clinical trial aims to evaluate the impact of fructose intake on liver lipogenesis in subjects with different genetic risk categories for NAFLD [36]. In a case control study, the combination of distinct gene variants related to oxidative stress mechanisms (glutathione S-transferase theta 1-GSTT1, glutathione S-transferase mu 1-GSTM1, sulfotransferase family 1A member 1-SULT1A1, cytochrome P450 2E1-CYP2E1 and cytochrome P450 1A1-CYP1A1) with high fruit/grilled food consumption increased the risk for NAFLD development [37]. In line with these results, previous studies have shown that high fructose diet promotes hepatic steatosis, oxidative stress and inflammation, leading to hepatocyte apoptosis [38]. The pathophysiology of fructose induced-NAFLD via oxidative stress encompasses several mechanisms, such as nonenzymatic reactions of fructose and ROS generation, hepatic phosphate deficiency and the production of harmful metabolites (e.g., methylglyoxal) [39]. In addition, the severity of liver injury by fructose may be mediated by the induced degree of mitochondrial dysfunction and oxidative damage [40]. On the other hand, the hepatic deleterious effects of fructose may be counteracted by some nutrients that prevent oxidative stress and increase the expression of antioxidant defense enzymes [41–45]. Dietary advanced glycation end products compounds found in grilled food have also been postulated to aggravate NAFLD via liver injury induced by chronic oxidative stress, and pharmacological and dietary strategies targeting the implied pathways could help to ameliorate NAFLD [46]. Therefore, the interaction between fructose/grilled food consumption and SNPs involved in oxidative stress may be crucial in NAFLD pathogenesis and resolution.

2.2. Lipids

In addition to carbohydrate overfeeding, dietary fat pattern may interrelate with some genotypes. In this sense, Santoro et al., showed that the interaction between PNPLA3 I148M and a high ratio of omega-6/omega-3 polyunsaturated fatty acid (PUFA) intake was associated with higher serum levels of alanine transaminase (ALT) and hepatic fat accumulation [47]. Jones et al., reported that the intake of several dietary types of unsaturated fat, including omega-6, was associated with liver fibrosis by PNPLA3 rs738409 variants [48]. Furthermore, the interaction between SH2B1 rs7359397 T allele and high protein/low fiber and monounsaturated fatty acid (MUFA) consumption may be associated with NAFLD severity [49].

Growing body of evidence supports that disturbances in cholesterol homeostasis contribute to the pathophysiology of NAFLD/NASH [50]. Beyond hepatic accumulation of fatty acids and triglycerides, an increase in free cholesterol deposition in the liver leads to hepatocyte injury [51]. Atherogenic dyslipidemia, a common feature of the metabolic syndrome, may facilitate this fact [52]. Remarkably, high cholesterol atherogenic diets may interact with SNPs involved in cholesterol metabolism. In a study including women that received a high cholesterol Western-type diet, the microsomal triglyceride transfer protein

(MTTP)-493 T/T variant was associated with higher fasting levels of plasma cholesterol and higher cholesterol absorption status, whereas these levels decreased to values comparable to G carriers after 3 months of low-fat diet [53]; this variant was related to an increased risk of NAFLD compared with G/G carriers [54]. TM6SF2 C > T polymorphism implies a less atherogenic lipoprotein profile and postprandial cholesterol redistribution from smaller atherogenic lipoprotein subfractions to larger VLDL subfractions in subjects with NAFLD [55]; however, specific interactions with high cholesterol diets remain unexplored. Similarly, SREBP-1c polymorphism is also closely implicated in cholesterol metabolism in NAFLD [56], yet dietary interactions have not been investigated.

2.3. Choline Deficiency in NAFLD

Choline is a key nutrient in NAFLD pathogenesis, as its deficiency is closely related to the onset and progression of this disease [57,58]. Susceptibility to choline deficiency and the subsequent increased risk of developing NAFLD may be influenced by specific polymorphisms in genes that regulate choline metabolism, such as PEMT [59,60]. In addition, a study showed that carriers of the 5,10-methylenetetrahydrofolate dehydrogenase (MTHFD)-1958A gene allele were more likely to develop NAFLD on a low-choline diet than non-carriers [61].

In light of the above, nutrient-gene interaction may play a crucial role in NAFLD pathogenesis, although large-scale, long-term prospective clinical studies are needed to corroborate these associations.

3. Gene Polymorphism and Response to Lifestyle Interventions in NAFLD

3.1. Dietary Changes

Currently, the primary treatment for NAFLD is based on lifestyle modifications, including diet and physical activity to achieve weight loss [62]. The role of nutritional intervention has been demonstrated to be essential for the prevention and management of NAFLD in a number of randomized controlled clinical trials [63–67]. Recent evidence also suggests that the presence of different SNPs combined with some dietary patterns may increase the effect of this approach. In a clinical trial performed within the Fatty Liver in Obesity (FLiO) Study, carriers of T allele of the SH2B1 rs7359397 genetic variant exhibited greater benefits in terms of hepatic health and liver status after two energy-restricted dietary patterns [68]. Interestingly, in a study performed in 140 Japanese patients with biopsy-proven NAFLD, the reduction in liver stiffness measurement after diet therapy for one year was greater among subjects with HSD17B13 rs6834314 GG variant [69]. Previously, in a pilot study conducted by Sevastianova et al., the homozygous subjects for the PNPLA3 rs738409 G allele experienced a more significant decrease in liver fat content in response to a 6-day hypocaloric low carbohydrate diet [70], and a post-hoc analysis of a randomized controlled trial including 154 patients revealed that this genotype was associated with a greater reduction in intrahepatic triglyceride content, body weight and waist-to-hip ratio after a dietitian-led lifestyle program based on a reduced caloric intake for 12 months [71]. Conversely, in a cohort study of 51 children, Koot et al., did not find any relationship between PNPLA3 rs738409 SNP and liver steatosis improvement in a 6-month intensive lifestyle treatment [72], and neither PNPLA3 nor TM6F2 variants were related to NAFLD improvement after a 4-month reduction of caloric intake, although these risk genotypes did not impair the response of dietetic intervention [73]. In addition to the aforementioned SNPs, the Gly385Arg polymorphism in fibroblast growth factor receptor 4 (FGFR4) was not linked to liver fat content or insulin sensitivity in 170 subjects with overweight/obesity at baseline, but it was associated with less decrease in liver fat accumulation and insulin sensitivity under healthy dietary conditions [74]. On the other hand, the presence of the STAT3 rs2293152 G genotype was associated with more beneficial changes after 24-week Mediterranean diet in an open-label study including 44 patients with NAFLD [75].

Thus, although further research is needed, some genetic variants associated with NAFLD development, severity and risk of progression may also confer an enhanced response to dietary intervention, and personalized dietary treatment depending on the presence of specific genetic polymorphism may constitute an attractive approach for NAFLD management. Furthermore, nutritional strategies based on the nutrient-induced insulin output ratio (NIOR) could help to select sensitive SNPs associated with fat and carbohydrate metabolism and design individualized nutrition plans for patients with NAFLD [76].

3.2. The Role of Omega-3 PUFA

Omega-3 PUFA supplementation might reduce liver fat, although well designed randomized controlled trials are required to assess their potential role in NAFLD [77,78]. In the last few years, dietary omega-3 PUFA and/or PUFA supplementation has also been related to NAFLD outcomes in the presence of some genetic determinants with mixed results (Table 1). On the one hand, Nobili et al., reported that I148M variant of PNPLA3 led to a decreased response to docosahexaenoic acid (DHA) supplementation in 60 children with NAFLD [79]. Moreover, in the WELCOME trial, the PNPLA3 148M/M genotype was associated with higher liver fat percentage and lower DHA tissue enrichment after 4 g DHA + eicosapentaenoic acid (EPA) supplementation for 15–18 months, although the TM6F2 E167K variant did not show significant associations [80]. Recently, an open-label study showed that short-term omega 3 PUFA intervention (DHA + EPA) did not change liver fat content regardless of the PNPLA3 148M variant [81]. In the EFFECT-I trial, PNPLA3 I148M did not influence the effects of omega-3 PUFA or fenofibrate on liver proton density fat fraction [82]. By contrast, a low omega-6 to omega-3 PUFA ratio diet reduced hepatic fat fraction in a significant higher percentage in the carriers of PNPLA3 148M/M genotype [83], and these results were concordant with those previously reported by Santoro et al. [33]. These findings may be explained by PNPLA3 rs738409 I148M-derived protein decreased ability in hydrolyzing omega-9 PUFA from glycerolipids; being omega-9 PUFA synthetized from omega-6 PUFA, omega-6 overload would increase intrahepatic triglyceride content [84]. Hence, further investigation is needed to elucidate the role of the interaction between omega-3 PUFA and PNPLA3 rs738409 in NAFLD and the study of alternative SNPs may help to find new relationships.

Table 1. Clinical studies assessing the role of the interaction between omega-3 PUFA and PNPLA3 rs738409 in NAFLD.

Study	Design (Sample Size)	Intervention (Time)	Result
Santoro et al., 2012 [47]	Cross-sectional study (127)	-	Higher HFF% and ALT levels in 148M/M variant presenting high dietary n-6/n-3 PUFA consumption
Nobili et al., 2013 [79]	RCT (60)	DHA 250–500 mg/day (24 months)	Lower response (steatosis) in I148M variant
Scorletti et al., 2015 [80]	RCT (85)	DHA + EPA 4 g/day (15–18 months)	Increased end of study liver fat % in 148M/M variant
Eriksson et al., 2018 [85]	RCT (84)	10 mg dapagliflozin/4 g n-3 PUFA/both (12 weeks)	Combined treatment induced greater response (PDFF) in I148M variant; n-3 PUFA treatment induced decreased response (PDFF) in I148M variant
Oscarsson et al., 2018 [82]	RCT (78)	200 mg fenofibrate/4 g n-3 PUFA (12 weeks)	No influence of I148M on the effects of n-3 PUFA supplementation (PDFF)
Kuttner et al., 2019 [81]	Open-label trial (20)	4 g n-3 PUFA (4 weeks)	No changes in transient elastography (CAP used to quantify liver fat) neither in the control group nor I148M
Van Name et al., 2020 [83]	Single-arm unblinded trial (20)	Low n-6/n-3 PUFA ratio (4:1) normocaloric diet (12 weeks)	Significant HFF% reduction in the 148M/M group

HFF%: hepatic fat fraction (%); ALT: alanine aminotransferase; n-6/n-3: omega-6/omega-3 ratio; PUFA: polyunsaturated fatty acids; RCT: randomized clinical trial; DHA: docosahexaenoic acid; EPA: eicosapentaenoic acid; PDFF: proton density fat fraction; CAP: controlled attenuation parameter.

3.3. Specific Nutrients

There is a growing interest in the potential benefits of natural supplements in the therapeutic landscape for NAFLD [86] and nutrigenetic approaches in this field may constitute an attractive option. In this sense, Mastiha, a natural product of the Mediterranean basin extracted from the *Pistacia lentiscus* tree, may reduce NASH and fibrosis via its anti-inflammatory, antioxidant and lipid-lowering properties, as well as the restoration of gut microbiota diversity [87,88]. The recent randomized trial MAST4HEALTH assessed the role of nutrigenetic interactions in the modulation of the anti-inflammatory and antioxidant effects of 6-months Mastiha supplementation on NAFLD [89]. In this study, several gene-by-Mastiha interactions were identified, and these associations were linked to levels of cytokines and antioxidant biomarkers after Mastiha treatment, some of them closely related to NAFLD pathogenesis [89]. Silymarin could also be effective in reducing transaminase levels in patients with NAFLD [90], however this effect may be attenuated in PNPLA3 G-allele carriers [91]. On the contrary, although Chia (*Salvia hispanica*), a source of omega-3 PUFA, antioxidants and fiber, may ameliorate NAFLD, no differences in response to this treatment have been found among PNPLA3 different SNPs [92]. In addition, in a pilot trial in subjects with obesity, supplementation with licorice (*Glycyrrhiza glabra*) resulted in significant changes in anthropometric parameters and insulin sensitivity only in those patients with the Pro/Pro SNP of the peroxisome proliferator-activated receptor gamma-2 (PPARγ2) [93]. Thus, given the potential benefits of licorice in NAFLD [94], genetic determinants may explain the variability in response to this nutrient. Folate serum levels may correlate with NASH severity [95], and folic acid supplementation has demonstrated to attenuate hepatic lipid accumulation and inflammation through the restoration of peroxisome proliferator-activated receptor alpha (PPARα), among other mechanisms [96]. Furthermore, the supplementation with folic acid in individuals with the high-risk variant MTHFD 1958A could attenuate signs of choline deficiency [61]. On the other hand, there are a number of nutraceuticals that could exert positive effects on NAFLD; however, their interaction with NAFLD-related SNPs is yet to be studied. In this regard, coenzyme Q10, as an activator of adenosin 5′ monophosphate activated protein kinase (AMPK), has been shown to alleviate NAFLD through the inhibition of lipogenesis and activation of fatty acid oxidation [97]. Paeoniflorin, a peony root component, improved biochemical and histological changes in NAFLD in animal models via insulin-sensitizing and antioxidant effects [98]. Resveratrol, a non-flavonoid phenol derived from grape skins, can attenuate insulin resistance and hepatic oxidative stress in NAFLD [42] and these effects may be mediated by changes in the gut microbiota, an essential component in NAFLD pathophysiology [99]. Supplementation with curcumin, extracted from *Curcuma longa* root, was associated with benefits on NAFLD through the amelioration of insulin resistance and lipid metabolism in both preclinical and clinical studies [100,101]. Berberine, an extract from the genus *Berberis* species, has a role on hepatic lipid metabolism and has been reported to be effective in NAFLD and related metabolic disorders [102]. In view of the foregoing, additional studies including gene-natural antioxidants/food supplements interaction might shed light on NAFLD personalized therapy.

3.4. Physical Activity

Physical exercise is one of the cornerstones of NAFLD therapy [103], however available data regarding potential interactions with gene polymorphisms remain scarce. In a case-control study conducted in 1027 Chinese children, physical activity was demonstrated to modulate the effect of PNPLA3 rs738409 variant: proportions of NAFLD increased with the presence of the G-allele only in participants with insufficient physical activity/sedentary behavior [104], and Muto et al., found similar results in a retrospective longitudinal study [105]. With regard to patients with NAFLD, some studies evaluated the impact of lifestyle intervention, including dietary modifications along with physical exercise recommendations [71,72,74] with different results, but the specific physical activity-gene interactions have not been evaluated to date.

4. Future Perspectives in NAFLD Treatment: Toward Personalized Therapies?

4.1. Bariatric Surgery and NAFLD

BS is considered the most effective treatment to achieve substantial weight loss, thus it constitutes an important therapeutic option for obesity and related comorbidities, including NAFLD [106]. In fact, BS is associated with NASH and fibrosis resolution in a significant number of patients, however a percentage of individuals do not experience enough histopathological improvement after this procedure [12]. Considerably, nutritional genomics play an essential part in personalized bariatric approaches, and the complex crosstalk between these two matters can generate reciprocal influences [107]. Different SNPs involved in the metabolic homeostasis are closely related to BS outcomes and, at the same time, BS induces both genetic and epigenetic modifications that have a major influence on metabolic pathways [108,109].

In this context, there is limited evidence with regard to the impact of gene polymorphism on BS outcomes in patients with NAFLD. In a prospective study including 84 individuals with obesity that underwent BS, PNPLA3 148M variant was associated with increased intrahepatic lipid accumulation before BS, but also with higher reduction of hepatic fat content and weight loss 12 months after the intervention [110]. Conversely, neither TM6F2 nor MBOAT7 showed significant associations [110]. Interestingly, several SNPs have been associated with lower hunger feelings and increased weight loss after BS, while other genetic determinants such as mitochondrial UCP2 have been proved to induce greater energy and carbohydrate intake after Roux-En-Y gastric bypass [111,112]. Hence, genetic determinants for predicting weight loss/regain after BS could be a useful tool to determine the success of this procedure, and NAFLD-related outcomes may be also affected by these SNPs.

4.2. Other Therapies

Glucose-lowering agents may be an effective treatment for NAFLD in patients with and without T2DM [62]. Among them, thiazolidinediones have shown several benefits, even in patients with advanced stages of NAFLD [113]. Remarkably, a substudy of 55 participants from a clinical trial to assess long-term efficacy of pioglitazone in NASH, identified SNPs associations with pioglitazone histologic response, including adenosine A1 receptor (ADORA1) rs903361, ATP binding cassette subfamily A member 1 (ABCA1) rs2230806, potassium voltage-gated channel subfamily Q member 1 (KCNQ1) rs2237895, PPARγ rs4135275 and PPARγ rs17817276, among others, and a genetic response score was designed based on the sum of response-associated alleles [114]. In the EFFECT-II study, 84 patients with T2DM and NAFLD were randomly assigned to 10 mg dapagliflozin/4 g omega-3 PUFA/a combination of both/placebo, and an interaction between PNPLA3 I184M (C/C vs. C/G + G/G) and reduction in liver fat content assessed by MRI was found across the active treatment groups [85] (Table 1). Moreover, the G allele carriers had an enhanced response to treatment only in the combined arm, what suggests synergistic effects between therapies in this genotype [85]. Additionally, in a retrospective study with 41 patients with NAFLD and T2DM the response to the dipeptidyl peptidase-4 inhibitor alogliptin was greater in PNPLA3 G-allele carriers [115], albeit in small study conducted in patients with T2DM, PNPLA3 GG genotype was linked to a diminished response to the glucagon-like peptide 1(GLP-1) receptor agonist exenatide in terms of reducing liver fat content [116].

SNPs may also regulate response to Vitamin E treatment in NAFLD. Gene polymorphism of cytochrome P450 4F2 might affect Vitamin E pharmacokinetics and could determine variability in its efficacy, as demonstrated a study with data from the PIVENS and TONIC clinical trials [117]. However, a retrospective study showed that liver stiffness reduction in patients with NAFLD taking Vitamin E was not influenced by PNPLA3 genotypes [118]. On the other hand, several genetic predictors of response to obeticholic acid in patients with NASH were identified in a pilot GWAS study, with the CELA3B rs75508464 variant with the most significant effect on NASH resolution [119].

Finally, the restoration of gut microbiota through the use of probiotics/symbiotics may constitute an interesting therapeutic approach in NAFLD [120]. Gut microbiota dysbiosis has a central role in NAFLD pathogenesis [121] and microbiota-derived metabolites (bile acids, short-chain fatty acids, branched-chain amino acids, etc.) are also important modulators of the disease [122]. Gut microbiome based metagenomic signature could be useful for the diagnosis of advanced stages of NAFLD [123], and gut microbiota-miRNA interactions have been reported to impact on NAFLD pathophysiology [124]. In animal models, the combination of blueberry juice and probiotics has been proved to improve NASH via increasing PPARα and reducing the levels of *SREBP-1* and *PNPLA3* [125]. Nevertheless, the potential interactions between probiotics/symbiotics and specific SNPs remain unknown.

5. Concluding Remarks

NAFLD is the most common cause of chronic liver disease globally and involves important clinical and socioeconomic implications. Gene polymorphism-nutrient interaction plays a central role in NAFLD pathogenesis and the effectiveness of lifestyle interventions, including dietary modifications, seems to be also modulated by different genetic determinants. In this review, a number of SNPs closely related to pathways involved in NAFLD (e.g., mitochondrial dysfunction, oxidative stress, lipid metabolism) and their interaction with both proven effective dietary patterns/food components and promising novel nutraceuticals for the treatment of NAFLD have been described. Since the variability in response to therapy in NAFLD may be explained by this fact, the assessment of key NAFLD-related SNPs in interventional studies should be considered. Moreover, gene-based personalized diet therapy may constitute a helpful option for the management of NAFLD, although more well-conducted large-scale, long-term trials assessing the influence of SNPs on the response to specific dietary approaches (e.g., Mediterranean diet, low-carbohydrate diet, intermittent fasting) and single nutrients are needed. Furthermore, these effects should be also evaluated in advanced stages of NAFLD. Finally, this review includes an integrative view of the emerging therapies and targets for NAFLD, pointing out the potential interplay between nutritional genomics, physical exercise, BS, pharmacotherapy and the gut microbiota in this pathology. Although recent studies have shown promising results in this regard, further investigation is warranted to determine its impact.

Author Contributions: Conceptualization, F.J.T., I.C.-P. and A.M.G.-P.; investigation, A.M.G.-P., I.C-P. and J.I.M.-M.; writing—original draft preparation, J.I.M.-M., A.M.G.-P. and I.C.-P.; writing—review and editing, I.C.-P. and A.M.G.-P.; visualization, I.C.-P. and A.M.G.-P.; supervision, F.J.T. All authors have read and agreed to the published version of the manuscript.

Funding: I.C.-P. was supported by Rio Hortega and now for Juan Rodes from the Spanish Ministry of Economy and Competitiveness (ISCIII) and cofounded by Fondo Europeo de Desarrollo Regional-FEDER (CM 17/00169, JR 19/00054). A.M.G.-P. was supported by a research contract from Servicio Andaluz de Salud (B-0033-2014). This study was supported by the "Centros de Investigación Biomédica en Red" (CIBER) of the Institute of Health Carlos III (ISCIII) (CB06/03/0018), and research grants from the ISCIII (PI18/01160) and co-financed by the European Regional Development Fund (ERDF).

Institutional Review Board Statement: Not applicable.

Informed Consent Statement: Not applicable.

Data Availability Statement: Not applicable.

Acknowledgments: Images in Figure 1 were obtained from smart.servier.com (access on 8 November 2021).

Conflicts of Interest: The authors declare no conflict of interest.

References

1. Younossi, Z.M.; Koenig, A.B.; Abdelatif, D.; Fazel, Y.; Henry, L.; Wymer, M. Global epidemiology of nonalcoholic fatty liver disease-Meta-analytic assessment of prevalence, incidence, and outcomes. *Hepatology* **2015**, *64*, 73–84. [CrossRef] [PubMed]
2. Brown, G.T.; Kleiner, D.E. Histopathological findings of non-alcoholic fatty liver disease and non-alcoholic steatohepatitis. *J. Med. Ultrason.* **2020**, *47*, 549–554. [CrossRef]
3. Younossi, Z.M.; Tampi, R.; Priyadarshini, M.; Nader, F.; Younossi, I.M.; Racila, A. Burden of Illness and Economic Model for Patients with Nonalcoholic Steatohepatitis in the United States. *Hepatology* **2019**, *69*, 564–572. [CrossRef] [PubMed]
4. Shin, D.; Kongpakpaisarn, K.; Bohra, C. Trends in the prevalence of metabolic syndrome and its components in the United States 2007–2014. *Int. J. Cardiol.* **2018**, *259*, 216–219. [CrossRef]
5. Eslam, M.; Newsome, P.N.; Sarin, S.K.; Anstee, Q.M.; Targher, G.; Romero-Gomez, M.; Zelber-Sagi, S.; Wong, V.W.-S.; Dufour, J.-F.; Schattenberg, J.M.; et al. A new definition for metabolic dysfunction-associated fatty liver disease: An international expert consensus statement. *J. Hepatol.* **2020**, *73*, 202–209. [CrossRef]
6. Berná, G.; Romero-Gomez, M. The role of nutrition in non-alcoholic fatty liver disease: Pathophysiology and management. *Liver Int.* **2020**, *40*, 102–108. [CrossRef]
7. Aron-Wisnewsky, J.; Vigliotti, C.; Witjes, J.; Le, P.; Holleboom, A.G.; Verheij, J.; Nieuwdorp, M.; Clément, K. Gut microbiota and human NAFLD: Disentangling microbial signatures from metabolic disorders. *Nat. Rev. Gastroenterol. Hepatol.* **2020**, *17*, 279–297. [CrossRef]
8. Stefan, N.; Häring, H.-U.; Cusi, K. Non-alcoholic fatty liver disease: Causes, diagnosis, cardiometabolic consequences, and treatment strategies. *Lancet Diabetes Endocrinol.* **2019**, *7*, 313–324. [CrossRef]
9. Powell, E.E.; Wong, V.W.-S.; Rinella, M. Non-alcoholic fatty liver disease. *Lancet* **2021**, *397*, 2212–2224. [CrossRef]
10. Koutoukidis, D.A.; Koshiaris, C.; Henry, J.A.; Noreik, M.; Morris, E.; Manoharan, I.; Tudor, K.; Bodenham, E.; Dunnigan, A.; Jebb, S.A.; et al. The effect of the magnitude of weight loss on non-alcoholic fatty liver disease: A systematic review and meta-analysis. *Metabolism* **2021**, *115*, 154455. [CrossRef]
11. Gonçalves, I.O.; Passos, E.; Rocha-Rodrigues, S.; Torrella, J.R.; Rizo, D.; Santos-Alves, E.; Portincasa, P.; Martins, M.J.; Ascensão, A.; Magalhães, J. Physical exercise antagonizes clinical and anatomical features characterizing Lieber-DeCarli diet-induced obesity and related metabolic disorders. *Clin. Nutr.* **2015**, *34*, 241–247. [CrossRef]
12. Lee, Y.; Doumouras, A.G.; Yu, J.; Brar, K.; Banfield, L.; Gmora, S.; Anvari, M.; Hong, D. Complete Resolution of Nonalcoholic Fatty Liver Disease After Bariatric Surgery: A Systematic Review and Meta-analysis. *Clin. Gastroenterol. Hepatol.* **2019**, *17*, 1040–1060.e11. [CrossRef] [PubMed]
13. Dongiovanni, P.; Valenti, L. Genetics of nonalcoholic fatty liver disease. *Metabolism* **2016**, *65*, 1026–1037. [CrossRef] [PubMed]
14. Sookoian, S.; Pirola, C.J. Meta-analysis of the influence of I148M variant of patatin-like phospholipase domain containing 3 gene (PNPLA3) on the susceptibility and histological severity of nonalcoholic fatty liver disease. *Hepatology* **2011**, *53*, 1883–1894. [CrossRef] [PubMed]
15. Trépo, E.; Romeo, S.; Zucman-Rossi, J.; Nahon, P. PNPLA3 gene in liver diseases. *J. Hepatol.* **2016**, *65*, 399–412. [CrossRef]
16. Romeo, S.; Kozlitina, J.; Xing, C.; Pertsemlidis, A.; Cox, D.; Pennacchio, L.A.; Boerwinkle, E.; Cohen, J.C.; Hobbs, H.H. Genetic variation in PNPLA3 confers susceptibility to nonalcoholic fatty liver disease. *Nat. Genet.* **2008**, *40*, 1461–1465. [CrossRef]
17. Li, B.-T.; Sun, M.; Li, Y.-F.; Wang, J.-Q.; Zhou, Z.-M.; Song, B.-L.; Luo, J. Disruption of the ERLIN–TM6SF2–APOB complex destabilizes APOB and contributes to non-alcoholic fatty liver disease. *PLoS Genet.* **2020**, *16*, e1008955. [CrossRef] [PubMed]
18. Mancina, R.M.; Dongiovanni, P.; Petta, S.; Pingitore, P.; Meroni, M.; Rametta, R.; Borén, J.; Montalcini, T.; Pujia, A.; Wiklund, O.; et al. The MBOAT7-TMC4 Variant rs641738 Increases Risk of Nonalcoholic Fatty Liver Disease in Individuals of European Descent. *Gastroenterology* **2016**, *150*, 1219–1230.e6. [CrossRef]
19. Gao, H.; Liu, S.; Zhao, Z.; Yu, X.; Liu, Q.; Xin, Y.; Xuan, S. Association of GCKR Gene Polymorphisms with the Risk of Nonalcoholic Fatty Liver Disease and Coronary Artery Disease in a Chinese Northern Han Population. *J. Clin. Transl. Hepatol.* **2019**, *7*, 297. [CrossRef]
20. Ma, Y.; Belyaeva, O.V.; Brown, P.M.; Fujita, K.; Valles, K.; Karki, S.; De Boer, Y.S.; Koh, C.; Chen, Y.; Du, X.; et al. 17-Beta Hydroxysteroid Dehydrogenase 13 Is a Hepatic Retinol Dehydrogenase Associated with Histological Features of Nonalcoholic Fatty Liver Disease. *Hepatology* **2019**, *69*, 1504–1519. [CrossRef]
21. Hooper, A.J.; Adams, L.A.; Burnett, J.R. Genetic determinants of hepatic steatosis in man. *J. Lipid Res.* **2011**, *52*, 593–617. [CrossRef]
22. Karkucinska-Wieckowska, A.; Simoes, I.C.M.; Kalinowski, P.; Lebiedzinska-Arciszewska, M.; Zieniewicz, K.; Milkiewicz, P.; Górska-Ponikowska, M.; Pinton, P.; Malik, A.N.; Krawczyk, M.; et al. Mitochondria, oxidative stress and nonalcoholic fatty liver disease: A complex relationship. *Eur. J. Clin. Investig.* **2021**, e13622. [CrossRef] [PubMed]
23. Al-Serri, A.; Anstee, Q.M.; Valenti, L.; Nobili, V.; Leathart, J.B.; Dongiovanni, P.; Patch, J.; Fracanzani, A.L.; Fargion, S.; Day, C.P.; et al. The SOD2 C47T polymorphism influences NAFLD fibrosis severity: Evidence from case-control and intra-familial allele association studies. *J. Hepatol.* **2012**, *56*, 448–454. [CrossRef] [PubMed]
24. Fares, R.; Petta, S.; Lombardi, R.; Grimaudo, S.; Dongiovanni, P.; Pipitone, R.M.; Rametta, R.; Fracanzani, A.L.; Mozzi, E.; Craxi, A.; et al. The UCP2 -866 G>A promoter region polymorphism is associated with nonalcoholic steatohepatitis. *Liver Int.* **2015**, *35*, 1574–1580. [CrossRef]
25. Lu, M.-Y.; Huang, J.-F.; Liao, Y.-C.; Bai, R.-K.; Trieu, R.B.; Chuang, W.-L.; Yu, M.-L.; Juo, S.-H.H.; Wong, L.-J. Mitochondrial polymorphism 12361A>G is associated with nonalcoholic fatty liver disease. *Transl. Res.* **2012**, *159*, 58–59. [CrossRef]

26. Eslam, M.; George, J. Genetic contributions to NAFLD: Leveraging shared genetics to uncover systems biology. *Nat. Rev. Gastroenterol. Hepatol.* **2019**, *17*, 40–52. [CrossRef]
27. Smagris, E.; BasuRay, S.; Li, J.; Huang, Y.; Lai, K.V.; Gromada, J.; Cohen, J.C.; Hobbs, H.H. Pnpla3I148M knockin mice accumulate PNPLA3 on lipid droplets and develop hepatic steatosis. *Hepatology* **2015**, *61*, 108–118. [CrossRef]
28. Schröder, T.; Kucharczyk, D.; Bär, F.; Pagel, R.; Derer, S.; Jendrek, S.T.; Sünderhauf, A.; Brethack, A.-K.; Hirose, M.; Möller, S.; et al. Mitochondrial gene polymorphisms alter hepatic cellular energy metabolism and aggravate diet-induced non-alcoholic steatohepatitis. *Mol. Metab.* **2016**, *5*, 283–295. [CrossRef] [PubMed]
29. Meroni, M.; Longo, M.; Rametta, R.; Dongiovanni, P. Genetic and Epigenetic Modifiers of Alcoholic Liver Disease. *Int. J. Mol. Sci.* **2018**, *19*, 3857. [CrossRef]
30. Moore, J.B.; Gunn, P.J.; Fielding, B.A. The Role of Dietary Sugars and de novo Lipogenesis in Non-Alcoholic Fatty Liver Disease. *Nutrients* **2014**, *6*, 5679–5703. [CrossRef]
31. Davis, J.N.; Lê, K.-A.; Walker, R.W.; Vikman, S.; Spruijt-Metz, N.; Weigensberg, M.J.; Allayee, H.; Goran, M.I. Increased hepatic fat in overweight Hispanic youth influenced by interaction between genetic variation in PNPLA3 and high dietary carbohydrate and sugar consumption. *Am. J. Clin. Nutr.* **2010**, *92*, 1522–1527. [CrossRef]
32. Nobili, V.; Liccardo, D.; Bedogni, G.; Salvatori, G.; Gnani, D.; Bersani, I.; Alisi, A.; Valenti, L.; Raponi, M. Influence of dietary pattern, physical activity, and I148M PNPLA3 on steatosis severity in at-risk adolescents. *Genes Nutr.* **2014**, *9*, 392. [CrossRef] [PubMed]
33. Santoro, N.; Caprio, S.; Pierpont, B.; Van Name, M.; Savoye, M.; Parks, E. Hepatic De Novo Lipogenesis in Obese Youth Is Modulated by a Common Variant in the GCKR Gene. *J. Clin. Endocrinol. Metab.* **2015**, *100*, E1125–E1132. [CrossRef]
34. Chung, M.; Ma, J.; Patel, K.; Berger, S.; Lau, J.; Lichtenstein, A.H. Fructose, high-fructose corn syrup, sucrose, and nonalcoholic fatty liver disease or indexes of liver health: A systematic review and meta-analysis. *Am. J. Clin. Nutr.* **2014**, *100*, 833–849. [CrossRef] [PubMed]
35. Todoric, J.; Di Caro, G.; Reibe, S.; Henstridge, D.C.; Green, C.R.; Vrbanac, A.; Ceteci, F.; Conche, C.; McNulty, R.; Shalapour, S.; et al. Fructose stimulated de novo lipogenesis is promoted by inflammation. *Nat. Metab.* **2020**, *2*, 1034–1045. [CrossRef] [PubMed]
36. Genetic-specific Effects of Fructose on Liver Lipogenesis—Full Text View—ClinicalTrials.gov. Available online: https://clinicaltrials.gov/ct2/show/NCT03783195?term=Liver+Lipogenesis&cond=Fructose&draw=2&rank=1 (accessed on 26 July 2021).
37. Miele, L.; Dall'Armi, V.; Cefalo, C.; Nedovic, B.; Arzani, D.; Amore, R.; Rapaccini, G.; Gasbarrini, A.; Ricciardi, W.; Grieco, A.; et al. A case–control study on the effect of metabolic gene polymorphisms, nutrition, and their interaction on the risk of non-alcoholic fatty liver disease. *Genes Nutr.* **2014**, *9*, 383. [CrossRef] [PubMed]
38. Choi, Y.; Abdelmegeed, M.A.; Song, B.-J. Diet high in fructose promotes liver steatosis and hepatocyte apoptosis in C57BL/6J female mice: Role of disturbed lipid homeostasis and increased oxidative stress. *Food Chem. Toxicol.* **2017**, *103*, 111–121. [CrossRef]
39. Jegatheesan, P.; De Bandt, J. Fructose and NAFLD: The Multifaceted Aspects of Fructose Metabolism. *Nutrients* **2017**, *9*, 230. [CrossRef] [PubMed]
40. García-Berumen, C.I.; Ortiz-Avila, O.; Vargas-Vargas, M.A.; Del Rosario-Tamayo, B.A.; Guajardo-López, C.; Saavedra-Molina, A.; Rodríguez-Orozco, A.R.; Cortés-Rojo, C. The severity of rat liver injury by fructose and high fat depends on the degree of respiratory dysfunction and oxidative stress induced in mitochondria. *Lipids Heal. Dis.* **2019**, *18*, 78. [CrossRef]
41. Cardoso, R.R.; Moreira, L.D.P.D.; Costa, M.A.d.C.; Toledo, R.C.L.; Grancieri, M.; Nascimento, T.P.D.; Ferreira, M.S.L.; da Matta, S.L.P.; Eller, M.R.; Martino, H.S.D.; et al. Kombuchas from green and black teas reduce oxidative stress, liver steatosis and inflammation, and improve glucose metabolism in Wistar rats fed a high-fat high-fructose diet. *Food Funct.* **2021**, *12*, 10813–10827. [CrossRef]
42. Bagul, P.K.; Middela, H.; Mattapally, S.; Padiya, R.; Bastia, T.; Madhusudana, K.; Reddy, B.R.; Chakravarty, S.; Banerjee, S.K. Attenuation of insulin resistance, metabolic syndrome and hepatic oxidative stress by resveratrol in fructose-fed rats. *Pharmacol. Res.* **2012**, *66*, 260–268. [CrossRef] [PubMed]
43. Suwannaphet, W.; Meeprom, A.; Yibchok-Anun, S.; Adisakwattana, S. Preventive effect of grape seed extract against high-fructose diet-induced insulin resistance and oxidative stress in rats. *Food Chem. Toxicol.* **2010**, *48*, 1853–1857. [CrossRef] [PubMed]
44. Tsai, H.-Y.; Wu, L.-Y.; Hwang, L.S. Effect of a Proanthocyanidin-Rich Extract from Longan Flower on Markers of Metabolic Syndrome in Fructose-Fed Rats. *J. Agric. Food Chem.* **2008**, *56*, 11018–11024. [CrossRef] [PubMed]
45. Polizio, A.H.; Gonzales, S.; Muñoz, M.C.; Peña, C.; Tomaro, M.L. Behaviour of the anti-oxidant defence system and heme oxygenase-1 protein expression in fructose-hypertensive rats. *Clin. Exp. Pharmacol. Physiol.* **2006**, *33*, 734–739. [CrossRef] [PubMed]
46. Leung, C.; Herath, C.B.; Jia, Z.; Andrikopoulos, S.; Brown, B.E.; Davies, M.; Rivera, L.R.; Furness, J.B.; Forbes, J.; Angus, P.W. Dietary advanced glycation end-products aggravate non-alcoholic fatty liver disease. *World J. Gastroenterol.* **2016**, *22*, 8026–8040. [CrossRef] [PubMed]
47. Santoro, N.; Savoye, M.; Kim, G.; Marotto, K.; Shaw, M.M.; Pierpont, B.; Caprio, S. Hepatic Fat Accumulation Is Modulated by the Interaction between the rs738409 Variant in the PNPLA3 Gene and the Dietary Omega6/Omega3 PUFA Intake. *PLoS ONE* **2012**, *7*, e37827. [CrossRef]

48. Jones, R.; Arenaza, L.; Rios, C.; Plows, J.; Berger, P.; Alderete, T.; Fogel, J.; Nayak, K.; Mohamed, P.; Hwang, D.; et al. PNPLA3 Genotype, Arachidonic Acid Intake, and Unsaturated Fat Intake Influences Liver Fibrosis in Hispanic Youth with Obesity. *Nutrients* **2021**, *13*, 1621. [CrossRef]
49. Perez-Diaz-Del-Campo, N.; Abete, I.; Cantero, I.; Marin-Alejandre, B.A.; Monreal, J.I.; Elorz, M.; Herrero, J.I.; Benito-Boillos, A.; Riezu-Boj, J.I.; Milagro, F.I.; et al. Association of the SH2B1 rs7359397 Gene Polymorphism with Steatosis Severity in Subjects with Obesity and Non-Alcoholic Fatty Liver Disease. *Nutrients* **2020**, *12*, 1260. [CrossRef]
50. Malhotra, P.; Gill, R.K.; Saksena, S.; Alrefai, W.A. Disturbances in Cholesterol Homeostasis and Non-alcoholic Fatty Liver Diseases. *Front. Med.* **2020**, *7*, 467. [CrossRef]
51. Ioannou, G.N.; Subramanian, S.; Chait, A.; Haigh, W.G.; Yeh, M.M.; Farrell, G.C.; Lee, S.P.; Savard, C. Cholesterol crystallization within hepatocyte lipid droplets and its role in murine NASH. *J. Lipid Res.* **2017**, *58*, 1067–1079. [CrossRef]
52. Chatrath, H.; Vuppalanchi, R.; Chalasani, N. Dyslipidemia in Patients with Nonalcoholic Fatty Liver Disease. *Semin. Liver Dis.* **2012**, *32*, 22–29. [CrossRef] [PubMed]
53. Wolff, E.; Vergnes, M.-F.; Defoort, C.; Planells, R.; Portugal, H.; Nicolay, A.; Lairon, D. Cholesterol absorption status and fasting plasma cholesterol are modulated by the microsomal triacylglycerol transfer protein −493 G/T polymorphism and the usual diet in women. *Genes Nutr.* **2010**, *6*, 71–79. [CrossRef] [PubMed]
54. Gouda, W.; Ashour, E.; Shaker, Y.; Ezzat, W. MTP genetic variants associated with non-alcoholic fatty liver in metabolic syndrome patients. *Genes Dis.* **2017**, *4*, 222–228. [CrossRef] [PubMed]
55. Musso, G.; Cipolla, U.; Cassader, M.; Pinach, S.; Saba, F.; De Michieli, F.; Paschetta, E.; Bongiovanni, D.; Framarin, L.; Leone, A.; et al. TM6SF2 rs58542926 variant affects postprandial lipoprotein metabolism and glucose homeostasis in NAFLD. mboxemphJ. Lipid Res. **2017**, *58*, 1221–1229. [CrossRef]
56. Musso, G.; Bo, S.; Cassader, M.; De Michieli, F.; Gambino, R. Impact of sterol regulatory element-binding factor-1c polymorphism on incidence of nonalcoholic fatty liver disease and on the severity of liver disease and of glucose and lipid dysmetabolism. *Am. J. Clin. Nutr.* **2013**, *98*, 895–906. [CrossRef]
57. Guerrerio, A.L.; Colvin, R.M.; Schwartz, A.K.; Molleston, J.P.; Murray, K.F.; Diehl, A.; Mohan, P.; Schwimmer, J.; Lavine, J.E.; Torbenson, M.S.; et al. Choline intake in a large cohort of patients with nonalcoholic fatty liver disease. *Am. J. Clin. Nutr.* **2012**, *95*, 892–900. [CrossRef]
58. Corbin, K.D.; Zeisel, S.H. Choline metabolism provides novel insights into nonalcoholic fatty liver disease and its progression. *Curr. Opin. Gastroenterol.* **2012**, *28*, 159–165. [CrossRef]
59. Da Costa, K.-A.; Kozyreva, O.G.; Song, J.; Galanko, J.A.; Fischer, L.M.; Zeisel, S.H. Common genetic polymorphisms affect the human requirement for the nutrient choline. *FASEB J.* **2006**, *20*, 1336–1344. [CrossRef]
60. Dong, H.; Wang, J.; Li, C.; Hirose, A.; Nozaki, Y.; Takahashi, M.; Ono, M.; Akisawa, N.; Iwasaki, S.; Saibara, T.; et al. The phosphatidylethanolamine N-methyltransferase gene V175M single nucleotide polymorphism confers the susceptibility to NASH in Japanese population. *J. Hepatol.* **2007**, *46*, 915–920. [CrossRef]
61. Kohlmeier, M.; da Costa, K.-A.; Fischer, L.M.; Zeisel, S.H. Genetic variation of folate-mediated one-carbon transfer pathway predicts susceptibility to choline deficiency in humans. *Proc. Natl. Acad. Sci. USA* **2005**, *102*, 16025–16030. [CrossRef]
62. EASL-EASD-EASO. Clinical Practice Guidelines for the management of non-alcoholic fatty liver disease. *J. Hepatol.* **2016**, *64*, 1388–1402. [CrossRef]
63. Pintó, X.; Fanlo-Maresma, M.; Corbella, E.; Corbella, X.; Mitjavila, M.T.; Moreno, J.J.; Casas, R.; Estruch, R.; Corella, D.; Bulló, M.; et al. A Mediterranean Diet Rich in Extra-Virgin Olive Oil Is Associated with a Reduced Prevalence of Nonalcoholic Fatty Liver Disease in Older Individuals at High Cardiovascular Risk. *J. Nutr.* **2019**, *149*, 1920–1929. [CrossRef] [PubMed]
64. Marin-Alejandre, B.A.; Abete, I.; Cantero, I.; Monreal, J.I.; Elorz, M.; Herrero, J.I.; Benito, A.; Quiroga, J.; Martinez-Echeverria, A.; Uriz-Otano, J.I.; et al. The Metabolic and Hepatic Impact of Two Personalized Dietary Strategies in Subjects with Obesity and Nonalcoholic Fatty Liver Disease: The Fatty Liver in Obesity (FLiO) Randomized Controlled Trial. *Nutrients* **2019**, *11*, 2543. [CrossRef] [PubMed]
65. Johari, M.I.; Yusoff, K.; Haron, J.; Nadarajan, C.; Ibrahim, K.N.; Wong, M.S.; Hafidz, M.I.A.; Chua, B.E.; Hamid, N.; Arifin, W.N.; et al. A Randomised Controlled Trial on the Effectiveness and Adherence of Modified Alternate-day Calorie Restriction in Improving Activity of Non-Alcoholic Fatty Liver Disease. *Sci. Rep.* **2019**, *9*, 11232. [CrossRef] [PubMed]
66. Skytte, M.J.; Samkani, A.; Petersen, A.D.; Thomsen, M.N.; Astrup, A.; Chabanova, E.; Frystyk, J.; Holst, J.J.; Thomsen, H.S.; Madsbad, S.; et al. A carbohydrate-reduced high-protein diet improves HbA1c and liver fat content in weight stable participants with type 2 diabetes: A randomised controlled trial. *Diabetologia* **2019**, *62*, 2066–2078. [CrossRef] [PubMed]
67. Razavi Zade, M.; Telkabadi, M.H.; Bahmani, F.; Salehi, B.; Farshbaf, S.; Asemi, Z. The effects of DASH diet on weight loss and metabolic status in adults with non-alcoholic fatty liver disease: A randomized clinical trial. *Liver Int.* **2016**, *36*, 563–571. [CrossRef]
68. Perez-Diaz-Del-Campo, N.; Marin-Alejandre, B.A.; Cantero, I.; Monreal, J.I.; Elorz, M.; Herrero, J.I.; Benito-Boillos, A.; Riezu-Boj, J.I.; Milagro, F.I.; Tur, J.A.; et al. Differential response to a 6-month energy-restricted treatment depending on SH2B1 rs7359397 variant in NAFLD subjects: Fatty Liver in Obesity (FLiO) Study. *Eur. J. Nutr.* **2021**, *60*, 3043–3057. [CrossRef]
69. Seko, Y.; Yamaguchi, K.; Tochiki, N.; Yano, K.; Takahashi, A.; Okishio, S.; Kataoka, S.; Okuda, K.; Umemura, A.; Moriguchi, M.; et al. The Effect of Genetic Polymorphism in Response to Body Weight Reduction in Japanese Patients with Nonalcoholic Fatty Liver Disease. *Genes* **2021**, *12*, 628. [CrossRef]

70. Sevastianova, K.; Kotronen, A.; Gastaldelli, A.; Perttilä, J.; Hakkarainen, A.; Lundbom, J.; Suojanen, L.; Orho-Melander, M.; Lundbom, N.; Ferrannini, E.; et al. Genetic variation in PNPLA3 (adiponutrin) confers sensitivity to weight loss-induced decrease in liver fat in humans. *Am. J. Clin. Nutr.* **2011**, *94*, 104–111. [CrossRef]
71. Shen, J.; Wong, G.L.-H.; Chan, H.L.-Y.; Chan, R.S.; Chan, H.-Y.; Chu, W.; Cheung, B.H.-K.; Yeung, D.K.-W.; Li, L.S.; Sea, M.M.-M.; et al. PNPLA3 gene polymorphism and response to lifestyle modification in patients with nonalcoholic fatty liver disease. *J. Gastroenterol. Hepatol.* **2015**, *30*, 139–146. [CrossRef]
72. Koot, B.G.P.; Van Der Baan-Slootweg, O.H.; Vinke, S.; Bohte, A.E.; Tamminga-Smeulders, C.L.J.; Jansen, P.L.M.; Stoker, J.; Benninga, M.A. Intensive lifestyle treatment for non-alcoholic fatty liver disease in children with severe obesity: Inpatient versus ambulatory treatment. *Int. J. Obes.* **2015**, *40*, 51–57. [CrossRef] [PubMed]
73. Krawczyk, M.; Stachowska, E.; Milkiewicz, P.; Lammert, F.; Milkiewicz, M. Reduction of Caloric Intake Might Override the Prosteatotic Effects of the PNPLA3 p.I148M and TM6SF2 p.E167K Variants in Patients with Fatty Liver: Ultrasound-Based Prospective Study. *Digestion* **2016**, *93*, 139–148. [CrossRef] [PubMed]
74. Lutz, S.Z.; Hennige, A.M.; Peter, A.; Kovarova, M.; Totsikas, C.; Machann, J.; Kröber, S.M.; Sperl, B.; Schleicher, E.; Schick, F.; et al. The Gly385(388)Arg Polymorphism of the FGFR4 Receptor Regulates Hepatic Lipogenesis under Healthy Diet. *J. Clin. Endocrinol. Metab.* **2019**, *104*, 2041–2053. [CrossRef] [PubMed]
75. Kaliora, A.C.; Gioxari, A.; Kalafati, I.P.; Diolintzi, A.; Kokkinos, A.; Dedoussis, G.V. The Effectiveness of Mediterranean Diet in Nonalcoholic Fatty Liver Disease Clinical Course: An Intervention Study. *J. Med. Food* **2019**, *22*, 729–740. [CrossRef] [PubMed]
76. Stachowska, E.; Ryterska, K.; Maciejewska, D.; Banaszczak, M.; Milkiewicz, P.; Milkiewicz, M.; Gutowska, I.; Ossowski, P.; Kaczorowska, M.; Jamioł-Milc, D.; et al. Nutritional Strategies for the Individualized Treatment of Non-Alcoholic Fatty Liver Disease (NAFLD) Based on the Nutrient-Induced Insulin Output Ratio (NIOR). *Int. J. Mol. Sci.* **2016**, *17*, 1192. [CrossRef] [PubMed]
77. Parker, H.M.; Johnson, N.A.; Burdon, C.A.; Cohn, J.S.; O'Connor, H.T.; George, J. Omega-3 supplementation and non-alcoholic fatty liver disease: A systematic review and meta-analysis. *J. Hepatol.* **2012**, *56*, 944–951. [CrossRef]
78. He, X.-X.; Wu, X.-L.; Chen, R.-P.; Chen, C.; Liu, X.-G.; Wu, B.-J.; Huang, Z.-M. Effectiveness of Omega-3 Polyunsaturated Fatty Acids in Non-Alcoholic Fatty Liver Disease: A Meta-Analysis of Randomized Controlled Trials. *PLoS ONE* **2016**, *11*, e0162368. [CrossRef] [PubMed]
79. Nobili, V.; Bedogni, G.; Donati, B.; Alisi, A.; Valenti, L. The I148M Variant of PNPLA3 Reduces the Response to Docosahexaenoic Acid in Children with Non-Alcoholic Fatty Liver Disease. *J. Med. Food* **2013**, *16*, 957–960. [CrossRef]
80. Scorletti, E.; West, A.; Bhatia, L.; Hoile, S.P.; McCormick, K.G.; Burdge, G.; Lillycrop, K.; Clough, G.F.; Calder, P.; Byrne, C.D. Treating liver fat and serum triglyceride levels in NAFLD, effects of PNPLA3 and TM6SF2 genotypes: Results from the WELCOME trial. *J. Hepatol.* **2015**, *63*, 1476–1483. [CrossRef]
81. Kuttner, C.-S.; Mancina, R.; Wagenpfeil, G.; Lammert, F.; Stokes, C. Four-Week Omega-3 Supplementation in Carriers of the Prosteatotic PNPLA3 p.I148M Genetic Variant: An Open-Label Study. *Lifestyle Genom.* **2019**, *12*, 10–17. [CrossRef]
82. Oscarsson, J.; Önnerhag, K.; Risérus, U.; Sundén, M.; Johansson, L.; Jansson, P.-A.; Moris, L.; Nilsson, P.M.; Eriksson, J.W.; Lind, L. Effects of free omega-3 carboxylic acids and fenofibrate on liver fat content in patients with hypertriglyceridemia and non-alcoholic fatty liver disease: A double-blind, randomized, placebo-controlled study. *J. Clin. Lipidol.* **2018**, *12*, 1390–1403.e4. [CrossRef] [PubMed]
83. Van Name, M.A.; Savoye, M.; Chick, J.M.; Galuppo, B.T.; Feldstein, A.E.; Pierpont, B.; Johnson, C.; Shabanova, V.; Ekong, U.; Valentino, P.L.; et al. A Low ω-6 to ω-3 PUFA Ratio (n−6:n−3 PUFA) Diet to Treat Fatty Liver Disease in Obese Youth. *J. Nutr.* **2020**, *150*, 2314–2321. [CrossRef] [PubMed]
84. Huang, Y.; Cohen, J.C.; Hobbs, H.H. Expression and Characterization of a PNPLA3 Protein Isoform (I148M) Associated with Nonalcoholic Fatty Liver Disease. *J. Biol. Chem.* **2011**, *286*, 37085–37093. [CrossRef] [PubMed]
85. Eriksson, J.W.; Lundkvist, P.; Jansson, P.-A.; Johansson, L.; Kvarnström, M.; Moris, L.; Miliotis, T.; Forsberg, G.-B.; Risérus, U.; Lind, L.; et al. Effects of dapagliflozin and n-3 carboxylic acids on non-alcoholic fatty liver disease in people with type 2 diabetes: A double-blind randomised placebo-controlled study. *Diabetologia* **2018**, *61*, 1923–1934. [CrossRef]
86. Cicero, A.F.G.; Colletti, A.; Bellentani, S. Nutraceutical Approach to Non-Alcoholic Fatty Liver Disease (NAFLD): The Available Clinical Evidence. *Nutrients* **2018**, *10*, 1153. [CrossRef]
87. Kannt, A.; Papada, E.; Kammermeier, C.; D'Auria, G.; Jiménez-Hernández, N.; Stephan, M.; Schwahn, U.; Madsen, A.N.; Oster-gaard, M.V.; Dedoussis, G.; et al. Mastiha (*Pistacia lentiscus*) Improves Gut Microbiota Diversity, Hepatic Steatosis, and Disease Activity in a Biopsy-Confirmed Mouse Model of Advanced Non-Alcoholic Steatohepatitis and Fibrosis. *Mol. Nutr. Food Res.* **2019**, *63*, e1900927. [CrossRef] [PubMed]
88. Amerikanou, C.; Kanoni, S.; Kaliora, A.C.; Barone, A.; Bjelan, M.; D'Auria, G.; Gioxari, A.; Gosalbes, M.J.; Mouchti, S.; Stathopoulou, M.G.; et al. Effect of Mastiha supplementation on NAFLD: The MAST4HEALTH Randomised, Controlled Trial. *Mol. Nutr. Food Res.* **2021**, *65*, 2001178. [CrossRef]
89. Kanoni, S.; Kumar, S.; Amerikanou, C.; Kurth, M.J.; Stathopoulou, M.G.; Bourgeois, S.; Masson, C.; Kannt, A.; Cesarini, L.; Kontoe, M.-S.; et al. Nutrigenetic Interactions Might Modulate the Antioxidant and Anti-Inflammatory Status in Mastiha-Supplemented Patients with NAFLD. *Front. Immunol.* **2021**, *12*, 1688. [CrossRef]

90. Kalopitas, G.; Antza, C.; Doundoulakis, I.; Siargkas, A.; Kouroumalis, E.; Germanidis, G.; Samara, M.; Chourdakis, M. Impact of Silymarin in individuals with nonalcoholic fatty liver disease: A systematic review and meta-analysis. *Nutrients* **2021**, *83*, 111092. [CrossRef] [PubMed]
91. Aller, R.; Laserna, C.; Rojo, M.Á.; Mora, N.; Sánchez, C.G.; Pina, M.; Sigüenza, R.; Primo, D.; Izaola, O.; De Luis, D. Role of the PNPLA3 polymorphism rs738409 on silymarin + vitamin E response in subjects with non-alcoholic fatty liver disease. *Rev. Esp. Enferm. Dig.* **2018**, *110*, 634–640. [CrossRef]
92. Medina-Urrutia, A.; Lopez-Uribe, A.R.; El Hafidi, M.; González-Salazar, M.D.C.; Posadas-Sánchez, R.; Jorge-Galarza, E.; Del Valle-Mondragón, L.; Juárez-Rojas, J.G. Chia (*Salvia hispanica*)-supplemented diet ameliorates non-alcoholic fatty liver disease and its metabolic abnormalities in humans. *Lipids Health Dis.* **2020**, *19*, 1–9. [CrossRef] [PubMed]
93. Namazi, N.; Alizadeh, M.; Mirtaheri, E.; Farajnia, S. The Effect of Dried Glycyrrhiza Glabra L. Extract on Obesity Management with Regard to PPAR-γ2 (Pro12Ala) Gene Polymorphism in Obese Subjects Following an Energy Restricted Diet. *Adv. Pharm. Bull.* **2017**, *7*, 221–228. [CrossRef] [PubMed]
94. Hajiaghamohammadi, A.; Ziaee, A.; Samimi, R. The Efficacy of Licorice Root Extract in Decreasing Transaminase Activities in Non-alcoholic Fatty Liver Disease: A Randomized Controlled Clinical Trial. *Phytother. Res.* **2012**, *26*, 1381–1384. [CrossRef] [PubMed]
95. Mahamid, M.; Mahroum, N.; Bragazzi, N.L.; Shalaata, K.; Yavne, Y.; Adawi, M.; Amital, H.; Watad, A. Folate and B12 Levels Correlate with Histological Severity in NASH Patients. *Nutrients* **2018**, *10*, 440. [CrossRef]
96. Xin, F.-Z.; Zhao, Z.-H.; Zhang, R.-N.; Pan, Q.; Gong, Z.-Z.; Sun, C.; Fan, J.-G. Folic acid attenuates high-fat diet-induced steatohepatitis via deacetylase SIRT1-dependent restoration of PPARα. *World J. Gastroenterol.* **2020**, *26*, 2203–2220. [CrossRef] [PubMed]
97. Chen, K.; Chen, X.; Xue, H.; Zhang, P.; Fang, W.; Chen, X.; Ling, W. Coenzyme Q10 attenuates high-fat diet-induced non-alcoholic fatty liver disease through activation of the AMPK pathway. *Food Funct.* **2019**, *10*, 814–823. [CrossRef]
98. Ma, Z.; Chu, L.; Liu, H.; Wang, W.; Li, J.; Yao, W.; Yi, J.; Gao, Y. Beneficial effects of paeoniflorin on non-alcoholic fatty liver disease induced by high-fat diet in rats. *Sci. Rep.* **2017**, *7*, srep44819. [CrossRef]
99. Du, F.; Huang, R.; Lin, D.; Wang, Y.; Yang, X.; Huang, X.; Zheng, B.; Chen, Z.; Huang, Y.; Wang, X.; et al. Resveratrol Improves Liver Steatosis and Insulin Resistance in Non-alcoholic Fatty Liver Disease in Association with the Gut Microbiota. *Front. Microbiol.* **2021**, *12*, 611323. [CrossRef]
100. Lee, E.S.; Kwon, M.-H.; Kim, H.M.; Woo, H.B.; Ahn, C.M.; Chung, C.H. Curcumin analog CUR5-8 ameliorates nonalcoholic fatty liver disease in mice with high-fat diet-induced obesity. *Metabolism* **2020**, *103*, 154015. [CrossRef]
101. Cicero, A.F.G.; Sahebkar, A.; Fogacci, F.; Bove, M.; Giovannini, M.; Borghi, C. Effects of phytosomal curcumin on anthropometric parameters, insulin resistance, cortisolemia and non-alcoholic fatty liver disease indices: A double-blind, placebo-controlled clinical trial. *Eur. J. Nutr.* **2019**, *59*, 477–483. [CrossRef]
102. Yan, H.-M.; Xia, M.-F.; Wang, Y.; Chang, X.-X.; Yao, X.-Z.; Rao, S.-X.; Zeng, M.-S.; Tu, Y.-F.; Feng, R.; Jia, W.-P.; et al. Efficacy of Berberine in Patients with Non-Alcoholic Fatty Liver Disease. *PLoS ONE* **2015**, *10*, e0134172. [CrossRef]
103. Katsagoni, C.N.; Georgoulis, M.; Papatheodoridis, G.; Panagiotakos, D.B.; Kontogianni, M.D. Effects of lifestyle interventions on clinical characteristics of patients with non-alcoholic fatty liver disease: A meta-analysis. *Metabolism* **2017**, *68*, 119–132. [CrossRef] [PubMed]
104. Wang, S.; Song, J.; Shang, X.; Chawla, N.; Yang, Y.; Meng, X.; Wang, H.; Ma, J. Physical activity and sedentary behavior can modulate the effect of the PNPLA3 variant on childhood NAFLD: A case-control study in a Chinese population. *BMC Med. Genet.* **2016**, *17*, 90. [CrossRef] [PubMed]
105. Muto, N.; Oniki, K.; Kudo, M.; Obata, Y.; Sakamoto, Y.; Tokumaru, N.; Izuka, T.; Watanabe, T.; Otake, K.; Ogata, Y.; et al. A Pilot Study Assessing the Possible Combined Effect of Physical Activity and *PNPLA3* rs738409 Polymorphism on the Risk for Non-Alcoholic Fatty Liver Disease in the Japanese Elderly General Population. *Diabetes Metab. Syndr. Obes. Targets Ther.* **2020**, *ume 13*, 333–341. [CrossRef]
106. Chang, S.-H.; Stoll, C.R.T.; Song, J.; Varela, J.E.; Eagon, C.J.; Colditz, G. The Effectiveness and Risks of Bariatric Surgery. *JAMA Surg.* **2014**, *149*, 275–287. [CrossRef] [PubMed]
107. Nicoletti, C.F.; Cortes-Oliveira, C.; Pinhel, M.A.S.; Nonino, C.B. Bariatric Surgery and Precision Nutrition. *Nutrients* **2017**, *9*, 974. [CrossRef] [PubMed]
108. Nicoletti, C.F.; Nonino, C.B.; de Oliveira, B.A.P.; Pinhel, M.A.D.S.; Mansego, M.L.; Milagro, F.I.; Zulet, M.A.; Martinez, J.A. DNA Methylation and Hydroxymethylation Levels in Relation to Two Weight Loss Strategies: Energy-Restricted Diet or Bariatric Surgery. *Obes. Surg.* **2015**, *26*, 603–611. [CrossRef] [PubMed]
109. Ortega, F.J.; Vilallonga, R.; Xifra, G.; Sabater-Masdeu, M.; Ricart, W.; Fernández-Real, J.M. Bariatric surgery acutely changes the expression of inflammatory and lipogenic genes in obese adipose tissue. *Surg. Obes. Relat. Dis.* **2016**, *12*, 357–362. [CrossRef]
110. Krawczyk, M.; Jiménez-Agüero, R.; Alustiza, J.M.; Emparanza, J.I.; Perugorria, M.J.; Bujanda, L.; Lammert, F.; Banales, J.M. PNPLA3 p.I148M variant is associated with greater reduction of liver fat content after bariatric surgery. *Surg. Obes. Relat. Dis.* **2016**, *12*, 1838–1846. [CrossRef]
111. Bandstein, M.; Mwinyi, J.; Ernst, B.; Thurnheer, M.; Schultes, B.; Schiöth, H.B. A genetic variant in proximity to the gene LYPLAL1 is associated with lower hunger feelings and increased weight loss following Roux-en-Y gastric bypass surgery. *Scand. J. Gastroenterol.* **2016**, *51*, 1050–1055. [CrossRef]

112. Nicoletti, C.F.; Kimura, B.M.; Oliveira, B.; De Pinhel, M.A.S.; Salgado, W.; Marchini, J.S.; Nonino, C.B. Role of UCP2 polymorphisms on dietary intake of obese patients who underwent bariatric surgery. *Clin. Obes.* **2016**, *6*, 354–358. [CrossRef] [PubMed]
113. Musso, G.; Cassader, M.; Paschetta, E.; Gambino, R. Thiazolidinediones and Advanced Liver Fibrosis in Nonalcoholic Steatohepatitis. *JAMA Intern. Med.* **2017**, *177*, 633–640. [CrossRef] [PubMed]
114. Kawaguchi-Suzuki, M.; Cusi, K.; Bril, F.; Gong, Y.; Langaee, T.; Frye, R.F. A Genetic Score Associates with Pioglitazone Response in Patients with Non-alcoholic Steatohepatitis. *Front. Pharmacol.* **2018**, *9*, 752. [CrossRef]
115. Kan, H.; Hyogo, H.; Ochi, H.; Hotta, K.; Fukuhara, T.; Kobayashi, T.; Naeshiro, N.; Honda, Y.; Kawaoka, T.; Tsuge, M.; et al. Influence of the rs738409 polymorphism in patatin-like phospholipase 3 on the treatment efficacy of non-alcoholic fatty liver disease with type 2 diabetes mellitus. *Hepatol. Res.* **2015**, *46*, E146–E153. [CrossRef] [PubMed]
116. Chen, Y.; Yan, X.; Xu, X.; Yuan, S.; Xu, F.; Liang, H. PNPLA3 I148M is involved in the variability in anti-NAFLD response to exenatide. *Endocrine* **2020**, *70*, 517–523. [CrossRef]
117. Athinarayanan, S.; Wei, R.; Zhang, M.; Bai, S.; Traber, M.; Yates, K.; Cummings, O.W.; Molleston, J.; Liu, W.; Chalasani, N. Genetic Polymorphism of Cytochrome P450 4F2, Vitamin E Level and Histological Response in Adults and Children with Nonalcoholic Fatty Liver Disease Who Participated in PIVENS and TONIC Clinical Trials. *PLoS ONE* **2014**, *9*, e95366. [CrossRef]
118. Fukui, A.; Kawabe, N.; Hashimoto, S.; Murao, M.; Nakano, T.; Shimazaki, H.; Kan, T.; Nakaoka, K.; Ohki, M.; Takagawa, Y.; et al. Vitamin E reduces liver stiffness in nonalcoholic fatty liver disease. *World J. Hepatol.* **2015**, *7*, 2749–2756. [CrossRef]
119. Gawrieh, S.; Guo, X.; Tan, J.; Lauzon, M.; Taylor, K.D.; Loomba, R.; Cummings, O.W.; Pillai, S.; Bhatnagar, P.; Kowdley, K.V.; et al. A Pilot Genome-Wide Analysis Study Identifies Loci Associated with Response to Obeticholic Acid in Patients with NASH. *Hepatol. Commun.* **2019**, *3*, 1571–1584. [CrossRef]
120. Sharpton, S.R.; Maraj, B.; Harding-Theobald, E.; Vittinghoff, E.; Terrault, N.A. Gut microbiome–targeted therapies in nonalcoholic fatty liver disease: A systematic review, meta-analysis, and meta-regression. *Am. J. Clin. Nutr.* **2019**, *110*, 139–149. [CrossRef]
121. Caussy, C.; Tripathi, A.; Humphrey, G.; Bassirian, S.; Singh, S.; Faulkner, C.; Bettencourt, R.; Rizo, E.; Richards, L.; Xu, Z.Z.; et al. A gut microbiome signature for cirrhosis due to nonalcoholic fatty liver disease. *Nat. Commun.* **2019**, *10*, 1406. [CrossRef]
122. Lee, G.; You, H.J.; Bajaj, J.S.; Joo, S.K.; Yu, J.; Park, S.; Kang, H.; Park, J.H.; Kim, J.H.; Lee, D.H.; et al. Distinct signatures of gut microbiome and metabolites associated with significant fibrosis in non-obese NAFLD. *Nat. Commun.* **2020**, *11*, 4982. [CrossRef] [PubMed]
123. Loomba, R.; Seguritan, V.; Li, W.; Long, T.; Klitgord, N.; Bhatt, A.; Dulai, P.S.; Caussy, C.; Bettencourt, R.; Highlander, S.K.; et al. Gut Microbiome-Based Metagenomic Signature for Non-invasive Detection of Advanced Fibrosis in Human Nonalcoholic Fatty Liver Disease. *Cell Metab.* **2017**, *25*, 1054–1062. [CrossRef]
124. Blasco-Baque, V.; Coupé, B.; Fabre, A.; Handgraaf, S.; Gourdy, P.; Arnal, J.F.; Courtney, M.; Schuster-Klein, C.; Guardiola, B.; Tercé, F.; et al. Associations between hepatic miRNA expression, liver triacylglycerols and gut microbiota during metabolic adaptation to high-fat diet in mice. *Diabetologia* **2017**, *60*, 690–700. [CrossRef] [PubMed]
125. Ren, T.; Zhu, J.; Zhu, L.; Cheng, M. The Combination of Blueberry Juice and Probiotics Ameliorate Non-Alcoholic Steatohepatitis (NASH) by Affecting SREBP-1c/PNPLA-3 Pathway via PPAR-α. *Nutrients* **2017**, *9*, 198. [CrossRef] [PubMed]

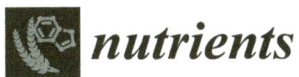

Systematic Review

Vitamin D and Type 1 Diabetes Risk: A Systematic Review and Meta-Analysis of Genetic Evidence

Liana Najjar [1], Joshua Sutherland [1], Ang Zhou [1,2] and Elina Hyppönen [1,2,*]

[1] Australian Centre for Precision Health, Unit of Clinical and Health Sciences, University of South Australia, P.O. Box 2471, Adelaide, SA 5001, Australia; najly002@mymail.unisa.edu.au (L.N.); joshua.sutherland@mymail.unisa.edu.au (J.S.); Ang.Zhou@unisa.edu.au (A.Z.)
[2] South Australian Health and Medical Research Institute, Adelaide, SA 5000, Australia
* Correspondence: elina.hypponen@unisa.edu.au; Tel.: +61-(08)-83022518

Abstract: Several observational studies have examined vitamin D pathway polymorphisms and their association with type 1 diabetes (T1D) susceptibility, with inconclusive results. We aimed to perform a systematic review and meta-analysis assessing associations between selected variants affecting 25-hydroxyvitamin D [25(OH)D] and T1D risk. We conducted a systematic search of Medline, Embase, Web of Science and OpenGWAS updated in April 2021. The following keywords "vitamin D" and/or "single nucleotide polymorphisms (SNPs)" and "T1D" were selected to identify relevant articles. Seven SNPs (or their proxies) in six genes were analysed: *CYP2R1* rs10741657, *CYP2R1* (low frequency) rs117913124, *DHCR7/NADSYN1* rs12785878, *GC* rs3755967, *CYP24A1* rs17216707, *AMDHD1* rs10745742 and *SEC23A* rs8018720. Seven case-control and three cohort studies were eligible for quantitative synthesis (*n* = 10). Meta-analysis results suggested no association with T1D (range of pooled ORs for all SNPs: 0.97–1.02; *p* > 0.01). Heterogeneity was found in *DHCR7/NADSYN1* rs12785878 (I^2: 64.8%, *p* = 0.02). Sensitivity analysis showed exclusion of any single study did not alter the overall pooled effect. No association with T1D was observed among a Caucasian subgroup. In conclusion, the evidence from the meta-analysis indicates a null association between selected variants affecting serum 25(OH)D concentrations and T1D.

Keywords: diabetes mellitus; type 1; meta-analysis; polymorphism; single nucleotide; vitamin D; 25-hydroxyvitamin D; CYP2R1

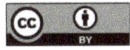

1. Introduction

Type 1 diabetes (T1D) is a chronic autoimmune disease, resulting from autoimmune degradation of pancreatic ß-cells leading to the inability to produce and/or use insulin [1]. T1D patients carry a genetic susceptibility to autoimmune disease development, with first-degree relatives of those affected also carrying an increased risk of developing the disease [2,3]. Undiagnosed or untreated T1D can result in hyperglycaemia, increasing the risk of developing microvascular and macrovascular injuries/health complications, such as nephropathy, ischemic heart disease and stroke [4]. Estimates of those with T1D below age 20 had risen to over a million in 2017, with evidence of increasing incidence worldwide [5]. Presently, there are no established treatments identified for the prevention of T1D and the search for genetic and environmental triggers remains ongoing.

Emerging evidence suggests low vitamin D status may play a role in T1D predisposition. Vitamin D is a steroid prohormone, with nutrition status approximated via serum 25-hydroxyvitamin D [25(OH)D] concentrations [6]. Notably, 25(OH)D deficiency is strongly associated with skeletal pathology, however, in the advent of vitamin D receptors being discovered throughout the body, there now is a greater acknowledgment of broader disorders associated with deficiency, including autoimmune issues, such as T1D and multiple sclerosis [7,8]. Recent evidence indicates an important role for active vitamin D [1,25(OH)2D] in immune regulation [9]. Mechanistic explanations for 1,25(OH)2D include immunomodulatory action leading to cytokine regulation, reducing the likelihood of destruction of pancreatic ß-cells [10]. Another potential mechanism is through direct protection of pancreatic ß-cells, serving to preserve barrier exclusion of pathogens, likely significant in the prevention of autoimmune disorders [11]. Such mechanistic insight has underpinned novel immune-modulatory concepts for the prevention of T1D.

Association between serum 25(OH)D concentrations and T1D risk is supported by evidence from in vitro and animal experiments [12–14], as well as human observational studies [15–18] and ecological correlation [19]. In animal studies, oral administration of the activated form of vitamin D was found to protect nonobese diabetic mice from T1D [12–14], while human observational studies have shown reduced levels of serum 25(OH)D are associated with increased risk of T1D [15,17]. In the aetiology of T1D observational studies have also shown support of vitamin D supplementation in being inversely associated with T1D [16,18,20]. Animal experimental data, therefore, indicate low 25(OH)D concentrations may be involved in T1D predisposition, however, a causal role of impaired vitamin D metabolism in the aetiology of T1D in humans is yet to be implicated, and stronger forms of evidence—less effected by confounding or reverse causation—are required.

Using selected vitamin D related genetic variants, it is possible in a genetic epidemiological setting to establish evidence of an etiological role of 25(OH)D in T1D pathophysiology. Since 25(OH)D synthesis is regulated by genes, single nucleotide polymorphisms (SNPs) may alter the bioavailability and target effects of vitamin D metabolites. Large-scale genome-wide association studies (GWAS) have identified several SNPs from genes influencing 25(OH)D levels; *CYP2R1*, *DHCR7/NADSY1*, *GC*, *CYP24A1*, *AMDHD1* and *SEC23A*, which have been used as genetic instrumental variants in this study [21,22].

As individual studies may not have enough statistical power to identify an association between selected genetic variants affecting serum 25(OH)D concentrations and T1D, a meta-analysis is a useful statistical tool to pool data from published studies, where increasing the statistical power can give more accurate estimates of effect sizes. In this study, we perform a systematic review and meta-analysis of all existing studies reporting an association between selected 25(OH)D related genetic variants (exposure) and T1D risk (outcome) in humans (population). This topic provides a further scientific understanding of T1D pathophysiology and the potentiality of preventing T1D through increases in 25(OH)D concentrations.

2. Materials and Methods

This systematic review and meta-analysis followed the Preferred Reporting Items for Systematic Reviews and Meta-Analyses (PRISMA) guidelines [23]. Registration: PROSPERO (ID CRD42021224844), https://www.crd.york.ac.uk/prospero/ (accessed on 10 January 2021).

2.1. Search Strategy

A search was conducted in four databases: Ovid Medline (1964-present), Ovid Embase (1947-present), Web of Science (1975-present), IEU OpenGWAS (2020-present) from inception to April 2021. The primary search terms were as follows: humans, single nucleotide polymorphism, genetic variation, type 1 diabetes mellitus and vitamin D. The selection of articles in Medline and Web of Science was performed using Medical Subject Headings (MeSH) to define these descriptors. The selection of articles in Embase was performed using Emtree (Embase subject headings) to define these descriptors. Boolean operators (e.g., OR, AND, NOT) were also combined with keywords and subject headings. An initial pilot search was undertaken to improve inclusion clarity of study inclusion and exclusion, improving accuracy and consistency. The strategy was developed by one reviewer (L.N.) and proofread for syntax, spelling and overall structure by two reviewers (E.H. and J.S.). As part of the development process, we used two relevant, existing studies [24,25] for validation purposes, testing if our search strategy could identify them. The set of search terms was slightly modified between databases due to different system procedural limitations, however, the overall approach remained as consistent as possible across each database. The selection of studies through OpenGWAS, as well as the UK Biobank, was prepared using R 4.0.2 software, conducting an SNP-based search for the selected genetic variants and their proxies ($r^2 > 0.8$), locating any additional studies fitting the inclusion criteria. Full search strategies are presented in Supplementary Tables S1–S4.

2.2. Inclusion and Exclusion Criteria

Studies testing exposure of selected genetic variants or their proxies with $r^2 > 0.8$ influencing 25(OH)D pathways for association with T1D status and 25(OH)D concentrations, were of interest. Eligible studies met the population, exposure, outcome (PEO) approach [26] as follows:

1. Population: human of any gender and age, race and geographical distribution.
2. Exposure: a biological approach to the selection of genetic variants was used, including variants having a biological link to the exposure. Seven vitamin D related SNPs were selected: *CYP2R1* (common variant) rs10741657, *CYP2R1* (rare variant/low frequency) rs117913124, *DHCR7/NADSYN1* rs12785878, *GC* rs3755967, *CYP24A1* rs17216707, *AMDHD1* rs10745742, *SEC23A* rs8018720. Of these selected SNPs, six are common variants identified based on the results of a recent GWAS for 25(OH)D concentration [21] and one is a low-frequency synonymous coding variant seen with a much larger effect on 25(OH)D concentration [22]. Strong genome-wide associations with 25(OH)D were found in genes located upstream (*DHCR7/NADSY1* and both *CYP2R1* variants), and two downstream (*CYP24A1* and *GC*) of the 25(OH)D metabolite biochemical pathway. Two genes outside the vitamin D metabolism pathway (*AMDHD1* and *SEC23A*) were also found to be significant variants and hence were included. 25(OH)D related proxies not directly present in the recent GWAS were also included if found in high linkage disequilibrium ($r^2 > 0.8$) using the Ldproxy function in LD link (https://ldlink.nci.nih.gov, accessed on 12 April 2021).
3. Outcome: the primary outcome measure, T1D, was defined by the World Health Organization criteria: diabetes symptoms (polyuria, polydipsia and insulin deficiency), accompanied by exogenous insulin usage once T1D had been diagnosed [27]. T1D could be self-reported or doctor-diagnosed when confirming cases.
4. Study design: peer-reviewed genetic association, cohort, cross-section, or case-control observational studies and Mendelian randomization (MR) studies, as well as clinical trials and unpublished cohort studies.
5. A sample size of at least 50 cases and 50 controls were mandatory for sufficient data extraction. Where there were multiple publications from the same study population, the most recent highest quality results with the largest sample size were used.
6. The publication reported genotype distribution in both cases and controls in order to estimate an odds ratio (OR) with a 95% confidence interval (CI).

The following exclusion criteria were also used:

1. Conference papers.
2. Other types of diabetes.

No language, publication status, or publication date limitations were imposed.

2.3. Study Selection and Data Extraction

Literature was searched in duplicate independently by two authors (L.N. and J.S.), and approved by a third author (E.H.). After excluding duplicates, article selection was carried out in two passes. In the first pass, title and abstract screening occurred for the selection of relevant papers meeting the eligibility criteria. In the second pass, proposed articles from the first pass were screened in full text for compliance with inclusion criteria. To ensure literature saturation, reference lists of obtained studies from original database searches were manually scanned for potential unidentified additional studies by one author

(L.N.), with eligibility confirmed by a second author (J.S.). Furthermore, OpenGWAS was used to identify unpublished studies, locating one FinnGen cohort study sharing summary-level data fitting the search parameters. Datasets were also identified in the UK Biobank, a large-scale prospective cohort study.

Data were extracted independently by two authors (L.N. and J.S.) using a predetermined data extraction template. The following data were extracted from the articles included in this systematic review: first author; region/demographic information; publication year; study design characteristics; participant characteristics, including gender and ethnicity if reported; the number of cases and controls studied; mean age (or range) at the onset of T1D in cases; outcome measure, diagnostic criteria of T1D; mean age (or range) of the control group; how the controls were selected; genotyping methods, genotype distribution, and allele frequency in cases and controls; all reported patient outcome measures; key findings; protocol availability and funding sources. Corresponding authors were contacted by e-mail for missing or unreported data a maximum of three attempts, to avoid any assumptions made from unclear information. All disagreements were resolved by consensus, or with the input of a third author (E.H. or A.Z.).

2.4. Statistical Analysis

All mentioned statistical analyses were performed with STATA 16.0 software (Stata Corporation, College Station, TX, USA) and R 4.0.2 software by two authors (L.N. and A.Z.). For each variant, OR per vitamin D-increasing allele was extracted from individual studies for the meta-analysis, as per the SUNLIGHT consortium [21]. If a study did not contain the selected vitamin D variant, the result of its proxy ($r^2 > 0.8$) was extracted and used to estimate the related effect. In studies where the OR per vitamin-D-increasing allele was not reported, we estimated the allelic effect from the contingency table of T1D distribution by SNP genotypes, where OR was computed by dividing the odds of T1D in the heterozygotes (i.e., with 1 25-hydroxyvitamin D increasing allele) by that in the homozygotes (i.e., with 0 25-hydroxyvitamin D increasing allele). Meta-analysis was performed using the random-effects model (REM, restricted maximum likelihood method) [28]. Heterogeneity between studies was assessed using Cochran's Q test the I^2 statistic, with heterogeneity considered to be substantial if the p-value for the Cochran's Q test < 0.05 or $I^2 > 50\%$. All p-values were for two-tailed tests, and <0.05 was considered statistically significant.

We conducted sensitivity analyses by removing a single study at a time, evaluating the integrity of the results. Subgroup analysis was performed by restricting the sample to the Caucasian population, to examine the possible effects of population stratification. Initial protocol pre-specified plan for further MR analyses, which were not conducted as it was considered redundant given clear results.

2.5. Risk of Bias and Credibility of the Evidence Assessment

The methodological quality of eligible studies was evaluated using Critical Appraisal Skills Program tools for cohort and case-control studies [29]. Two authors (L.N. and J.S.) independently completed risk of bias assessment and recorded supporting justification and information for each domain to optimise the tool's value (met; partially met; not met; unclear). The domains were: Are the results of the study valid? Were the cases recruited in an acceptable way? Was the exposure accurately measured to minimise bias? Have authors taken account of the potential confounding factors in the design and/or in their analysis? How precise are the results? (size of confidence intervals). Results were compared by categorising each study for study quality (risk of bias) judgement (low, some concerns, high). Articles were judged as 'low' when five or more domains were met. Conversely, articles were judged as 'high' when three or more domains were unmet. Disagreements were resolved by a third author (E.H.). Outcome reporting bias was assessed by comparing outcomes specified in protocols, with outcomes reported in corresponding publications. Where protocols were not available, outcomes specified in the methods and results sections of publications were compared.

Two reviewers assessed the risk of bias due to missing results in a synthesis (L.N. and A.Z.). Potential publication bias was assessed by examining for asymmetry using Begg's funnel plot for each SNP [30]. If publication bias was present, the plot would be asymmetric, indicating a deficiency in publications with negative results. No further formal assessment of publication bias, such as Egger's test was performed, due to insufficient studies [31].

3. Results

3.1. Study Selection

Initially, 290 potential studies were identified from the search. Figure 1 shows a flowchart of the study selection process based on the PRISMA statement [23]. After the initial pass, 58 were excluded as duplicates. 212 were excluded after reading the title and abstract because of evident irrelevance. In the second pass, the full text of the 20 studies selected in the first pass were read and 10 studies were excluded for not meeting the search criteria. Two articles were excluded because they did not provide sufficient data for the calculation of Ors with 95% CI [32,33]. Three papers were excluded because they were family-based [34–36]. Two papers were excluded as they assessed associations between polymorphisms not in linkage disequilibrium with the selected variants [37,38]. Two papers did not investigate the association between the selected variants and T1D, investigating a different outcome [39,40]. Only one study was excluded due to using the same sample population [24]. Therefore, 10 studies were included in this systematic review.

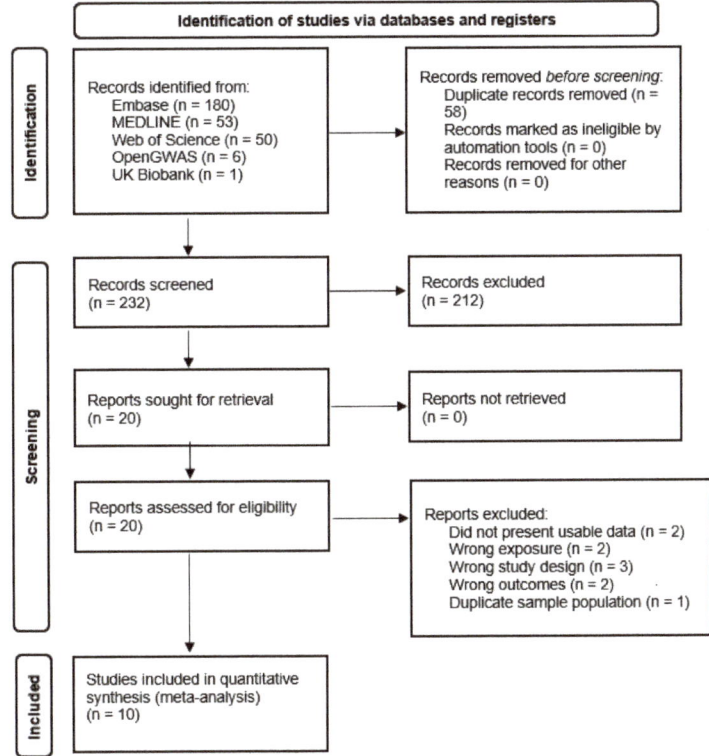

Figure 1. Flowchart illustrating the literature search and study selection.

3.2. Characteristics of Included Studies

The summary characteristics of included studies are shown in Table 1. The studies were published between 1999 to 2021, conducted in different geographical locations. Of the 10 included studies, seven were case-control studies [25,40–44], and three had a cohort design [45–47]. Most studies focused on T1D in childhood, as indicated by the mean age of onset in cases. Appropriate genotyping methods and diagnostic criteria were used in all included studies. Of the studies selected, six studies [40–43,47] fulfilled the WHO diagnostic criteria for T1D, while the majority of the remaining studies [25,44–46,48] indirectly captured criteria by description from multiple case sample populations. Polymerase chain reaction-restriction fragment length polymorphism (PCR-RFLP) was used by half the included studies as the genotyping method.

Similarly, none of the eligible studies endeavoured to control for vitamin D dietary intake through infancy and/or childhood, a known risk factor of T1D. However, when study quality was assessed, all included studies presented with a low risk of bias using the CASP tools, with no deviation from the Hardy-Weinberg equilibrium in controls reported in all case-control studies, and only some studies presenting with one item partially unmet (Supplementary Table S5).

Statistical methods to control confounding varied between studies. Most studies adjusted for different potential confounding factors, such as age, sex, genotype batch, geographical origin and BMI (see Table 1). Two remaining papers were matched case-control studies to control for known potential confounding variables. Hussein et al. [41], matched by age and ethnic origin, while Mahmoud et al. [42] matched by gender. Six studies [40,43–47] did not report OR results directly, and some, but not all, of the studies, generated adjusted ORs.

Table 1. Characteristics of observational studies evaluating the association between vitamin D genetic variants and type 1 diabetes included in the meta-analysis.

Author, Year	Study Details		Participant Characteristics					Polymorphism Details				Findings
	Country	Study Design	Ethnicity	n Cases/n Controls	Mean Age of Cases/ Controls (Year)	Mean Age of Onset in Cases (Years)	T1D Diagnostic Criteria	Genotyping	Adjusted Factors	Gene	Variant	EA [a]	Relevant Key Findings
Manousaki et al., 2021 [45]	Canada, United Kingdom, United States	Cohort	European	9338/15,705	NI	NI	Multiple criteria	PCR-RFLP	Age, sex, season of 25OHD measurement, genotype batch, genotype array, assessment centre (proxy for latitude)	CYP2R1 CYP2R1 (low frequency) DHCR7/ NADSYN1 GC CYP24A1 AMDHD1 SEC23A	rs10741657 rs117913124 rs12785878 rs3755967 [b] rs17216707 rs10745742 rs8018720	A G T C [c] T T G	No association of individual SNPs with T1D.
Almeida et al., 2020 [25]	Portugal	Case-control	Caucasian Portuguese	350/490	29.0/32.2	17.2	Classic clinical presentation [d]	PCR-RFLP	Age at bleed, sex, BMI, month of bleed, geographical region 25OHD and 1α,25(OH)2D levels. (25OHD measurement obtained in same season)	CYP2R1 DHCR7/ NADSYN1 GC	rs10741657 rs12785878 rs3755967 [b]	A T C [c]	No association of individual SNP with T1D.
Nam et al., 2019 [44]	Korea	Case-control	Korean	96/156	14.7/14.0	NI	Classic clinical presentation [d]	PCR		CYP2R1	rs10741657	A	No association of individual SNP with T1D.
Hussein et al., 2012 [41]	Egypt	Matched case-control	Egyptian	120/120	11.7/11.1	NI	WHO and ADA	PCR-RFLP	Nil	CYP2R1	rs10741657	A	An association of GG genotype of CYP2R1 polymorphism (coded by 25OHD decreasing alleles) with risk of T1D in Egyptian children [OR = 2.6, 95% CI = 1.1–6.1, p = 0.03]. A synergistic effect of multiple risk alleles between GG genotype of CYP2R1 and CC genotype of CYP27B1 and T1D risk found.
Mahmoud et al., 2011 [42]	Egypt	Matched case-control	Egyptian	59/65	13/>24	7.5	WHO	PCR-RFLP	Nil	GC	rs3755967 [b]	C [c]	No association between VDBP polymorphisms with T1D.

Table 1. Cont.

Author; Year	Study Details			Participant Characteristics				Polymorphism Details				Findings
	Country	Study Design	Ethnicity	n Cases/n Controls	Mean Age of Cases/ Controls (Year)	Mean Age of Onset in Cases (Years)	T1D Diagnostic Criteria	Genotyping	Adjusted Factors	Gene	Variant	EA [a]	Relevant Key Findings
Blanton et al., 2011 [45]	United States	Case-control	American	1705/2033	NI	12.9	Classic clinical presentation [d]	TaqMan PCR Assays	Sex, onset of T1D, HLA risk	GC	rs3755967 [b]	C [c]	No association between VDBP polymorphisms with T1D detected. An association of the phenotype of lower VDBP levels with T1D. An association of the 'G' allele of CYP2R1 common variant
Ramos-Lopez et al., 2007 [40]	Germany	Case-control	German	284/294	NI	11.5	WHO	PCR-RFLP	25(OH)D3 levels	CYP2R1	rs10741657	A	polymorphisms (coded by 25(OH)D decreasing alleles) with T1D risk.
Klupa et al., 1999 [43]	United States	Case-control	European	181/163	36.2/52.55	10.9	WHO	PCR	Nil; sensitivity confirmed via stratification by obesity and age at examination	GC	rs3755967 [b]	C [c]	No association of individual SNP with T1D.
FinnGen [46]	Finland	Cohort	Finnish	1143– 1267/82,381– 82,655	NI	NI	Strict definition (Minimal/absent insulin production by pancreas)	Illumina and Affymetrix Chip Arrays	Sex, age, 10 PCs, genotyping batch	CYP2R1 CYP2R1 (low frequency) DHCR7/ NADSYN1 GC CYP24A1 AMDHD1 SEC23A	rs10741657 rs117913124 [b] rs12785878 rs3755967 rs17216707 rs10745742 rs8018720	A G [c] T C T T G	NI
UK Biobank [47]	United Kingdom	Cohort	Caucasian British	3074– 3221/370,277– 387,397	NI	NI	WHO	UK Biobank Axiom Array	Age, sex, birth location, assessment centre, SNP array, pc1-pc40, account for relatedness	CYP2R1 CYP2R1 (low frequency) DHCR7/ NADSYN1 GC CYP24A1 AMDHD1 SEC23A	rs10741657 rs117913124 rs12785878 rs3755967 rs17216707 rs10745742 rs8018720	A G T C T T G	NI

Abbreviation: 25(OH)D, 25-Hydroxyvitamin D; n, number; T1D, type 1 diabetes; NI, not informed; ADA, American Diabetes Association; WHO, World Health Organization; PCR, polymerase chain reactions; PCR-RFLP, polymerase chain reaction-restricted fragment length polymorphism; SNP, single nucleotide polymorphism; Vit D, vitamin D; EA, effect allele; OR, odds ratio; VDBP, vitamin D binding protein. [a] Each effect allele represents the 25(OH)D concentration increasing allele, as defined by Sunlight Consortium [21]. [b] Identified using LDproxy, coded by 25(OH)D concentration decreasing alleles (see methods) [c] Effect allele direction reversed based on 25(OH)D concentration increasing, as defined by Sunlight Consortium (see methods) [21]. [d] Low/undetectable serum C-peptide and presence of 1+ pancreatic autoantibodies.

3.3. Findings from the Meta-Analysis

All specified polymorphisms (namely rs10741657 G/A (*CYP2R1*), rs117913124 A/G (*CYP2R1* low frequency), rs12785878 G/T (*DHCR7/NADSYN1*), rs3755967 T/C (*GC*), rs17216707 C/T (*CYP24A1*), rs10745742 C/T (*AMDHD1*), rs8018720 C/G (*SEC23A*) were reported in three or more studies and taken forward to the meta-analyses. Associations between the SNPs and T1D, using individual and pooled OR estimates, are displayed in Figure 2 and Supplementary Figure S1.

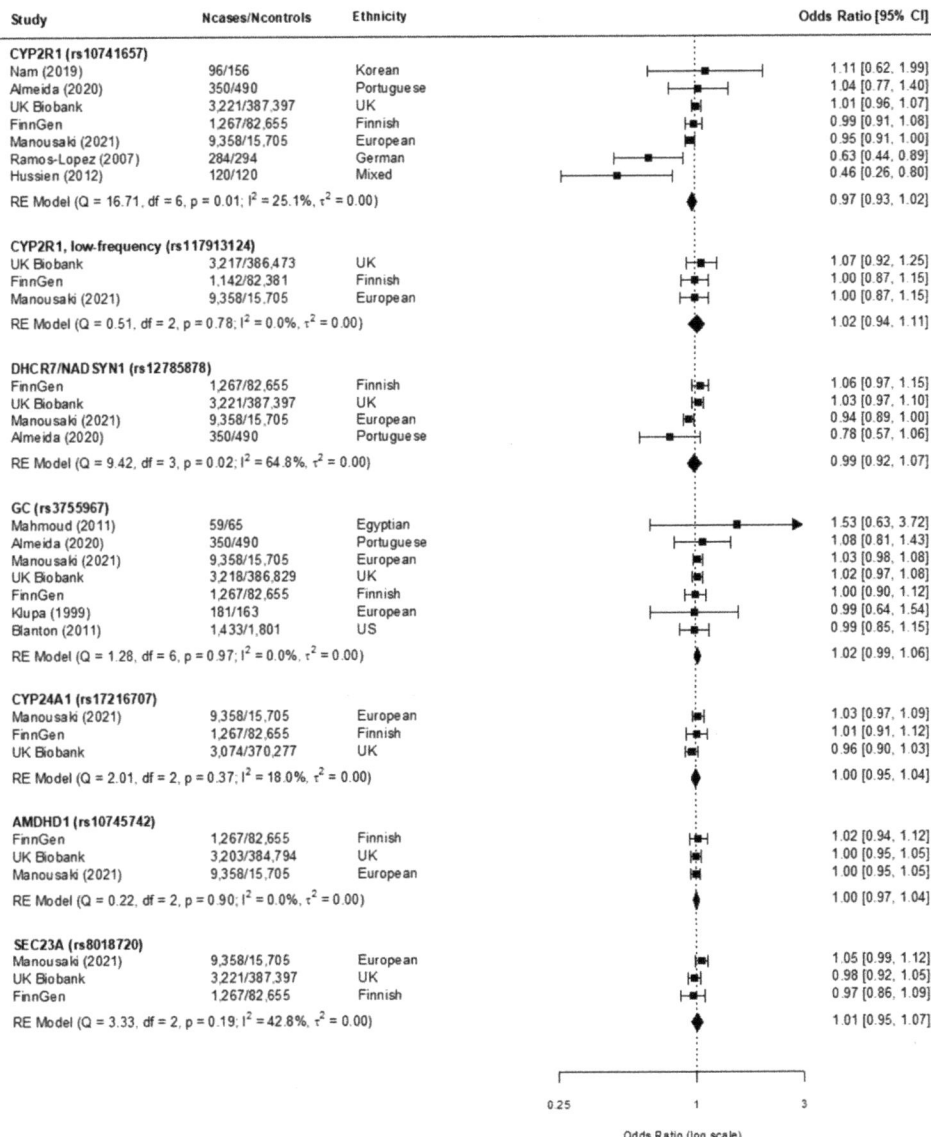

Figure 2. Meta-analysis for the association between selected genetic variants affecting serum 25-hydroxyvitamin concentrations and type 1 diabetes with the random effects model (variants coded by 25-hydroxyvitamin D increasing alleles). Squares represent the individual odds ratio estimate. Diamonds show the pooled effect. Horizontal bars represent the 95% confidence intervals.

For rs10741657 G/A (*CYP2R1*), the reported ORs ranged from 0.46 to 1.11 (Figure 2). The random-effects pooled OR was 0.97 (95% CI 0.93, 1.02; $p = 0.01$) with little heterogeneity among the studies ($I^2 = 25.1\%$). For rs117913124 A/G (*CYP2R1* low frequency), the ORs ranged from 1.00 to 1.07 (Figure 2) with a pooled OR of 1.02 (95% CI 0.94, 1.11; $p = 0.78$; I = 0.0%). For rs12785878 G/T (*DHCR7/NADSYN1*), the ORs ranged from 0.78 to 1.06 (Figure 2), with a pooled OR of 0.99 (95% CI 0.92, 1.07; $p = 0.02$). There was evidence of moderate between-study heterogeneity ($I^2 = 64.8\%$). For rs3755967 T/C (*GC*), the OR ranged from 0.99 to 1.53 (Figure 2), with a pooled OR of 1.02 and no sign of heterogeneity (95% CI 0.99, 1.06; $p = 0.97$; I = 0.0%). In the evaluation for publication bias, asymmetry in Begg's funnel plot was observed for *GC* rs3755967 (Supplementary Figure S2). For rs17216707 C/T (*CYP24A1*), the OR ranged from 0.96 to 1.03 (Figure 2). The random-effects model pooled OR was 1.00 (95% CI 0.95, 1.04, $p = 0.37$), with little indication of heterogeneity ($I^2 = 18.0\%$). For rs10745742 C/T (*AMDHD1*), the OR ranged from 1.00 to 1.02 (Figure 2) with a pooled OR of 1.00 (95% CI 0.97, 1.04; $p = 0.90$). Again, there was no sign of heterogeneity ($I^2 = 0.0\%$). For rs8018720 C/G (*SEC23A*), the OR ranged from 0.97 to 1.05 (Figure 2). The REM yielded a pooled OR of 1.01 (95% CI 0.95, 1.07, $p = 0.19$) with little heterogeneity among the studies ($I^2 = 42.8\%$). In view of these individual estimates, under the studied models no statistically significant associations between any of the seven SNPs alone (or their proxies) and T1D were found. Other than in rs3755967 (*GC*), no other asymmetry in Begg's funnel plot was observed. No outcome reporting bias was detected in any of the studies.

Furthermore, a sensitivity analysis was also performed to assess the influence of each study using the leave-one-out method. The pooled ORs were not changed materially and remained not significant, indicating good stability of results (range of pooled OR: 0.97–1.02). A subgroup analysis performed on the Caucasian population found no manifestations of association, with no major changes in primary outcomes (Supplementary Figure S1). Analyses showed all seven selected polymorphisms (or their proxies) were not associated with T1D risk under the studied models (range of pooled OR: 0.98–1.02).

4. Discussion

4.1. Main Findings

Our extensive systematic review and meta-analysis did not provide support for an association between 25(OH)D related variants and T1D. Our review identified 10 studies for inclusion, which were all relatively high quality, presenting only minor systematic flaws in methodology. However, evidence from published studies was inconsistent, and for most polymorphisms, only a handful of studies were found. Many of the studies were small, limiting the statistical power of each meta-analysis, and preventing robust sensitivity analyses to evaluate associations by possible sources of heterogeneity, such as geographic location, and ancestry.

To the best of our knowledge, our study is the largest and most comprehensive systematic review and meta-analysis on the topic. The largest of the previous studies was a recently published MR study [45], which also provided a null finding, and from which raw data were included in this study. We conducted leave-one-out analyses, which suggested limited impact by any single study, alleviating concerns for bias caused by the inclusion of smaller or early studies. Furthermore, ethnicity is believed to have a major role in vitamin D synthesis (and possibly metabolism), however, subgroup analysis on Caucasian participants also provided no evidence for an association between the selected 25(OH)D related genetic variants and T1D.

From publications included in our review, those studies which found evidence for an association with T1D risk, tended to be comparatively small, while the association could not be confirmed in the large genetic databases. For example, Ramos-Lopez et al. [40] found an association of the *CYP2R1* common variant polymorphisms with T1D in 578 German participants, providing early support for the causal role of 25(OH)D in the pathogenesis of T1D. Hussein et al. [41] also found an association in an Egyptian sample (n cases = 120) between the *CYP2R1* common variant with risk of T1D. Smaller study over-estimates of effect can yield asymmetric funnel plots that can be explained by a restrictive study population [49]. However, the two smaller studies reporting an association included in this paper, had a matched case-control design, suggesting a possibility they were more carefully designed than the larger database based studies. For example, case ascertainment in the database studies typically had diagnoses confirmed by self-report or hospitalisation. Furthermore, despite including participants from diverse ethnic groups, Hussein and colleagues, had an ethnicity-matched control sample [41]. In contrast, recent larger studies in the European population including between 350 and 9358 cases [25,45,46], as well as our analyses including 3221 cases (387,397 controls) from the UK Biobank, did not find evidence for an association between any of the selected genetic variants and T1D. While we did not find evidence for publication bias, there was possible asymmetry in Begg's funnel plot for *GC* rs3755967 (Supplementary Figure S2). However, its interpretation should be taken as merely an evaluation of whether smaller studies gave different results to larger studies, as further formal testing for publication bias would have been largely underpowered due to the limited number of studies.

High heterogeneity was found in the meta-analysis *DHCR7/NADSYN1* rs12785878 polymorphism, (I^2 = 64.8%), which was unanticipated given the studies included in the analyses of this variant were all of European ancestry, with adjustments for confounding factors. However, DHCR7 affects skin synthesis of vitamin D following exposure to UVB radiation from the sunlight and may be particularly sensitive to subtle variations in population structure. Variants affecting vitamin D metabolism have been shown to display population-specific patterns in frequency [50], and are believed to have contributed to adaptations during the evolutionary history which has allowed individuals to avoid severe vitamin D deficiency [51]. This has been seen in earlier vitamin D related genetic meta-analyses, which have allowed for the examination of population stratification. Notably, a large meta-analysis found the *BsmI* polymorphism in the vitamin D-receptor gene was only associated with T1D in those with Asian ancestry [52]. Differing environmental factors, such as geographical differences in diet and sun exposure, may also play a role to aggravate or compensate susceptibility conferred by variants in these genes [53].

4.2. Considerations of Alternative Explanation for Observed Results

Vitamin D status is mainly determined by lifestyle factors, such as exposure to sunlight, dietary supplementation and intake, as well as personal characteristics including obesity and age. Indeed, common genetic variants typically have modest effects, and they only account for a small amount of the variation in 25(OH)D levels [54]. Therefore, even if variation in 25(OH)D concentrations is important for T1D, but only at the very extreme (such as clinical deficiency), this type of genetic instrument may not be able to pick up an association, especially if most of the population investigated has relatively normal concentrations. The influence of genetic variations may also be affected by interactions with other genes and by environmental factors.

Given the limited number of studies, we were unable to assess ethnic differences in the association between 25(OH)D variants and T1D. Given ethnicity may affect the function and expression of vitamin D related genes [50,52,53], it is possible that we may have missed associations that are only seen in a particular population group.

4.3. Strengths and Limitations

Our study benefits from the systematic way in which results have been summarised, our comprehensive search strategy and the inclusion of grey literature. The design captures lifetime differences in 25(OH)D levels, rather than a single vitamin D measurement. Our study also has some limitations requiring consideration. Despite including information from the largest available databases to supplement all published data, available information remains limited. The relatively small number of included studies prevented us from undertaking analysis to examine the associations in diverse ethnic groups or to account for other population characteristics. There was little to no information from populations that were vitamin D deficient. For example, the FinnGen study in Finland commenced in 2017, after the National Nutrition Council had launched the national food fortification of vitamin D (2002) [55]. Therefore, we are unable to exclude weak associations or associations that are only relevant in the context of very low 25(OH)D concentrations. We did not have access to individual level data for most of the studies, therefore, adjustments strategies could not be harmonised. Results could be limited by the absence of dietary information for all study participants, as studies have shown an association between vitamin D genes can vary due to diet, or even past sun exposure [56]. Furthermore, evidence participants of the UK Biobank are not representative of the UK population, having a healthy volunteer selection bias [57]. Thus, we are only able to investigate for a causal effect within the constraints of each study, which may have contributed to the null finding.

4.4. Guidelines for Future Research

Investigating for smaller causal effects may be important for public health, due to a high prevalence of low 25(OH)D concentrations in many populations. Findings need to be elucidated by conducting larger scale epidemiological investigations, exploiting the potential for vitamin D related genetic variants as a risk factor for T1D, to confirm or refute the study findings. Furthermore, said studies will need to investigate the role of 25(OH)D related genetic variants in the context of clinical deficiency, where even subtle increases in concentrations may help, providing a more comprehensive understanding of the association between variants affecting serum 25(OH)D concentration and T1D.

5. Conclusions

Results from this meta-analysis showed no large effect of a genetically determined reduction in 25(OH)D concentrations by selected polymorphisms on T1D risk, despite the strong association seen in some observational studies. Although the hypothesis that a different SNP distribution from vitamin D related genes is associated with T1D was not confirmed by this study, small effects cannot be discounted. To make conclusive estimates in complex diseases, such as T1D, further characterization of complex interactions between genetic and environmental factors, like the included variants affecting serum 25(OH)D concentrations, need to be considered.

Supplementary Materials: The following are avaiable online at https://www.mdpi.com/2072-6643/13/12/4260/s1, Supplementary Figure S1. Funnel plot analysis for publication bias; Supplementary Figure S2. Subgroup analysis of Caucasian participants for the association between selected genetic variants affecting serum 25-hydroxyvitamin concentrations and type 1 diabetes with the random effects model (coded by 25-hydroxyvitamin D increasing alleles). Squares represent the individual odds ratio estimate. Diamonds show the pooled effect. Horizontal bars represent the 95% confidence intervals; Supplementary Table S1. Ovid: MEDLINE search strategy—the database coverage was 1946 to present, and the database was last searched on 1 April 2021; Supplementary Table S2. Ovid: Embase Classic and Embase search strategy—the database coverage was 1947 to present, and the database was last searched on 1 April 2021; Supplementary Table S3. Web of Science search strategy—the database coverage was 1947 to present, and the database was last searched on 1 April 2021; Supplementary Table S4. OpenGWAS search strategy –annotated R script using R package. The database coverage was 2020 to present, and the database was last searched on 1 April 2021; Supplementary Table S5. Quality assessment of the included studies: summary of critical appraisal using CASP tools; Supplementary Material S1 Author ICMJE disclosure forms.

Author Contributions: L.N.: Conceptualization, Methodology, Software, Validation, Formal analysis, Investigation, Data curation, Writing—original draft preparation, Writing—reviewing and editing, Visualization, Project administration. E.H.: Conceptualization, Methodology, Resources, Writing—reviewing and editing, Supervision, Project administration, Funding acquisition. A.Z.: Conceptualization, Methodology, Software, Formal analysis, Writing—reviewing and editing, Supervision. J.S.: Investigation, Writing—reviewing and editing, Supervision. All authors have read and agreed to the published version of the manuscript.

Funding: This research was in part supported by National Health and Medical Research Council, Australia (GNT11123603).

Institutional Review Board Statement: Not applicable.

Informed Consent Statement: Not applicable.

Data Availability Statement: Not applicable, due to being systematic review with meta-analyses. All data is available in primary studies.

Acknowledgments: We want to acknowledge the participants and investigators of the FinnGen study, and all the participants and investigators of the UK Biobank.

Conflicts of Interest: The authors declare no potential duality of interest associated with this study. All authors have completed the ICMJE uniform disclosure form (see Supplementary Materials).

Abbreviations

Abbreviations
25(OH)D: 25-Hydroxyvitamin D; CI, confidence interval; CASP, Critical Appraisal Skills Program; GWAS, genome wide association study; MR, Mendelian randomization; MeSH, Medical Subject Headings; OR, odds ratio; PEO, Population, Exposure and Outcomes approaches; PRISMA, Preferred Reporting Items for Systematic Reviews and Meta-Analyses; SNP, single nucleotide polymorphism; T1D, type 1 diabetes.

References

1. Paschou, S.A.; Papadopoulou-Marketou, N.; Chrousos, G.P.; Kanaka-Gantenbein, C. On type 1 diabetes mellitus pathogenesis. *Endocr. Connect.* **2018**, *7*, R38–R46. [CrossRef]
2. Cernea, S.; Dobreanu, M.; Raz, I. Prevention of type 1 diabetes: Today and tomorrow. *Diabetes/Metab. Res. Rev.* **2010**, *26*, 602–605. [CrossRef]
3. Huber, A.; Menconi, F.; Corathers, S.; Jacobson, E.M.; Tomer, Y. Joint Genetic Susceptibility to Type 1 Diabetes and Autoimmune Thyroiditis: From Epidemiology to Mechanisms. *Endocr. Rev.* **2008**, *29*, 697–725. [CrossRef]
4. World Health Organization. *Global Report on Diabetes*; World Health Organization: Geneva, Switzerland, 2016. Available online: http://apps.who.int/iris/bitstream/handle/10665/204871/9789241565257_eng.pdf;jsessionid=CCC2429A03D7EF6D638C05F6F008A3C2?sequence=1 (accessed on 8 July 2020).
5. International Diabetes Federation. IDF Diabetes Atlas 8th Edition. 2017. Available online: http://www.diabetesatlas.org/across-the-globe.html (accessed on 10 February 2020).
6. Pike, J.W.; Christakos, S. Biology and Mechanisms of Action of the Vitamin D Hormone. *Endocrinol. Metab. Clin. N. Am.* **2017**, *46*, 815–843. [CrossRef]
7. Jiang, X.; Kiel, D.P.; Kraft, P. The genetics of vitamin D. *Bone* **2019**, *126*, 59–77. [CrossRef] [PubMed]
8. Wang, Y.; Zhu, J.; DeLuca, H.F. Where is the vitamin D receptor? *Arch. Biochem. Biophys.* **2012**, *523*, 123–133. [CrossRef]
9. Infante, M.; Ricordi, C.; Sanchez, J.; Clare-Salzler, M.J.; Padilla, N.; Fuenmayor, V.; Chavez, C.; Alvarez, A.; Baidal, D.; Alejandro, R.; et al. Influence of Vitamin D on Islet Autoimmunity and Beta-Cell Function in Type 1 Diabetes. *Nutrients* **2019**, *11*, 2185. [CrossRef] [PubMed]
10. Hayes, C.E.; Nashold, F.E.; Spach, K.M.; Pedersen, L.B. The immunological functions of the vitamin D endocrine system. *Cell. Mol. Boil.* **2003**, *49*, 277–300.
11. Hewison, M.; Zehnder, D.; Chakraverty, R.; Adams, J.S. Vitamin D and barrier function: A novel role for extra-renal 1α-hydroxylase. *Mol. Cell. Endocrinol.* **2004**, *215*, 31–38. [CrossRef] [PubMed]
12. Mathieu, C.; Waer, M.; Laureys, J.; Rutgeerts, O.; Bouillon, R. Prevention of autoimmune diabetes in NOD mice by 1,25 dihydroxyvitamin D3. *Diabetol.* **1994**, *37*, 552–558. [CrossRef] [PubMed]
13. Casteels, K.; Waer, M.; Bouillon, R.; Depovere, J.; Valckx, D.; Laureys, J.; Mathieu, C. 1,25-Dihydroxyvitamin D3 restores sensitivity to cyclophosphamide-induced apoptosis in non-obese diabetic (NOD) mice and protects against diabetes. *Clin. Exp. Immunol.* **1998**, *112*, 181–187. [CrossRef] [PubMed]
14. Zella, J.B.; DeLuca, H.F. Vitamin D and autoimmune diabetes. *J. Cell. Biochem.* **2003**, *88*, 216–222. [CrossRef]
15. Delvin, E.; Souberbielle, J.-C.; Viard, J.-P.; Salle, B. Role of vitamin D in acquired immune and autoimmune diseases. *Crit. Rev. Clin. Lab. Sci.* **2014**, *51*, 232–247. [CrossRef]
16. Hyppönen, E.; Läärä, E.; Reunanen, A.; Jarvelin, M.-R.; Virtanen, S. Intake of vitamin D and risk of type 1 diabetes: A birth-cohort study. *Lancet* **2001**, *358*, 1500–1503. [CrossRef]
17. Littorin, B.; Blom, P.; Schölin, A.; Arnqvist, H.J.; Blohmé, G.; Bolinder, J.; Ekbom-Schnell, A.; Eriksson, J.W.; Gudbjörnsdottir, S.; Nyström, L.; et al. Lower levels of plasma 25-hydroxyvitamin D among young adults at diagnosis of autoimmune type 1 diabetes

compared with control subjects: Results from the nationwide Diabetes Incidence Study in Sweden (DISS). *Diabetologia* **2006**, *49*, 2847–2852. [CrossRef]
18. Zipitis, C.S.; Akobeng, A.K. Vitamin D supplementation in early childhood and risk of type 1 diabetes: A systematic review and meta-analysis. *Arch. Dis. Child.* **2008**, *93*, 512–517. [CrossRef] [PubMed]
19. Dahlquist, G.; Mustonen, L. Childhood Onset Diabetes—Time Trends and Climatological Factors. *Int. J. Epidemiol.* **1994**, *23*, 1234–1241. [CrossRef] [PubMed]
20. Gregoriou, E.; Mamais, I.; Tzanetakou, I.; Lavranos, G.; Chrysostomou, S. The Effects of Vitamin D Supplementation in Newly Diagnosed Type 1 Diabetes Patients: Systematic Review of Randomized Controlled Trials. *Rev. Diabet. Stud.* **2017**, *14*, 260–268. [CrossRef]
21. Jiang, X.; O'Reilly, P.; Aschard, H.; Hsu, Y.-H.; Richards, J.B.; Dupuis, J.; Ingelsson, E.; Karasik, D.; Pilz, S.; Berry, D.; et al. Genome-wide association study in 79,366 European-ancestry individuals informs the genetic architecture of 25-hydroxyvitamin D levels. *Nat. Commun.* **2018**, *9*, 1–12. [CrossRef]
22. Manousaki, D.; Dudding, T.; Haworth, S.; Hsu, Y.-H.; Liu, C.-T.; Medina-Gomez, C.; Voortman, T.; van der Velde, N.; Melhus, H.; Robinson-Cohen, C.; et al. Low-Frequency Synonymous Coding Variation in CYP2R1 Has Large Effects on Vitamin D Levels and Risk of Multiple Sclerosis. *Am. J. Hum. Genet.* **2017**, *101*, 227–238. [CrossRef] [PubMed]
23. Moher, D.; Liberati, A.; Tetzlaff, J.; Altman, D.G. Preferred Reporting Items for Systematic Reviews and Meta-Analyses: The PRISMA Statement. *J. Clin. Epidemiol.* **2009**, *62*, 1006–1012. [CrossRef]
24. Cooper, J.D.; Smyth, D.J.; Walker, N.M.; Stevens, H.; Burren, O.S.; Wallace, C.; Greissl, C.; Ramos-Lopez, E.; Hyppönen, E.; Dunger, D.B.; et al. Inherited Variation in Vitamin D Genes Is Associated With Predisposition to Autoimmune Disease Type 1 Diabetes. *Diabetes* **2011**, *60*, 1624–1631. [CrossRef] [PubMed]
25. Almeida, J.T.; Rodrigues, D.; Guimarães, J.; Lemos, M.C. Vitamin D Pathway Genetic Variation and Type 1 Diabetes: A Case–Control Association Study. *Genes* **2020**, *11*, 897. [CrossRef] [PubMed]
26. Moola, S.; Munn, Z.; Sears, K.; Sfetcu, R.; Currie, M.; Lisy, K.; Tufanaru, C.; Qureshi, R.; Mattis, P.; Mu, P. Conducting systematic reviews of association (etiology). *Int. J. Evid.-Based Health* **2015**, *13*, 163–169. [CrossRef]
27. World Health Organization. *Diabetes*; World Health Organization: Geneva, Switzerland, 2020. Available online: https://www.who.int/news-room/fact-sheets/detail/diabetes (accessed on 8 July 2020).
28. DerSimonian, R.; Laird, N. Meta-analysis in clinical trials revisited. *Contemp. Clin. Trials* **2015**, *45*, 139–145. [CrossRef] [PubMed]
29. CASP. *CASP Checklists*; CASP: Oxford, UK, 2020. Available online: https://casp-uk.net/ (accessed on 8 July 2020).
30. Begg, C.B.; Mazumdar, M. Operating Characteristics of a Rank Correlation Test for Publication Bias. *Biometrics* **1994**, *50*, 1088–1101. [CrossRef] [PubMed]
31. Egger, M.; Smith, G.D.; Schneider, M.; Minder, C. Bias in meta-analysis detected by a simple, graphical test. *BMJ* **1997**, *315*, 629–634. [CrossRef]
32. Frederiksen, B.N.; Kroehl, M.; Fingerlin, T.E.; Wong, R.; Steck, A.K.; Rewers, M.; Norris, J.M. Association between Vitamin D Metabolism Gene Polymorphisms and Risk of Islet Autoimmunity and Progression to Type 1 Diabetes: The Diabetes Autoimmunity Study in the Young (DAISY). *J. Clin. Endocrinol. Metab.* **2013**, *98*, E1845–E1851. [CrossRef]
33. Thorsen, S.U.; Mortensen, H.B.; Carstensen, B.; Fenger, M.; Thuesen, B.; Husemoen, L.; Bergholdt, R.; Brorsson, C.A.; Pociot, F.; Linneberg, A.; et al. No association between type 1 diabetes and genetic variation in vitamin D metabolism genes: A Danish study. *Pediatr. Diabetes* **2013**, *15*, 416–421. [CrossRef] [PubMed]
34. Pani, M.A.; Donner, H.; Herwig, J.; Usadel, K.H.; Badenhoop, K. Vitamin D Binding Protein Alleles and Susceptibility for Type 1 Diabetes in Germans. *Autoimmunity* **1999**, *31*, 67–72. [CrossRef]
35. Miettinen, M.E.; Smart, M.; Kinnunen, L.; Mathews, C.; Harjutsalo, V.; Surcel, H.-M.; Lamberg-Allardt, C.; Tuomilehto, J.; Hitman, G.A. Maternal VDR variants rather than 25-hydroxyvitamin D concentration during early pregnancy are associated with type 1 diabetes in the offspring. *Diabetology* **2015**, *58*, 2278–2283. [CrossRef]
36. Tapia, G.; Mårild, K.; Dahl, S.R.; Lund-Blix, N.A.; Viken, M.K.; Lie, B.A.; Njølstad, P.R.; Joner, G.; Skrivarhaug, T.; Cohen, A.S.; et al. Maternal and Newborn Vitamin D–Binding Protein, Vitamin D Levels, Vitamin D Receptor Genotype, and Childhood Type 1 Diabetes. *Diabetes Care* **2019**, *42*, 553–559. [CrossRef]
37. Bailey, R.; Cooper, J.D.; Zeitels, L.; Smyth, D.J.; Yang, J.H.M.; Walker, N.M.; Hyppönen, E.; Dunger, D.B.; Ramos-Lopez, E.; Badenhoop, K.; et al. Association of the Vitamin D Metabolism Gene *CYP27B1* with Type 1 Diabetes. *Diabetes* **2007**, *56*, 2616–2621. [CrossRef] [PubMed]
38. Norris, J.M.; Lee, H.-S.; Frederiksen, B.; Erlund, I.; Uusitalo, U.; Yang, J.; Lernmark, Å.; Simell, O.; Toppari, J.; Rewers, M.; et al. Plasma 25-Hydroxyvitamin D Concentration and Risk of Islet Autoimmunity. *Diabetes* **2017**, *67*, 146–154. [CrossRef]
39. Mcgovern, A.P.; Hine, J.; De Lusignan, S. The incidence of infection is higher in older people with poor glycemic control. *Diabetes* **2016**, *65*, A360–A431. [CrossRef]
40. Ramos-Lopez, E.; Brück, P.; Jansen, T.; Herwig, J.; Badenhoop, K. CYP2R1 (vitamin D 25-hydroxylase) gene is associated with susceptibility to type 1 diabetes and vitamin D levels in Germans. *Diabetes/Metab. Res. Rev.* **2007**, *23*, 631–636. [CrossRef]
41. Hussein, A.G.; Mohamed, R.H.; Alghobashy, A.A. Synergism of CYP2R1 and CYP27B1 polymorphisms and susceptibility to type 1 diabetes in Egyptian children. *Cell. Immunol.* **2012**, *279*, 42–45. [CrossRef] [PubMed]
42. Aakre, K.M.; Watine, J.; Bunting, P.S.; Sandberg, S.; Oosterhuis, W.P. Diabetes mellitus and metabolic syndrome. *Clin. Chem. Lab. Med.* **2011**, *49*. [CrossRef]

43. Klupa, T.; Malecki, M.; Hanna, L.; Sieradzka, J.; Frey, J.; Warram, J.H.; Sieradzki, J.; Krolewski, A.S. Amino acid variants of the vitamin D-binding protein and risk of diabetes in white Americans of European origin. *Eur. J. Endocrinol.* **1999**, *141*, 490–493. [CrossRef]
44. Nam, H.; Rhie, Y.; Lee, K. Vitamin D level and gene polymorphisms in Korean children with type 1 diabetes. *Pediatr. Diabetes* **2019**, *20*, 750–758. [CrossRef]
45. Manousaki, D.; Harroud, A.; Mitchell, R.E.; Ross, S.; Forgetta, V.; Timpson, N.J.; Smith, G.D.; Polychronakos, C.; Richards, J.B. Vitamin D levels and risk of type 1 diabetes: A Mendelian randomization study. *PLoS Med.* **2021**, *18*, e1003536. [CrossRef]
46. FinnGen. FinnGen Documentation of R5 Release. FinnGen: Finland. 2021. Available online: https://finngen.gitbook.io/documentation/ (accessed on 21 June 2021).
47. UK Biobank. *Access Matter: Representativeness of UK Biobank Resource*; UK Biobank: Stockport, UK, 2021. Available online: https://www.ukbiobank.ac.uk/ (accessed on 14 August 2021).
48. Blanton, D.; Han, Z.; Bierschenk, L.; Linga-Reddy, M.P.; Wang, H.; Clare-Salzler, M.; Haller, M.; Schatz, D.; Myhr, C.; She, J.-X.; et al. Reduced Serum Vitamin D-Binding Protein Levels Are Associated With Type 1 Diabetes. *Diabetes* **2011**, *60*, 2566–2570. [CrossRef]
49. Terrin, N.; Schmid, C.; Lau, J. In an empirical evaluation of the funnel plot, researchers could not visually identify publication bias. *J. Clin. Epidemiol.* **2005**, *58*, 894–901. [CrossRef]
50. Jones, P.; Lucock, M.; Chaplin, G.; Jablonski, N.G.; Veysey, M.; Scarlett, C.; Beckett, E. Distribution of variants in multiple vitamin D-related loci (DHCR7/NADSYN1, GC, CYP2R1, CYP11A1, CYP24A1, VDR, RXRα and RXRγ) vary between European, East-Asian and Sub-Saharan African-ancestry populations. *Genes Nutr.* **2020**, *15*, 1–11. [CrossRef] [PubMed]
51. Kuan, V.; Martineau, A.R.; Griffiths, C.J.; Hyppönen, E.; Walton, R. DHCR7 mutations linked to higher vitamin D status allowed early human migration to Northern latitudes. *BMC Evol. Biol.* **2013**, *13*, 1–10. [CrossRef]
52. Zhang, J.; Li, W.; Liu, J.; Wu, W.; Ouyang, H.; Zhang, Q.; Wang, Y.; Liu, L.; Yang, R.; Liu, X.; et al. Polymorphisms in the vitamin D receptor gene and type 1 diabetes mellitus risk: An update by meta-analysis. *Mol. Cell. Endocrinol.* **2012**, *355*, 135–142. [CrossRef]
53. Bouillon, R. Genetic and Racial Differences in the Vitamin D Endocrine System. *Endocrinol. Metab. Clin. N. Am.* **2017**, *46*, 1119–1135. [CrossRef]
54. Berry, D.; Hypponen, E. Determinants of vitamin D status: Focus on genetic variations. *Curr. Opin. Nephrol. Hypertens.* **2011**, *20*, 331–336. [CrossRef]
55. Raulio, S.; Erlund, I.; Männistö, S.; Sarlio-Lähteenkorva, S.; Sundvall, J.; Tapanainen, H.; Vartiainen, E.; Virtanen, S. Successful nutrition policy: Improvement of vitamin D intake and status in Finnish adults over the last decade. *Eur. J. Public Health* **2016**, *27*, 268–273. [CrossRef]
56. Mäkinen, M.; Simell, V.; Mykkänen, J.; Ilonen, J.; Veijola, R.; Hyöty, H.; Knip, M.; Simell, O.; Toppari, J.; Hermann, R. An Increase in Serum 25-Hydroxyvitamin D Concentrations Preceded a Plateau in Type 1 Diabetes Incidence in Finnish Children. *J. Clin. Endocrinol. Metab.* **2014**, *99*, E2353–E2356. [CrossRef]
57. Fry, A.; Littlejohns, T.J.; Sudlow, C.; Doherty, N.; Adamska, L.; Sprosen, T.; Collins, R.; Allen, N.E. Comparison of Sociodemographic and Health-Related Characteristics of UK Biobank Participants with Those of the General Population. *Am. J. Epidemiol.* **2017**, *186*, 1026–1034. [CrossRef] [PubMed]

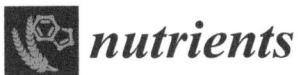

Article

Vitamin D Receptor (*VDR*) Gene Polymorphisms Modify the Response to Vitamin D Supplementation: A Systematic Review and Meta-Analysis

Ricardo Usategui-Martín [1,2,*], Daniel-Antonio De Luis-Román [3,4,5], José María Fernández-Gómez [6], Marta Ruiz-Mambrilla [7] and José-Luis Pérez-Castrillón [4,5,8,*]

1. IOBA, University of Valladolid, 47011 Valladolid, Spain
2. Cooperative Health Network for Research (RETICS), Oftared, National Institute of Health Carlos III, ISCIII, 47011 Madrid, Spain
3. Department of Endocrinology, Clinical University Hospital, 47002 Valladolid, Spain; dluisro@saludcastillayleon.es
4. Department of Medicine, Faculty of Medicine, University of Valladolid, 47002 Valladolid, Spain
5. Instituto de Endocrinología y Nutrición (IENVA), University of Valladolid, 47002 Valladolid, Spain
6. Department of Cell Biology, Histology and Pharmacology, Faculty of Medicine, University of Valladolid, 47002 Valladolid, Spain; josefg@med.uva.es
7. Department of Surgery, Faculty of Medicine, University of Valladolid, 47002 Valladolid, Spain; martamaria.ruiz@uva.es
8. Department of Internal Medicine, Río Hortega University Hospital, 47002 Valladolid, Spain
* Correspondence: ricardo.usategui@uva.es (R.U.-M.); joseluis.perez@uva.es (J.-L.P.-C.)

Citation: Usategui-Martín, R.; De Luis-Román, D.-A.; Fernández-Gómez, J.M.; Ruiz-Mambrilla, M.; Pérez-Castrillón, J.-L. Vitamin D Receptor (*VDR*) Gene Polymorphisms Modify the Response to Vitamin D Supplementation: A Systematic Review and Meta-Analysis. *Nutrients* 2022, 14, 360. https://doi.org/10.3390/nu14020360

Academic Editor: Andrea Fabbri

Received: 16 December 2021
Accepted: 13 January 2022
Published: 15 January 2022

Publisher's Note: MDPI stays neutral with regard to jurisdictional claims in published maps and institutional affiliations.

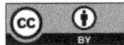

Copyright: © 2022 by the authors. Licensee MDPI, Basel, Switzerland. This article is an open access article distributed under the terms and conditions of the Creative Commons Attribution (CC BY) license (https://creativecommons.org/licenses/by/4.0/).

Abstract: The vitamin D receptor (VDR), a member of the nuclear receptor superfamily of transcriptional regulators, is crucial to calcitriol signalling. VDR is regulated by genetic and environmental factors and it is hypothesised that the response to vitamin D supplementation could be modulated by genetic variants in the *VDR* gene. The best studied polymorphisms in the *VDR* gene are ApaI (rs7975232), BsmI (rs1544410), TaqI (rs731236) and FokI (rs10735810). We conducted a systematic review and meta-analysis to evaluate the response to vitamin D supplementation according to the BsmI, TaqI, ApaI and FokI polymorphisms. We included studies that analysed the relationship between the response to vitamin D supplementation and the genotypic distribution of these polymorphisms. We included eight studies that enrolled 1038 subjects. The results showed no significant association with the BsmI and ApaI polymorphisms ($p = 0.081$ and $p = 0.63$) and that the variant allele (Tt+tt) of the TaqI polymorphism and the FF genotype of the FokI variant were associated with a better response to vitamin D supplementation ($p = 0.02$ and $p < 0.001$). In conclusion, the TaqI and FokI polymorphisms could play a role in the modulation of the response to vitamin D supplementation, as they are associated with a better response to supplementation.

Keywords: vitamin D receptor; VDR; vitamin D; polymorphisms; TaqI; FokI; vitamin D supplementation

1. Introduction

The vitamin D receptor (VDR), a member of the nuclear receptor superfamily of transcriptional regulators, plays a crucial role in calcitriol or 1-alfa,25-dihidroxicolecalciferol (1α,25(OH)2D) signalling. VDR is activated by binding with 1α,25(OH)2D, which forms a heterodimer with the retinoid X receptor (RXR). The 1α,25(OH)2D-VDR-RXR complex migrates to the nucleus to regulate the transcription of genes involved in vitamin D effects including phosphorous and calcium metabolism, cell proliferation and the control of innate and adaptive immunity [1–3].

The *VDR* gene is located on chromosome 12 (12q13.11) and more than 900 allelic variants in the *VDR* locus have been reported. The best studied *VDR* gene polymorphisms are ApaI (rs7975232), BsmI (rs1544410), TaqI (rs731236) and FokI (rs10735810). ApaI, TaqI and BsmI are silent genetic variants that increase mRNA stability. The FokI polymorphism is located on exon 2 and results in a protein shortened by three amino acids [4–6]. These genetic variants have been associated with a predisposition to chronic diseases such as type 2 diabetes, cancer, autoimmune diseases, cardiovascular alterations, rheumatic arthritis and metabolic bone diseases [7–10].

VDR regulation is determined by genetic and environmental factors [11]. The principal environmental factors associated with VDR regulation are diet, exposure to sunlight, infections and pollution [12–15]. It has been postulated that these environmental factors could modify vitamin D levels which regulate the receptor. The mechanism is not clearly understood but it is hypothesised that it may be through epigenetic mechanisms [16]. Other factors involved in VDR regulation are the intake of the vitamin D precursor and the production and activity of the ligand. Genetic factors could modulate the influence of environmental factors on VDR regulation [11]. In this scenario, it has been reported that the response to vitamin D supplementation differs widely between individuals and one hypothesis is that genetic variants in the *VDR* gene are important in the response to vitamin D supplementation. The polymorphisms in the *VDR* gene could modify the VDR activity and therefore could be the explanation for the different response to vitamin D supplementation [4–6,17]. Various authors have examined how genetic variants in the *VDR* gene are associated with the response to vitamin D supplementation, and the many genetic association studies show contradictory results [18–21]. Therefore, our objective was to conduct a systematic review and meta-analysis to evaluate the response to vitamin D supplementation according to the BsmI, TaqI, ApaI and FokI polymorphisms in the *VDR* gene.

2. Material and Methods

2.1. Inclusion Criteria and Search Strategy

To analyse the influence of *VDR* genetic variants on the response to vitamin D supplementation, studies including serum vitamin D levels before and after supplementation according to the genetic distribution of the BsmI, TaqI, ApaI and FokI *VDR* polymorphisms were considered eligible for inclusion.

This systematic review and meta-analysis were performed in accordance with the PRISMA guidelines [22] (Supplementary Material Table S1). We included studies evaluating the response to vitamin D supplementation according to genetic variants in the *VDR* gene. To identify eligible studies, we conducted a computer-based search in the PubMed, Web of Science, Scopus and Embase electronic databases up to November 2021. Potentially relevant articles were searched for using the following terms in combination with Medical Subject Headings (MeSH) terms and text words: "Vitamin D receptor", "VDR", "BsmI", "TaqI", "ApaI", "FokI", "polymorphism", "mutations", "variants", "cholecalciferol", "vitamin D", "supplementation" and "vitamin D supplementation". No language restrictions were applied. The references of selected articles were scanned to identify additional relevant articles. The MedLine option "related articles" and review articles on the topic were also used to supplement the search.

2.2. Data Extraction

Bibliographic research and data extraction were conducted independently by three investigators (RUM, DDLR and JMFG). Differences were resolved by consensus with the senior author (JLPC). We extracted the authors names, the publication year, demographic information (age and sex), the follow-up time after vitamin D supplementation and serum vitamin D levels before and after supplementation according to the *VDR* gene polymorphisms.

2.3. Statistical Analysis

Independent meta-analyses were carried out to compare baseline and post-supplementation serum vitamin D levels according to the genetic distribution of the *VDR* polymorphisms included. Sub-analyses by age and sex were also carried out. Meta-analysis was only carried out when ≥3 studies were available. We analysed all polymorphisms under a dominant model for the minor alleles.

As previously described [23–25], meta-analyses were carried out using RevMan 5.0 software [26]. The difference between baseline and post-supplementation status and their 95% confidence interval (CI) were estimated for each study. Random-effects model was used to calculate the p-values (DerSimonian and Laird method). A p-value < 0.05 was considered statistically significant. To analyse the heterogeneity of the studies we applied Cochran's Q-statistic (p < 0.10 indicated heterogeneity across studies). Inconsistency in the meta-analysis was estimated using the I^2 statistic and this represented the percentage of the observed between-study variability due to heterogeneity. The following cut-off points were applied: (I^2 = 0–25%, no heterogeneity; I^2 = 25–50%, moderate heterogeneity; I^2 = 50–75%, large heterogeneity; I^2 = 75–100%, extreme heterogeneity). To assess publication bias, Begger's funnel plot was examined based on visual inspection. Asymmetry suggested publication bias. Finally, sensitivity analyses to examine the effect of excluding individual studies were carried out.

3. Results

3.1. Identification and Selection of Relevant Studies

Figure 1 shows the flow chart of the studies selected for inclusion in the meta-analysis. We initially identified 215 candidate articles for inclusion. After removing duplicates, the abstracts of 131 articles were reviewed and 103 were excluded. Thus, a total of 28 full text studies were assessed for eligibility. Of these, 20 articles were excluded because they did not contain the necessary information to carry out the meta-analysis (Supplementary Material Table S2). Therefore, eight studies that fulfilled the inclusion criteria were finally included in the meta-analysis [20,27–33]. The response to vitamin D supplementation according to the BsmI polymorphism in the *VDR* gene was analysed in six studies [20,27–30,32]. Five studies analysed the vitamin D response according to the genotypic distribution of the TaqI genetic variant [27–30,32]. The influence of the ApaI polymorphism was studied in four articles [27,29,30,32]. Finally, the influence of the FokI polymorphism in the response to vitamin D supplementation was analysed in five studies [27,29–31,33].

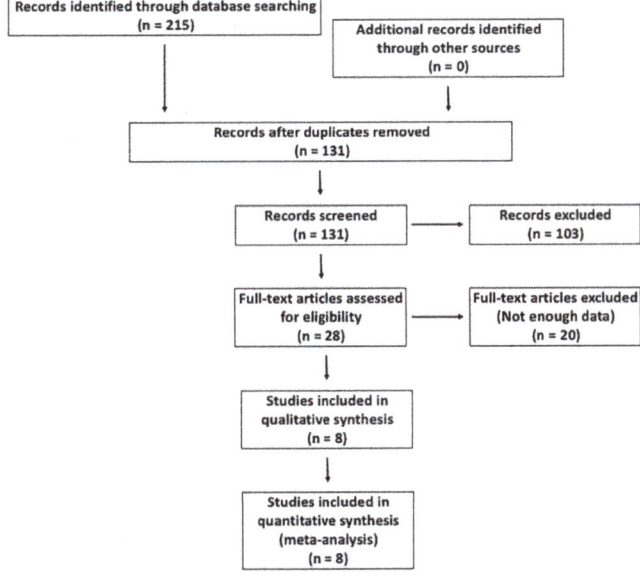

Figure 1. Flow chart of the studies selected for inclusion in the meta-analysis.

3.2. Study Characteristics

The studies included in the meta-analysis enrolled 1038 subjects. Detailed demographic characteristics are shown in Table 1. The mean age of the subjects included was 36.1 (10.2) years with a range of 10 to 78 years. Two studies included subjects aged <18 years [28,33] and one study only specified that subjects were aged >18 years [27]. There was a higher prevalence of women than men (77.8% vs. 8.6%). One article did not report the sex of the subjects [31]. The mean follow-up time after vitamin D supplementation was 7.4 (4.9) months. Baseline and post-supplementation serum vitamin D levels according to the BsmI, TaqI, ApaI and FokI polymorphisms in the *VDR* gene are summarized in Table 2. In the case of BsmI polymorphism, two studies associated the variant genotype with better response to vitamin D supplementation [27,30], two studies with worse response [20,32] and two studies did not show statistically significant association [28,29]. Five studies statistically associated the variant genotype of TaqI polymorphism with response to vitamin D supplementation [27–30,32]. Two studies associated the genotypic distribution of ApaI polymorphism with the response to supplementation [29,32]. For the FokI polymorphism, four articles showed association with response to vitamin D supplementation [27,30,31,33]. All studies used genomic DNA extracted from nucleated peripheral blood cells, and genotyping was performed using polymerase chain reaction-restriction fragment length polymorphism (PCR-RFLP).

Table 1. Characteristics of the studies included in the meta-analysis.

Authors, Year	N	Age [Years (SD)]	Gender [n (%)] Women	Gender [n (%)] Men	Country	Vitamin D Dose	Follow-Up Time
Graafmans et al., 1997	81	78 (5)	81 (100%)	0 (0%)	Netherlands	400 IU/24 h	12 months
Arabi et al., 2009	167	10 to 17	167 (100%)	0 (0%)	Lebanon	1100 IU/24 h	12 months
Neyestani et al., 2013	140	29 to 67	-	-	Iran	1000 IU/24 h	3 months
Sanwalka et al., 2015	102	11.2 (0.5)	102 (100%)	0 (0%)	India	333 IU/24 h	12 months
Al-Daghri et al., 2017	199	>18	114 (57.2%)	90 (42.8%)	Saudi Arabia	2000 IU/24 h	12 months
Mohseni et al., 2018	26	47.7 (8.0)	26 (100%)	0 (0%)	Iran	7000 IU/24 h	2 months
Pérez-Alonso et al., 2019	142	55 (4)	142 (100%)	0 (0%)	Spain	800 IU/24 h	3 months
Kazemian et al., 2020	176	48.6 (8.7)	176 (100%)	0 (0%)	Iran	4000 IU/24 h	3 months

SD: standard deviation, IU: international units.

3.3. Meta-Analysis of the Association between Gene Variants in the VDR Gene and the Response to Vitamin D Supplementation

The results of the meta-analysis are shown in Figure 2. The results showed that the BsmI genetic variant was not significantly associated with the response to vitamin D supplementation ($p = 0.81$, Figure 2A). In the case of the TaqI polymorphism, the variant allele (Tt+tt genotype) was significantly associated with a better response to vitamin D supplementation ($p = 0.02$, Figure 2B). There was no significant association between the ApaI variant and the response to vitamin D supplementation ($p = 0.63$, Figure 2C). Finally, subjects carrying the FF genotype of the FokI polymorphism in the *VDR* gene responded better to vitamin D supplementation than subjects with the variant allele (Ff+ff) ($p < 0.001$, Figure 2D).

When a meta-analysis includes fewer than 10 articles, the power of the test for funnel plot asymmetry is too low to distinguish the probability of real asymmetry [34]. Even so, we examined publication bias by visual inspection using Begger's funnel plot (Supplementary Material Figure S1) and it appeared to be symmetrical, although there was some uncertainty regarding the degree of symmetry.

The results were not modified by excluding articles that included only subjects aged <18 years or only analysing articles including females. Sub-analyses on the basis of ethnicity could not be carried out because the selected articles did not include this information. After sensitivity analysis, the exclusion of individual studies did not alter the results.

Table 2. Baseline and post-supplementation vitamin D levels according to the BsmI, TaqI, ApaI and FokI polymorphisms in the vitamin D receptor (*VDR*) gene.

Authors, Year	Vitamin D Levels BEFORE Supplementation, ng/mL [Mean (SD)]								Vitamin D Levels AFTER Supplementation, ng/mL [Mean (SD)]							
	rs1544410 (BsmI)		rs731236 (TaqI)		rs7975232 (ApaI)		rs10735810 (FokI)		rs1544410 (BsmI)		rs731236 (TaqI)		rs7975232 (ApaI)		rs10735810 (FokI)	
	BB	Bd+dd	TT	Tt+tt	AA	Aa+aa	FF	Ff+ff	BB	Bd+dd	TT	Tt+tt	AA	Aa+aa	FF	Ff+ff
Graafmans et al., 1997	26 (7.5)	29.2 (8.5)	-	-	-	-	-	-	30.1 (10.1)	25.75 (14.8)	-	-	-	-	-	-
Arabi et al., 2009	14.3 (9.4)	14.25 (7.9)	14.0 (8.5)	13.9 (7.7)	-	-	-	-	27.64 (14.5)	26.11 (12.3)	23.39 (15.6)	29.64 (15.5)	-	-	-	-
Neyestani et al., 2013	-	-	-	-	-	-	38.1 (21.5)	37.9 (16.7)	-	-	-	-	-	-	73.6 (25)	65 (24.3)
Sanwalka et al., 2015	-	-	-	-	-	-	27.77 (3.1)	22.8 (2.04)	-	-	-	-	-	-	61.72 (6.2)	47.02 (8.9)
Al-Daghri et al., 2017	31.1 (14)	34 (11.1)	31.9 (12.7)	33.8 (11.6)	35.1 (9.5)	33.3 (12.4)	33 (12.4)	34.8 (11.1)	50.1 (14.7)	55.6 (17.3)	51.2 (13.6)	55.4 (17.8)	56.2 (13.3)	54 (18.2)	57.4 (17.3)	47.9 (13.8)
Mohseni et al., 2018	9.0 (1.4)	12.75 (1.4)	16.5 (4.6)	12.2 (1.5)	13.6 (1.3)	13.6 (2.7)	13.0 (1.0)	11.2 (1.4)	11.0 (1.4)	16.7 (4.3)	11.5 (1.2)	14.6 (1.5)	14.8 (3.2)	14.6 (3.1)	28.0 (12)	15.3 (3.1)
Pérez-Alonso et al., 2019	21 (10)	24.5 (9)	25 (9)	23 (9.5)	23 (10)	24 (9)	-	-	28 (9)	30.5 (10)	31 (8)	30 (9)	29 (9.5)	31.1 (9.5)	-	-
Kazemian et al., 2020	30.2 (11.4)	41.7 (16.9)	31.8 (10.4)	37.4 (11.3)	40.9 (14.2)	31.35 (11.4)	34.4 (12.4)	30.8 (9.4)	99.3 (34)	131.2 (29)	105.3 (31.5)	118.9 (29.4)	111 (21.4)	98.3 (23)	114.9 (34)	107.8 (23)

SD: standard deviation.

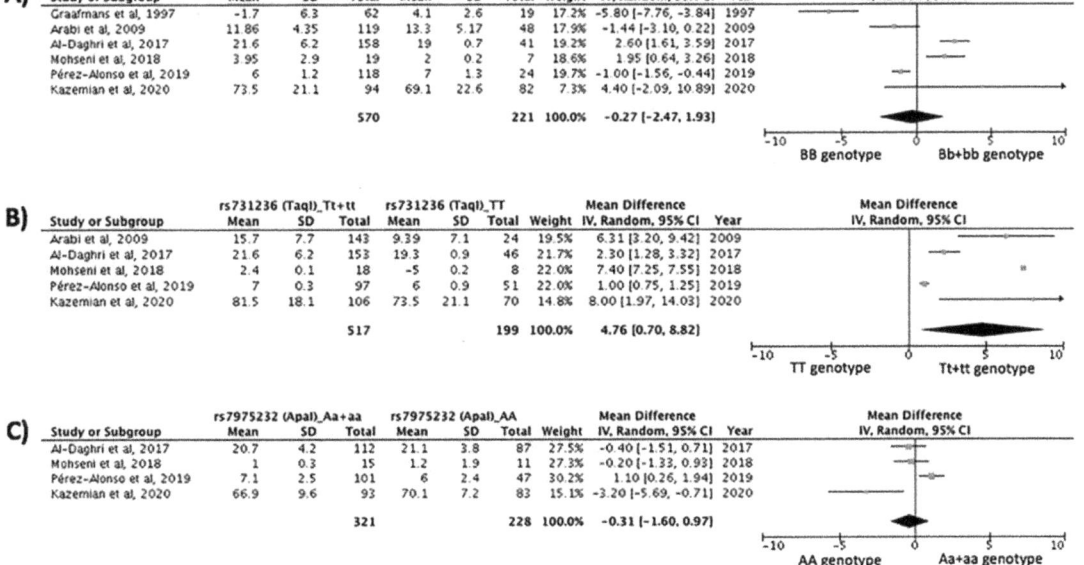

Figure 2. *Cont.*

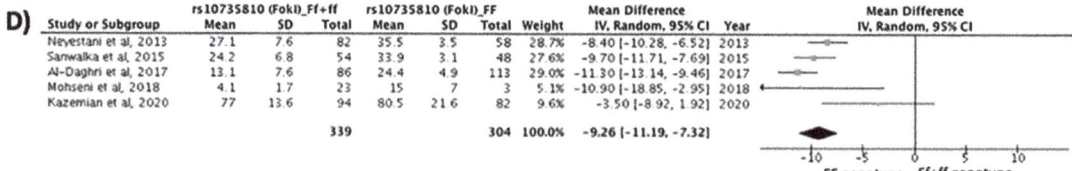

Figure 2. Meta-analysis of the association between gene variants in the vitamin D receptor *(VDR)* gene and the response to vitamin D supplementation. (**A**) Association between the BsmI polymorphism and the response to vitamin D supplementation. Test for overall effect: $Z = 0.24$ ($p = 0.81$). Test for heterogeneity: $\chi 2 = 6.31$ ($p < 0.001$), $I2 = 9.4\%$. (**B**) Association between the TaqI polymorphism and the response to vitamin D supplementation. Test for overall effect: $Z = 2.30$ ($p = 0.02$). Test for heterogeneity: $\chi 2 = 19.47$ ($p < 0.001$), $I2 = 10\%$. (**C**) Association between the ApaI polymorphism and the response to vitamin D supplementation. Test for overall effect: $Z = 0.48$ ($p = 0.63$). Test for heterogeneity: $\chi 2 = 1.24$ ($p = 0.004$), $I2 = 7.7\%$. (**D**) Association between the FokI polymorphism and the response to vitamin D supplementation. Test for overall effect: $Z = 9.39$ ($p < 0.001$). Test for heterogeneity: $\chi 2 = 2.47$ ($p = 0.04$), $I2 = 5.9\%$.

4. Discussion

The relationship between genetic variants in the *VDR* gene and the response to vitamin D supplementation remains unclear. Thus, we carried out a systematic review and meta-analysis to evaluate the response to supplementation according to the genotype distribution of the BsmI, TaqI, ApaI and FokI polymorphisms in the *VDR* gene. The results showed that the variant allele of the TaqI polymorphism and the FF genotype of the FokI variant were associated with a better response to vitamin D supplementation. The BsmI and ApaI polymorphisms were not associated with the response to vitamin D supplementation.

Calcitriol signalling is crucial in bone metabolism as it is involved in calcium absorption, parathormone secretion and, therefore, bone resorption and cellular differentiation. Vitamin D deficiency has been associated with bone metabolism alterations [35–37]. Therefore, vitamin D intake as a preventive nutritional treatment of osteoporosis plays an important role in improving health status [38,39], but the efficacy of supplementation varies widely between subjects [18–20]. One explanatory hypothesis is that genetic variants in *VDR* could modulate the response to vitamin D supplementation. Our results showed that carrying the variant allele of the TaqI polymorphism was associated with a better response to vitamin D supplementation. TaqI is a silent polymorphism located in the 3′ *VDR* gene region and has been associated with an increase in mRNA stability [4–6]. A previous meta-analysis associated the TaqI genetic variant with the risk of bone fracture [10]. This may be in line with our results, as the TaqI polymorphism may modify the response to vitamin D supplementation and thus could modify the risk of bone fracture. However, other factors besides vitamin D levels are involved in the susceptibility to bone fracture [40]. Our meta-analysis also associated the FF genotype of the FokI polymorphism with a better response to vitamin D supplementation. The FokI polymorphism is located on exon 2 and the F allele has been associated with the translation of a more active protein [17]. The greater activity of VDR could be associated with a better response to vitamin D supplementation. In addition, the F allele of the FokI genetic variant has also been associated with better calcium absorption, higher bone mineral density and a reduced risk of vertebral bone fractures [41–44]. Therefore, it seems clear that the F allele of the FokI polymorphism is associated with greater VDR activity, improving the response to vitamin D and calcium supplementation and being associated with the risk of bone fracture. Finally, we also performed sub analysis by age and sex due to it having been reported that vitamin D metabolism is affected by these factors [45,46]. Our results were not modified when analysing according to age and gender. In this sense, we hypothesise that differences in vitamin D absorption caused by sex and age are probably more notable in subjects with the same genotype, and as our sample is very heterogeneous we do not observe differences.

This study had some limitations. Firstly, a general limitation of meta-analyses of genetic association studies—contradictory results and heterogeneity in the studies included—is quite common and reflects the true genetic heterogeneity of the different samples or hidden stratification of the population. Only a small number of studies were eligible for inclusion in our study and there was a lack of information in some, so they could not be included in the meta-analysis. Furthermore, several of the studies had low sample sizes with wide variations. Finally, the exposure to sunlight is one of the environmental factors which is crucial in VDR regulation [11]. Thus, it could have been interesting to analyse the results obtained as a function of sunlight exposure, but this could not be done because only one included paper reported this information [32]. Even with these limitations, this meta-analysis contributes significantly to our understanding the crucial role of *VDR* gene polymorphisms in the modulation of the vitamin D supplementation response.

5. Conclusions

In conclusion, this meta-analysis advances our current understating of how *VDR* gene polymorphisms influence the response to vitamin D supplementation, providing moderate evidence that the variant allele of the TaqI polymorphism and the FF genotype of the FokI genetic variant were associated with a better response to vitamin D supplementation. Further research with a homogeneous design should be carried out to improve understanding of the role of *VDR* gene polymorphisms in the modulation of the response to vitamin D supplementation, and its possible clinical value.

Supplementary Materials: The following supporting information can be downloaded at: https://www.mdpi.com/article/10.3390/nu14020360/s1, Figure S1: Funnel plot of studies included in the meta-analysis assessing the association of genetic variants in the vitamin D receptor (VDR) gene and the response to vitamin D supplementation. (A) BsmI polymorphism. (B) TaqI polymorphism. (C) ApaI polymorphism. (D) FokI polymorphism; Table S1: PRISMA checklist; Table S2: Reasons for exclusion the articles not included in the meta-analysis.

Author Contributions: Conceptualization: J.-L.P.-C.; methodology: R.U.-M., D.-A.D.L.-R., J.M.F.-G., M.R.-M. and J.-L.P.-C.; formal analysis: R.U.-M.; investigation: R.U.-M., D.-A.D.L.-R., J.M.F.-G., M.R.-M. and J.-L.P.-C.; data curation: R.U.-M., D.-A.D.L.-R., J.M.F.-G. and J.-L.P.-C.; writing—original draft preparation: R.U.-M.; writing—review and editing: R.U.-M., D.-A.D.L.-R., J.M.F.-G., M.R.-M. and J.-L.P.-C.; supervision: J.-L.P.-C. All authors have read and agreed to the published version of the manuscript.

Funding: This research received no external funding.

Institutional Review Board Statement: Not applicable.

Informed Consent Statement: Not applicable.

Data Availability Statement: All data and results are available in this manuscript.

Acknowledgments: The authors thank the participants and researchers of the primary studies identified for this meta-analysis.

Conflicts of Interest: The authors declare no conflict of interest.

References

1. Long, M.D.; Sucheston-Campbell, L.E.; Campbell, M.J.; Vitamin, D. receptor and RXR in the post-genomic era. *J. Cell Physiol.* **2015**, *230*, 758–766. [CrossRef]
2. Haussler, M.R.; Whitfield, G.K.; Kaneko, I.; Haussler, C.A.; Hsieh, D.; Hsieh, J.-C.; Jurutka, P.W. Molecular Mechanisms of Vitamin D Action. *Calcif. Tissue Int.* **2013**, *92*, 77–98. [CrossRef]
3. Reschly, E.J.; Krasowski, M.D. Evolution and function of the NR1I nuclear hormone receptor subfamily (VDR, PXR, and CAR) with respect to metabolism of xenobiotics and endogenous compounds. *Curr. Drug Metab.* **2006**, *7*, 349–365. [CrossRef]
4. Uitterlinden, A.G.; Fang, Y.; Van Meurs, J.B.J.; Pols, H.A.P.; Van Leeuwen, J.P.T.M. Genetics and biology of vitamin D receptor polymorphisms. *Gene* **2004**, *338*, 143–156. [CrossRef] [PubMed]

5. Whitfield, G.K.; Remus, L.S.; Jurutka, P.W.; Zitzer, H.; Oza, A.K.; Dang, H.T.L.; Haussler, C.A.; Galligan, M.A.; Thatcher, M.L.; Dominguez, C.E.; et al. Functionally relevant polymorphisms in the human nuclear vitamin D receptor gene. *Mol. Cell. Endocrinol.* **2001**, *177*, 145–159. [CrossRef]
6. Barger-Lux, M.J.; Heaney, R.P.; Hayes, J.; DeLuca, H.F.; Johnson, M.L.; Gong, G. Vitamin D receptor gene polymorphism, bone mass, body size, and vitamin D receptor density. *Calcif. Tissue Int.* **1995**, *57*, 161–162. [CrossRef]
7. Li, L.; Wu, B.; Liu, J.-Y.; Yang, L.-B. Vitamin D receptor gene polymorphisms and type 2 diabetes: A meta-analysis. *Arch. Med. Res.* **2013**, *44*, 235–241. [CrossRef] [PubMed]
8. Lee, Y.H.; Bae, S.-C.; Choi, S.J.; Ji, J.D.; Song, G.G. Associations between vitamin D receptor polymorphisms and susceptibility to rheumatoid arthritis and systemic lupus erythematosus: A meta-analysis. *Mol. Biol. Rep.* **2011**, *38*, 3643–3651. [CrossRef]
9. Ortlepp, J.R.; Krantz, C.; Kimmel, M.; Von Korff, A.; Vesper, K.; Schmitz, F.; Mevissen, V.; Janssens, U.; Franke, A.; Hanrath, P. Additive effects of the chemokine receptor 2, vitamin D receptor, interleukin-6 polymorphisms and cardiovascular risk factors on the prevalence of myocardial infarction in patients below 65 years. *Int. J. Cardiol.* **2005**, *105*, 90–95. [CrossRef] [PubMed]
10. Ji, G.-R.; Yao, M.; Sun, C.-Y.; Li, Z.-H.; Han, Z. BsmI, TaqI, ApaI and FokI polymorphisms in the vitamin D receptor (VDR) gene and risk of fracture in Caucasians: A meta-analysis. *Bone* **2010**, *47*, 681–686. [CrossRef]
11. Saccone, D.; Asani, F.; Bornman, L. Regulation of the vitamin D receptor gene by environment, genetics and epigenetics. *Gene* **2015**, *561*, 171–180. [CrossRef] [PubMed]
12. Lamberg-Allardt, C. Vitamin D in foods and as supplements. *Prog. Biophys. Mol. Biol.* **2006**, *92*, 33–38. [CrossRef]
13. Holick, M.F. Vitamin D: A millenium perspective. *J. Cell. Biochem.* **2003**, *88*, 296–307. [CrossRef]
14. Agarwal, K.S.; Mughal, M.Z.; Upadhyay, P.; Berry, J.L.; Mawer, E.B.; Puliyel, J.M. The impact of atmospheric pollution on vitamin D status of infants and toddlers in Delhi, India. *Arch. Dis. Child.* **2002**, *87*, 111–113. [CrossRef] [PubMed]
15. Liu, P.T.; Stenger, S.; Li, H.; Wenzel, L.; Tan, B.H.; Krutzik, S.R.; Ochoa, M.T.; Schauber, J.; Wu, K.; Meinken, C. Toll-like receptor triggering of a vitamin D-mediated human antimicrobial response. *Science* **2006**, *311*, 1770–1773. [CrossRef]
16. Fetahu, I.S.; Höbaus, J.; Kállay, E. Vitamin D and the epigenome. *Front. Physiol.* **2014**, *5*, 164. [CrossRef] [PubMed]
17. Arai, H.; Miyamoto, K.; Taketani, Y.; Yamamoto, H.; Iemori, Y.; Morita, K.; Tonai, T.; Nishisho, T.; Mori, S.; Takeda, E. A vitamin D receptor gene polymorphism in the translation initiation codon: Effect on protein activity and relation to bone mineral density in Japanese women. *J. Bone Miner. Res.* **1997**, *12*, 915–921. [CrossRef]
18. Barry, E.L.; Rees, J.R.; Peacock, J.L.; Mott, L.A.; Amos, C.I.; Bostick, R.M.; Figueiredo, J.C.; Ahnen, D.J.; Bresalier, R.S.; Burke, C.A.; et al. Genetic variants in CYP2R1, CYP24A1, and VDR modify the efficacy of vitamin D3 supplementation for increasing serum 25-hydroxyvitamin D levels in a randomized controlled trial. *J. Clin. Endocrinol. Metab.* **2014**, *99*, E2133–E2137. [CrossRef]
19. Elnenaei, M.O.; Chandra, R.; Mangion, T.; Moniz, C. Genomic and metabolomic patterns segregate with responses to calcium and vitamin D supplementation. *Br. J. Nutr.* **2011**, *105*, 71–79. [CrossRef]
20. Graafmans, W.C.; Lips, P.; Ooms, M.E.; Van Leeuwen, J.P.; Pols, H.A.; Uitterlinden, A.G. The effect of vitamin D supplementation on the bone mineral density of the femoral neck is associated with vitamin D receptor genotype. *J. Bone Miner. Res.* **1997**, *12*, 1241–1245. [CrossRef]
21. Serrano, J.C.E.; De Lorenzo, D.; Cassanye, A.; Martín-Gari, M.; Espinel, A.; Delgado, M.A.; Pamplona, R.; Portero-Otin, M. Vitamin D receptor BsmI polymorphism modulates soy intake and 25-hydroxyvitamin D supplementation benefits in cardiovascular disease risk factors profile. *Genes Nutr.* **2013**, *8*, 561–569. [CrossRef] [PubMed]
22. Moher, D.; Liberati, A.; Tetzlaff, J.; Altman, D.G.; Group, T.P. Preferred Reporting Items for Systematic Reviews and Meta-Analyses: The PRISMA Statement. *PLoS Med.* **2009**, *6*, e1000097. [CrossRef] [PubMed]
23. Usategui-Martín, R.; Carbonell, C.; Novo-Veleiro, I.; Hernández-Pinchete, S.; Mirón-Canelo, J.A.; Chamorro, A.-J.; Marcos, M. Association between genetic variants in CYP2E1 and CTRC genes and susceptibility to alcoholic pancreatitis: A systematic review and meta-analysis. *Drug Alcohol Depend.* **2020**, *209*, 107873. [CrossRef] [PubMed]
24. Usategui-Martín, R.; Pastor-Idoate, S.; Chamorro, A.J.; Fernández, I.; Fernández-Bueno, I.; Marcos-Martín, M.; González-Sarmiento, R.; Carlos Pastor, J. Meta-analysis of the rs243865 MMP-2 polymorphism and age-related macular degeneration risk. *PLoS ONE* **2019**, *14*, e0213624. [CrossRef] [PubMed]
25. Valentín-Bravo, F.J.; García-Onrubia, L.; Andrés-Iglesias, C.; Valentín-Bravo, E.; Martín-Vallejo, J.; Pastor, J.C.; Usategui-Martín, R.; Pastor-Idoate, S. Complications associated with the use of silicone oil in vitreoretinal surgery: A systemic review and meta-analysis. *Acta Ophthalmol.* 2021. [CrossRef]
26. *Review Manager (RevMan) [Computer Program]*; Version 5.3; The Nordic Cochrane Centre, The Cochrane Collaboration: Copenhagen, UK, 2014.
27. Al-Daghri, N.M.; Mohammed, A.K.; Al-Attas, O.S.; Ansari, M.G.A.; Wani, K.; Hussain, S.D.; Sabico, S.; Tripathi, G.; Alokail, M.S. Vitamin D Receptor Gene Polymorphisms Modify Cardiometabolic Response to Vitamin D Supplementation in T2DM Patients. *Sci Rep.* **2017**, *7*, 8280. [CrossRef]
28. Arabi, A.; Zahed, L.; Mahfoud, Z.; El-Onsi, L.; Nabulsi, M.; Maalouf, J.; Fuleihan, G.E.-H. Vitamin D receptor gene polymorphisms modulate the skeletal response to vitamin D supplementation in healthy girls. *Bone* **2009**, *45*, 1091–1097. [CrossRef] [PubMed]
29. Kazemian, E.; Akbari, M.E.; Moradi, N.; Gharibzadeh, S.; Amouzegar, A.; Jamshidi-Naeini, Y.; Mondul, A.M.; Khademolmele, M.; Ghodoosi, N.; Zarins, K.R.; et al. Effect of vitamin D receptor polymorphisms on plasma oxidative stress and apoptotic biomarkers among breast cancer survivors supplemented vitamin D3. *Eur. J. Cancer Prev.* **2020**, *29*, 433–444. [CrossRef]

30. Mohseni, H.; Amani, R.; Hosseini, S.A.; Ekrami, A.; Ahmadzadeh, A.; Latifi, S.M. Genetic Variations in VDR could Modulate the Efficacy of Vitamin D3 Supplementation on Inflammatory Markers and Total Antioxidant Capacity among Breast Cancer Women: A Randomized Double Blind Controlled Trial. *Asian Pac. J. Cancer Prev.* **2019**, *20*, 2065–2072. [CrossRef] [PubMed]
31. Neyestani, T.R.; Djazayery, A.; Shab-Bidar, S.; Eshraghian, M.R.; Kalayi, A.; Shariátzadeh, N.; Khalaji, N.; Zahedirad, M.; Gharavi, A.; Houshiarrad, A.; et al. Vitamin D Receptor Fok-I polymorphism modulates diabetic host response to vitamin D intake: Need for a nutrigenetic approach. *Diabetes Care.* **2013**, *36*, 550–556. [CrossRef]
32. Pérez-Alonso, M.; Briongos, L.-S.; Ruiz-Mambrilla, M.; Velasco, E.A.; Olmos, J.M.; De Luis, D.; Dueñas-Laita, A.; Pérez-Castrillón, J.-L. Association Between Bat Vitamin D Receptor 3′ Haplotypes and Vitamin D Levels at Baseline and a Lower Response After Increased Vitamin D Supplementation and Exposure to Sunlight. *Int. J. Vitam. Nutr. Res.* **2020**, *90*, 290–294. [CrossRef]
33. Sanwalka, N.; Khadilkar, A.; Chiplonkar, S.; Khatod, K.; Phadke, N.; Khadilkar, V. Influence of Vitamin D Receptor Gene Fok1 Polymorphism on Bone Mass Accrual Post Calcium and Vitamin D Supplementation. *Indian J. Pediatr.* **2015**, *82*, 985–990. [CrossRef]
34. Cochrane Handbook for Systematic Reviews of Interventions. Available online: http://handbook-5-1.cochrane.org (accessed on 21 November 2021).
35. De Martinis, M.; Allegra, A.; Sirufo, M.M.; Tonacci, A.; Pioggia, G.; Raggiunti, M.; Ginaldi, L.; Gangemi, S. Vitamin D Deficiency, Osteoporosis and Effect on Autoimmune Diseases and Hematopoiesis: A Review. *Int. J. Mol. Sci.* **2021**, *22*, 8855. [CrossRef] [PubMed]
36. Priemel, M.; Von Domarus, C.; Klatte, T.O.; Kessler, S.; Schlie, J.; Meier, S.; Proksch, N.; Pastor, F.; Netter, C.; Streichert, T.; et al. Bone mineralization defects and vitamin D deficiency: Histomorphometric analysis of iliac crest bone biopsies and circulating 25-hydroxyvitamin D in 675 patients. *J. Bone Miner. Res.* **2010**, *25*, 305–312. [CrossRef] [PubMed]
37. Binkley, N. Does Low Vitamin D Status Contribute to "Age-Related" Morbidity? *J. Bone Miner. Res.* **2007**, *22*, V55–V58. [CrossRef]
38. Tang, B.M.P.; Eslick, G.D.; Nowson, C.; Smith, C.; Bensoussan, A. Use of calcium or calcium in combination with vitamin D supplementation to prevent fractures and bone loss in people aged 50 years and older: A meta-analysis. *Lancet* **2007**, *370*, 657–666. [CrossRef]
39. Chevalley, T.; Rizzoli, R.; Nydegger, V.; Slosman, D.; Rapin, C.H.; Michel, J.P.; Vasey, H.; Bonjour, J.-P. Effects of calcium supplements on femoral bone mineral density and vertebral fracture rate in vitamin-D-replete elderly patients. *Osteoporos. Int.* **1994**, *4*, 245–252. [CrossRef]
40. Boonen, S.; Lips, P.; Bouillon, R.; Bischoff-Ferrari, H.A.; Vanderschueren, D.; Haentjens, P. Need for additional calcium to reduce the risk of hip fracture with vitamin d supplementation: Evidence from a comparative metaanalysis of randomized controlled trials. *J. Clin. Endocrinol. Metab.* **2007**, *92*, 1415–1423. [CrossRef]
41. Moradi, S.; Khorrami-Nezhad, L.; Maghbooli, Z.; Hosseini, B.; Keshavarz, S.A.; Mirzaei, K. Vitamin D Receptor Gene Variation, Dietary Intake and Bone Mineral Density in Obese Women: A Cross Sectional Study. *J. Nutr. Sci. Vitaminol.* **2017**, *63*, 228–236. [CrossRef]
42. Abrams, S.A.; Griffin, I.J.; Hawthorne, K.M.; Chen, Z.; Gunn, S.K.; Wilde, M.; Darlington, G.; Shypailo, R.J.; Ellis, K.J. Vitamin D receptor Fok1 polymorphisms affect calcium absorption, kinetics, and bone mineralization rates during puberty. *J. Bone Miner. Res.* **2005**, *20*, 945–953. [CrossRef]
43. Ames, S.K.; Ellis, K.J.; Gunn, S.K.; Copeland, K.C.; Abrams, S.A. Vitamin D receptor gene Fok1 polymorphism predicts calcium absorption and bone mineral density in children. *J. Bone Miner. Res.* **1999**, *14*, 740–746. [CrossRef]
44. Moffett, S.P.; Zmuda, J.M.; Cauley, J.A.; Ensrud, K.; A Hillier, T.; Hochberg, M.C.; Li, J.; Cayabyab, S.; Lee, J.M.; Peltz, G.; et al. Association of the VDR Translation Start Site Polymorphism and Fracture Risk in Older Women. *J. Bone Miner. Res.* **2007**, *22*, 730–736. [CrossRef] [PubMed]
45. Gallagher, J.C. Vitamin D and Aging. *Endocrinol. Metab. Clin. N. Am.* **2013**, *42*, 319–332. [CrossRef] [PubMed]
46. Verdoia, M.; Schaffer, A.; Barbieri, L.; Di Giovine, G.; Marino, P.; Suryapranata, H.; De Luca, G. Impact of gender difference on vitamin D status and its relationship with the extent of coronary artery disease. *Nutr. Metab. Cardiovasc. Dis.* **2015**, *25*, 464–470. [CrossRef] [PubMed]

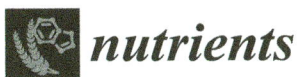

Article

Effects of Dietary Fat to Carbohydrate Ratio on Obesity Risk Depending on Genotypes of Circadian Genes

Jinyoung Shon [1], Yerim Han [1,2] and Yoon Jung Park [1,2,*]

1. Department of Nutritional Science and Food Management, Ewha Womans University, Seoul 03760, Korea; shon.jinyoung.layla@gmail.com (J.S.); hanyelim97@naver.com (Y.H.)
2. Graduate Program in System Health Science & Engineering, Ewha Womans University, Seoul 03760, Korea
* Correspondence: park.yoonjung@ewha.ac.kr; Tel.: +82-2-3277-6533

Abstract: Although the impacts of macronutrients and the circadian clock on obesity have been reported, the interactions between macronutrient distribution and circadian genes are unclear. The aim of this study was to explore macronutrient intake patterns in the Korean population and associations between the patterns and circadian gene variants and obesity. After applying the criteria, 5343 subjects (51.6% male, mean age 49.4 ± 7.3 years) from the Korean Genome and Epidemiology Study data and nine variants in seven circadian genes were analyzed. We defined macronutrient intake patterns by tertiles of the fat to carbohydrate ratio (FC). The very low FC (VLFC) was associated with a higher risk of obesity than the optimal FC (OFC). After stratification by the genotypes of nine variants, the obesity risk according to the patterns differed by the variants. In the female VLFC, the major homozygous allele of *CLOCK* rs11932595 and *CRY1* rs3741892 had a higher abdominal obesity risk than those in the OFC. The GG genotype of *PER2* rs2304672 in the VLFC showed greater risks for obesity and abdominal obesity. In conclusion, these findings suggest that macronutrient intake patterns were associated with obesity susceptibility, and the associations were different depending on the circadian clock genotypes of the *CLOCK*, *PER2*, and *CRY1* loci.

Keywords: macronutrient distribution; circadian gene; genetic variant; single nucleotide polymorphisms (SNPs); obesity

Citation: Shon, J.; Han, Y.; Park, Y.J. Effects of Dietary Fat to Carbohydrate Ratio on Obesity Risk Depending on Genotypes of Circadian Genes. *Nutrients* 2022, 14, 478. https://doi.org/10.3390/nu14030478

Academic Editors: Daniel-Antonio Luis Roman and Ana B. Crujeiras

Received: 30 December 2021
Accepted: 19 January 2022
Published: 22 January 2022

Publisher's Note: MDPI stays neutral with regard to jurisdictional claims in published maps and institutional affiliations.

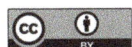

Copyright: © 2022 by the authors. Licensee MDPI, Basel, Switzerland. This article is an open access article distributed under the terms and conditions of the Creative Commons Attribution (CC BY) license (https://creativecommons.org/licenses/by/4.0/).

1. Introduction

The circadian clock governs 24 h rhythms and regulates the sleep–wake cycle. In mammals, circadian rhythms influence metabolism and physiological processes [1]. Furthermore, the circadian clock regulates glucose and fat metabolism and energy metabolism by coordinating the expression of clock-controlled genes [1,2]. The circadian core genes, including the circadian locomotor output cycle kaput (*CLOCK*), aryl hydrocarbon receptor nuclear translocator-like (*ARNTL*, also known as *BMAL1*), period homolog (*PER1*, *PER2*), and cryptochrome (*CRY1*, *CRY2*) regulate the circadian rhythm mechanism [1,3]. The ARNTL-CLOCK complex drives the transcription of *PER* and *CRY* genes by binding to enhancer elements. Increased proteins of PER and CRY inhibit ARNTL-CLOCK-mediated transcription. This transcription–translation negative feedback loop leads the circadian rhythm, which takes 24 h [3,4].

Multiple evidence from mouse models and human studies have reported a link between the risk of disease and clock genes [5–14]. Moreover, genetic variations of clock genes might play a role in metabolic disorders. Single nucleotide polymorphisms (SNPs) of *CLOCK* and *ARNTL* influence body weight control, the development of obesity, and susceptibility to metabolic diseases [12,13,15–20]. Additionally, the SNPs of circadian genes are associated with eating behavior and dietary intake, including carbohydrate, protein, and fat, and this association contributes to the modulation of physiological responses [21–25].

The master clock located in the hypothalamic suprachiasmatic nucleus can be regulated by the light–dark cycle [1,26,27], whereas peripheral clocks in peripheral tissues, such as the liver and heart, are entrained by other environmental factors [1,6,26]. Dietary nutrients are a crucial driver for oscillation of the peripheral circadian clock [28,29]. Several studies have reported an altered phase of the peripheral clock under time-restricted feeding conditions or high-fat diet feeding experiments [30–32]. Feeding mice with a high-fat diet induced reprogramming of the liver clock and changes in eating behavior [30,33,34]. Furthermore, substitution of a diet component with another component influenced phase shifts in the liver circadian clock [35]. The ketogenic diet, which comprises high-fat with low-carbohydrate and protein contents, affected the peripheral circadian clocks and drive tissue-specific oscillation of clock-controlled genes [36]. A low-carbohydrate and high-protein diet altered the expressions of circadian genes and key gluconeogenic regulatory genes, resulting in mild hypoglycemia [37]. These results indicate that dietary macronutrient composition is a strong factor for the regulation of peripheral clocks and clock-controlled genes involved in metabolic processes.

Dietary macronutrients are important to maintain health and physiological functions. In previous nutritional intervention studies, the results mainly focused on the effects of low-fat or low-carbohydrate diets on obesity-related features such as weight control [38–41]. However, most interventional diets that modify macronutrient distribution are based on an energy deficit or investigated over the short term, resulting in inconsistent metabolic outcomes. One of the most interesting studies carried out by Solon-Biet et al. investigated the effects of macronutritional challenges using a chronic ad libitum-fed mouse model [42]. Interestingly, a 'high-protein and low-carbohydrate diet' induced negative outcomes related to metabolic health and longevity. In contrast, a 'low-protein and high-carbohydrate diet' improved health and extended the lifespan. This suggests that results derived from dietary interventions are not consistent with actual responses under a long-term diet without calorie restriction. Moreover, given that the distributions of dietary macronutrients differ between populations, results from western-style intervention diets (e.g., low-protein and high-fat diet and low-carbohydrate diet) are hard to apply to Asian populations. Thus, the understanding of dietary macronutrient distribution must be considered in the context of population health improvement.

Several studies that investigated the effects of nutritional challenges on the circadian system reported that altered feeding cycles under an obesogenic diet were related to metabolic disorder [43,44]. Macronutrient intake and the timing of the caloric intake were related to the sleep cycle and influence of obesity risk [45,46]. Moreover, circadian clock gene SNPs and energy and fat intake were associated with metabolic health and obesity-related outcomes [23–25]. Collectively, these results suggest that dietary macronutrient intake and circadian genes contribute to susceptibility to metabolic diseases. However, the potential role of circadian gene SNPs and dietary macronutrient distribution was not investigated for its link to disease risk. Therefore, in this study, we defined Korean macronutrient intake patterns and analyzed the effects of an association between patterns and circadian clock gene variants and obesity risk.

2. Materials and Methods
2.1. Study Data and Subjects

This study used the Korean population data from the Korean Genome and Epidemiology Study (KoGES), provided by the Center for Genome Science, National Institute of Health, Korean Centers for Disease Control (KCDC) and Prevention, Chungcheongbuk-do, Korea [47]. A local community-based cohort was obtained from urban (Ansan) and rural (Ansung) regions, containing genomic, demographic, anthropometric, biochemical, clinical, and nutritional information. All participants provided written informed consent, and cohort data were surveyed every 2 years on a follow-up basis since 2001. We used the baseline examination dataset for this study. Among 10,038 subjects, 3253 were excluded due to missing data (Figure 1). Exclusion criteria (cancer, dementia, stroke, steroid drugs, insulin therapy, oral diabetes medication, thyroid drugs, and hormone replacement therapy) were applied for the elimination of effects derived from diseases and drugs on food intake. Finally, we investigated 5343 subjects aged 40~64 years, of which 2756 were male (mean age 48.9 ± 7.0 years), and 2587 were female (mean age 49.9 ± 7.6 years). The study was approved by the Institutional Review Board of Ewha Womans University, Seoul, Korea (IRB approval number: ewha-202105-0003-01).

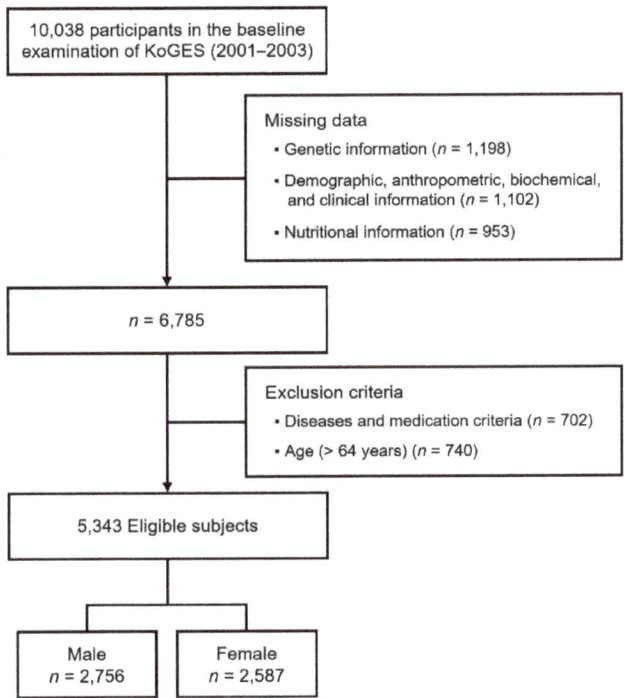

Figure 1. A flow chart of the study population.

2.2. Selection and Analysis of SNPs

Genomic DNA derived from blood samples was genotyped with the Affymetrix Genome-Wide Human SNP Array 5.0 kit (Affymetrix, Inc., Santa Clara, CA, USA) [48], and 1000 genome sequences were used for imputation [49]. After applying the Bayesian Robust Linear Modeling with Mahalanobis Distance (BRLMM) algorithm and standard quality control procedures, samples with a missing call rate >4%, heterozygosity >30%, gender incompatibility, or obtained from subjects who had cancer were excluded [50]. Among 352,228 SNPs, we selected 235 SNPs that were located in the loci of the circadian core genes *CLOCK*, *ARNTL*, *PER1*, *PER2*, *PER3*, *CRY1*, and *CRY2* (Figure 2). SNPs with a high missing genotype call rate (>5%), low minor allele frequency (MAF < 0.05), and low Hardy–Weinberg equilibrium (p value $< 1 \times 10^{-6}$) were excluded. We conducted linkage disequilibrium (LD)-based pruning ($r^2 > 0.2$); one SNP which had the highest MAF was selected from each LD block using PLINK software version 1.09 [51] and Haploview software version 4.1 (Broad Institute of MIT and Harvard, Cambridge, MA, USA) [52]. Utilizing the multitissue expression quantitative loci (eQTL) analysis from the Genotype Tissue Expression (GTEx) projects (release version 8) [53,54], we selected 9 SNPs related to circadian gene regulation (Tables 1 and A1, Figure 2). A recessive model was used for further investigation due to the small number of subjects of homozygous for the minor allele.

Table 1. The list of SNPs analyzed in this study.

Gene	SNP ID	Chromosome	Location	Alleles	MAF	HWE
CLOCK	rs11932595	4	55457430	A/G	0.1065	0.6955
	rs9312661	4	55476159	G/A	0.3604	0.2992
ARNTL	rs10766065	11	13256414	T/C	0.4983	0.9491
	rs9633835	11	13324046	A/G	0.4665	0.8643
PER2	rs2304672	2	238277948	G/C	0.0620	0.5825
CRY1	rs3741892	12	106993385	G/C	0.2321	0.4557
	rs11113192	12	107119148	G/C	0.2528	0.1215
	rs2541891	12	107184503	C/G	0.4131	0.3236
CRY2	rs7951225	11	45853841	A/T	0.3498	0.5747

MAF, minor allele frequency; HWE, Hardy–Weinberg equilibrium. Alleles are presented as major/minor allele.

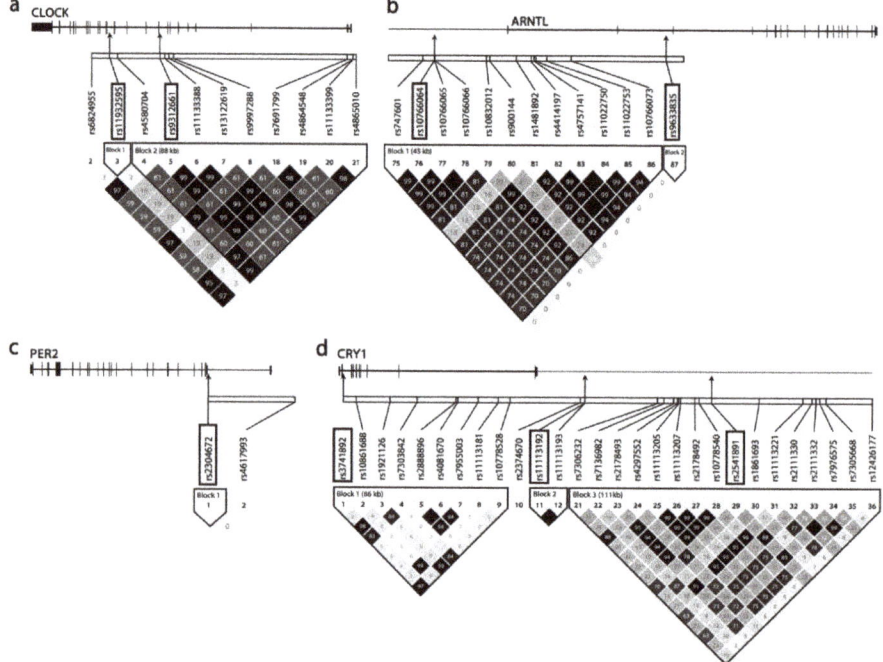

Figure 2. Pairwise linkage disequilibrium (LD) blocks for SNPs of the circadian gene locus. The horizontal white bar depicts DNA segmentation of circadian gene locus, CLOCK (**a**), ARNTL (**b**), PER2 (**c**), and CRY1 (**d**). Each diamond represents the magnitude of LD for a single pair of markers. The numbers inside the diamonds indicate the r^2 value. The blocks are shaded corresponding to the r^2 from no LD (white, $r^2 = 0$) to strong LD (black, $r^2 = 1.0$), and gray tones indicate intermediate. A part of SNPs included data was shown, and the black arrows indicate SNPs analyzed in this study.

2.3. Macronutrient Patterns

A validated semi-quantitative food frequency questionnaire with 103 food items was used for assessing dietary data [55]. The consumption frequency and portion size of items during the previous year were investigated. The sum of the nutrient intake from each food item was calculated to evaluate the average daily energy intake and nutrient intake of each individual. Macronutrient (carbohydrate, fat, and protein) intake was presented as the percentage of total energy intake. Given the protein intake was positively correlated with fat intake in this cohort population (data not shown), we defined fat to carbohydrate ratio (FC ratio) by dividing '% energy from fat' by '% energy from carbohydrate'. Subsequently, subjects were categorized by tertiles of the FC ratio: Very low FC (VLFC; the first tertile), Low FC (LFC; the second tertile), and Optimal FC (OFC; the third tertile).

2.4. Definitions of the Obesity and Abdominal Obesity

Anthropometric measurements were obtained (i.e., height, weight, waist circumference) by trained staff in cohort study [47]. In the present study, obesity was defined as a BMI ≥ 25 kg/m^2 according to Asia–Pacific BMI cut-off from the World Health Organization Report [56]. The abdominal obesity was defined as a waist circumference $\geq$90 cm for males and $\geq$85 cm for females according to the diagnostic criteria for Korea [57].

2.5. Statistical Analysis

Data were presented as the mean $\pm$ standard deviation, number, and percentage. ANOVA analysis with Tukey post hoc comparison test was used to identify group differences, and Welch's ANOVA with Games–Howell test was used to adjust for unequal variances. The Chi-square test was used to analyze categorical variables. Multiple logistic regression analysis was used for exploring the associations between genotypes and disease after adjustment for covariates, such as age, body mass index (BMI), sleep duration, alcohol intake, tobacco consumption, physical activity, energy intake, and number of regular meals. Statistical analyses were performed using SAS software version 9.4 (SAS Institute, Inc., Cary, NC, USA) and RStudio ver.1.2.1335 (RStudio Inc., Boston, MA, USA). A p-value of <0.05 was considered to be statistically significant. Bonferroni correction was applied to correct for multiple testing (Bonferroni corrected $p < 0.011$).

3. Results

3.1. General Characteristics and Nutritional Intake

The main characteristics of all the included participants are shown in Appendix B. After dividing subjects into tertiles of the FC ratio, the general characteristics according to groups were analyzed (Table 2). Subjects in the VLFC group (T1) were older than the LFC group (T2) and the OFC group (T3) (male VLFC: 50.8 $\pm$ 7.3 years, LFC: 48.6 $\pm$ 6.7 years, and OFC: 47.3 $\pm$ 6.4 years; female VLFC: 53.2 $\pm$ 7.5 years, LFC: 49.7 $\pm$ 7.5 years, and OFC: 46.9 $\pm$ 6.3 years). The VLFC showed had a lower BMI than other groups in males (24.7 $\pm$ 2.9 kg/m^2), whereas female VLFC had a higher BMI (25.3 $\pm$ 3.4 kg/m^2). In the VLFC group, the portion of rural subjects was greater than other groups (male VLFC: 43.2% and female VLFC: 58.2%). The proportion of urban subjects was highest in the OFC group (male OFC: 84.8% and female OFC 78.0%). The VLFC had a lower lean body mass and body fat than other groups in males (52.7 $\pm$ 5.8 kg and 15.1 $\pm$ 4.7 kg, respectively). In contrast, female VLFC had a lower lean body mass (39.8 $\pm$ 4.6 kg) and higher body fat (15.7 $\pm$ 4.9 kg). Furthermore, the female VLFC showed a higher waist to hip ratio (0.91 $\pm$ 0.05) compared to other groups.

The nutritional intake including total energy, carbohydrate, protein, and fat was highest in the OFC group and lowest in the VLFC group. However, carbohydrate intake did not differ by FC group in females. The VLFC group had a significantly higher % of energy from carbohydrate intake (78.2 $\pm$ 3.0% in females) and consequently a lower % of energy from protein and fat (11.7 $\pm$ 1.4% and 8.6 $\pm$ 2.0% in females, respectively) than in other groups (Appendix C). Considering that the Korean Acceptable Macronutrient Distribution Range (AMDR) for carbohydrate is 55~65%, for protein is 7~20%, and for fat is 15~30% of the energy intake for adults [58], the OFC group's proportion fitted the Korean AMDR.

Table 2. General characteristics and nutritional data by tertile of FC ratio.

Variables	Male VLFC (T1) (n = 918)	Male LFC (T2) (n = 919)	Male OFC (T3) (n = 919)	Male p	Male Post Hoc	Female VLFC (T1) (n = 862)	Female LFC (T2) (n = 863)	Female OFC (T3) (n = 862)	Female p	Female Post Hoc
General characteristics										
Age (year)	50.8 ± 7.3	48.6 ± 6.7	47.3 ± 6.4	<0.0001	A-B-C	53.2 ± 7.5	49.7 ± 7.5	46.9 ± 6.3	<0.0001	A-B-C
BMI (kg/m²)	24.2 ± 2.9	24.7 ± 2.9	24.6 ± 2.8	0.0030	A-B-B	25.3 ± 3.4	24.7 ± 3.1	24.6 ± 3.3	<0.0001	A-B-B
Residential area—Urban	522 (56.9)	728 (79.3)	779 (84.8)	<0.0001	-	361 (41.9)	590 (68.4)	672 (78)	<0.0001	-
Body composition [1]										
Lean body mass (kg)	52.7 ± 5.8	54.2 ± 6.1	54.6 ± 6.0	<0.0001	A-B-B	39.8 ± 4.6	40.2 ± 4.3	40.7 ± 4.3	0.0011	A-B-B
Lean body mass (%)	78.1 ± 5.0	77.8 ± 4.9	78.2 ± 4.6	0.2600	A-B-C	67.7 ± 5.5	68.5 ± 4.9	68.9 ± 5.3	0.0002	A-B-B
Body fat (kg)	15.1 ± 4.7	15.7 ± 4.9	15.5 ± 4.6	0.0354	A-B-B	19.4 ± 5.3	18.8 ± 4.9	18.8 ± 5.3	0.0375	A-B-B
Body fat (%)	21.9 ± 4.9	22.1 ± 4.9	21.8 ± 4.5	0.3834	A-B-B	32.4 ± 5.1	31.5 ± 4.9	31.1 ± 5.2	<0.0001	A-B-B
Waist to hip ratio	0.90 ± 0.04	0.90 ± 0.04	0.90 ± 0.04	0.1779	A-B-B	0.91 ± 0.05	0.90 ± 0.05	0.89 ± 0.05	<0.0001	A-B-B
Nutritional intake										
Energy (kcal/day)	1766.0 ± 509.6	1979.1 ± 423.3	2250.2 ± 527.9	<0.0001	A-B-C	1640.4 ± 522.7	1834.6 ± 473.7	2020.5 ± 614.5	<0.0001	A-B-C
Carbohydrate (g/day)	333.4 ± 99.3	344.0 ± 74.4	350.8 ± 82.3	0.0002	A-B-B	320.8 ± 103.4	330.8 ± 87.8	325.5 ± 100.0	0.095	A-A-A
Protein (g/day)	53.5 ± 16.4	67.9 ± 16.4	87.3 ± 24.3	<0.0001	A-B-C	47.8 ± 16.4	61.8 ± 16.9	76.9 ± 25.7	<0.0001	A-B-C
Fat (g/day)	21.4 ± 7.7	34.6 ± 8.4	53.1 ± 16.2	<0.0001	A-B-C	15.9 ± 6.6	27.7 ± 8.0	44.2 ± 16.9	<0.0001	A-B-C
% Energy from each macronutrient										
Carbohydrate	75.5 ± 3.1	69.5 ± 1.9	62.5 ± 4.1	<0.0001	A-B-C	78.2 ± 3.0	72.1 ± 2.1	64.5 ± 4.5	<0.0001	A-B-C
Protein	12.1 ± 1.5	13.7 ± 1.4	15.5 ± 2.0	<0.0001	A-B-C	11.7 ± 1.4	13.5 ± 1.6	15.3 ± 2.0	<0.0001	A-B-C
Fat	10.8 ± 2.2	15.7 ± 1.2	21.1 ± 2.9	<0.0001	A-B-C	8.6 ± 2.0	13.5 ± 1.3	19.6 ± 3.5	<0.0001	A-B-C
FC ratio	0.14 ± 0.03	0.23 ± 0.02	0.34 ± 0.08	<0.0001	A-B-C	0.11 ± 0.03	0.19 ± 0.02	0.31 ± 0.09	<0.0001	A-B-C
Number of regular meal (meal/day)	2.9 ± 0.3	2.9 ± 0.3	2.8 ± 0.4	<0.0001	A-B-C	2.9 ± 0.3	2.8 ± 0.4	2.7 ± 0.5	<0.0001	A-B-C
Alcohol intake (g/day)	16.0 ± 24.6	18.0 ± 26.5	24.8 ± 32.7	<0.0001	A-A-B	1.0 ± 4.0	1.2 ± 4.2	2.4 ± 7.6	<0.0001	A-A-B
Tobacco consumption (pack/year)	17.9 ± 17.2	16.4 ± 16.2	18.2 ± 17.3	0.0585	A-A-A	0.3 ± 2.7	0.3 ± 2.9	0.4 ± 2.4	0.9189	A-A-A
Sleep duration (h)	6.9 ± 1.2	6.7 ± 1.3	6.6 ± 1.3	0.0003	A-B-B	6.8 ± 1.4	6.6 ± 1.4	6.4 ± 1.4	<0.0001	A-B-C
Moderate physical activity [2]	314 (34.2)	322 (35.0)	392 (42.7)	0.0002	-	244 (28.3)	337 (39.0)	347 (40.3)	<0.0001	-

VLFC, Very low FC; LFC, Low FC; OFC, Optimal FC. Data are presented as mean ± standard deviation and number (percentage). ANOVA analysis with Tukey post hoc test and Welch's ANOVA with Games-Howell test for adjusting unequal variances. [1] Data were collected from subjects who completed body composition analysis; male: n = 725, n = 819, n = 844; female: n = 641, n = 739, and n = 761. [2] ≥30 min per day.

In contrast, the VLFC and LFC had an inadequate composition of macronutrients, which fell outside the AMDR with a higher carbohydrate and lower fat intake. Because the OFC had a macronutrionally balanced diet with optimal proportions, we designated the OFC as the reference group in our further analysis. The FC ratio was 0.14 ± 0.03, 0.23 ± 0.02, and 0.34 ± 0.08 for male VLFC, LFC, and OFC respectively; and 0.11 ± 0.03, 0.19 ± 0.02, and 0.31 ± 0.09 for female VLFC, LFC, and OFC respectively.

3.2. Risk of Obesity by Macronutrient Intake Patterns

The prevalence of disease according to the tertiles of the FC ratio is shown in Table 3. In males, the LFC group had an increased risk of obesity (odds ratio (OR): 1.29, 95% confidence interval (CI): 1.07–1.57) compared with the OFC group. There was no effect of patterns on the incidence of abdominal obesity in males. Interestingly, in females, the VLFC group showed greater odds of obesity and abdominal obesity than in the OFC group (OR: 1.50, 95% CI:1.20–1.86; OR: 1.84, 95% CI 1.36–2.48, respectively).

Table 3. The association between tertiles of FC ratio and prevalence of disease.

	Male	p	Female	p
Obesity [1]				
VLFC (T1)	1.15 (0.93–1.42)	0.205	1.50 (1.20–1.86)	0.000
LFC (T2)	1.29 (1.07–1.57)	0.010	1.12 (0.91–1.37)	0.281
OFC (T3)	1		1	
Abdominal obesity [2]				
VLFC (T1)	0.92 (0.64–1.33)	0.670	1.84 (1.36–2.48)	<0.0001
LFC (T2)	0.87 (0.54–1.40)	0.449	0.90 (0.67–1.20)	0.462
OFC (T3)	1		1	

All odds ratios (OR) and 95% confidence intervals (CI) were calculated by performing multiple logistic regression. [1] BMI ≥ 25 kg/m^2, odds ratio adjusted for age, sleep duration, energy intake, number of regular meals, alcohol intake, tobacco consumption, and moderate physical activity. [2] Waist circumference ≥ 90 cm for males and ≥ 85 cm for females, odds ratio adjusted for age, BMI, sleep duration, energy intake, number of regular meals, alcohol intake, tobacco consumption, and moderate physical activity.

3.3. Macronutrient Intake Patterns, Genetic Variants, and Risk of Obesity

To investigate the association of macronutrient composition and genetic variations of circadian clock genes, we stratified subjects by the genotypes of nine SNPs and analyzed the risk of obesity (Tables 4 and 5). The homozygous major allele of each SNP in the OFC was used as the reference group in the regression analysis, and the Bonferroni adjustment was used for multiple testing correction.

The risk of disease was increased in the VLFC group, particularly in females (Table 5). In the male VLFC group, the minor allele carriers of *CLOCK* rs9312661, *CRY2* rs7951225, and the GG genotype of *CRY1* rs11113192 showed increased risks of obesity; however, significances were diminished after the Bonferroni correction (Table 4). An interaction between *CRY1* rs11113192 and the FC on obesity was observed (p-interaction = 0.009); however, the significance disappeared after multiple corrections. No statistically significant differences were found for abdominal obesity.

Table 4. Prevalence of diseases by macronutrient intake patterns and genetic variants in males.

Gene	SNP		VLFC (T1)	LFC (T2)	OFC (T3)	p-Interaction	VLFC (T1)	LFC (T2)	OFC (T3)	p-Interaction
				Obesity [1]				Abdominal Obesity [2]		
CLOCK	rs11932595	AA	1.14 (0.90–1.44)	1.31 (1.06–1.63)	1	0.892	0.95 (0.63–1.43)	0.96 (0.66–1.39)	1	0.604
		GA/GG	1.41 (1.00–1.98)	1.46 (1.04–2.04)	1.21 (0.86–1.69)		1.18 (0.67–2.07)	0.93 (0.52–1.66)	1.45 (0.84–2.51)	
	rs9312661	AA	1.13 (0.83–1.54)	1.34 (0.99–1.80)	1	0.906	1.03 (0.59–1.77)	1.11 (0.67–1.84)	1	0.501
		GA/GG	1.35 (1.01–1.81)	1.47 (1.11–1.94)	1.16 (0.88–1.51)		1.11 (0.66–1.86)	0.95 (0.58–1.56)	1.27 (0.80–2.03)	
	rs10766065	TT	1.16 (0.79–1.71)	1.38 (0.96–2.00)	1	0.910	1.38 (0.71–2.68)	0.77 (0.40–1.47)	1	0.145
		CT/CC	1.21 (0.88–1.66)	1.34 (0.98–1.81)	1.06 (0.78–1.43)		1.08 (0.61–1.90)	1.24 (0.72–2.13)	1.33 (0.79–2.26)	
ARNTL	rs9633835	AA	1.24 (0.86–1.79)	1.40 (0.97–2.02)	1	0.839	0.74 (0.39–1.38)	0.79 (0.42–1.46)	1	0.700
		GA/GG	1.24 (0.90–1.70)	1.40 (1.03–1.89)	1.11 (0.83–1.50)		0.71 (0.41–1.22)	0.65 (0.39–1.08)	0.71 (0.43–1.17)	
PER2	rs2304672	GG	1.18 (0.94–1.47)	1.33 (1.09–1.64)	1	0.665	1.01 (0.69–1.49)	0.89 (0.62–1.28)	1	0.281
		CG/CC	1.04 (0.69–1.59)	1.15 (0.78–1.70)	1.11 (0.72–1.70)		0.57 (0.27–1.21)	0.96 (0.50–1.86)	1.21 (0.60–2.44)	
	rs3741892	GG	1.01 (0.77–1.31)	1.14 (0.89–1.47)	1	0.180	0.75 (0.48–1.19)	0.74 (0.48–1.13)	1	0.262
		CG/CC	1.12 (0.84–1.50)	1.24 (0.95–1.63)	0.81 (0.62–1.05)		0.76 (0.46–1.25)	0.69 (0.44–1.10)	0.60 (0.38–0.96)	
CRY1	rs11113192	GG	1.50 (1.14–1.97)	1.52 (1.17–1.96)	1	0.009	1.10 (0.68–1.77)	1.02 (0.65–1.60)	1	0.542
		CG/CC	1.06 (0.80–1.41)	1.37 (1.04–1.80)	1.28 (0.98–1.67)		1.17 (0.70–1.95)	1.14 (0.71–1.83)	1.50 (0.95–2.36)	
	rs2541891	CC	1.31 (0.94–1.84)	1.47 (1.06–2.03)	1	0.522	0.77 (0.43–1.38)	1.01 (0.58–1.75)	1	0.385
		GC/GG	1.09 (0.81–1.47)	1.23 (0.93–1.64)	1.02 (0.77–1.35)		1.18 (0.71–1.96)	0.95 (0.58–1.55)	1.16 (0.72–1.88)	
CRY2	rs7951225	AA	1.17 (0.86–1.60)	1.44 (1.07–1.92)	1	0.617	0.94 (0.55–1.61)	1.20 (0.73–1.96)	1	0.159
		TA/TT	1.35 (1.01–1.80)	1.44 (1.09–1.89)	1.20 (0.91–1.56)		0.92 (0.56–1.50)	0.68 (0.42–1.11)	1.01 (0.64–1.60)	

All odds ratios and 95% confidence intervals were calculated by performing multiple logistic regression. p-interaction: interaction between SNP and FC tertiles. Data in **bold** indicate statistically significant value after Bonferroni correction for multiple comparisons (corrected p-value: 0.05/45 = 0.001). [1] BMI ≥ 25 kg/m^2, odds ratio adjusted for age, sleep duration, energy intake, number of regular meals, alcohol intake, tobacco consumption, and moderate physical activity. [2] Waist circumference ≥ 90 cm for males, odds ratio adjusted for BMI and the same covariates as obesity.

Table 5. Prevalence of diseases by macronutrient intake patterns and genetic variants in females.

Gene	SNP		Obesity [1]				Abdominal Obesity [2]			
			VLFC (T1)	LFC (T2)	OFC (T3)	p-Interaction	VLFC (T1)	LFC (T2)	OFC (T3)	p-Interaction
CLOCK	rs11932595	AA	1.35 (1.06–1.71)	1.04 (0.83–1.30)	1	0.093	**1.84 (1.32–2.56)**	0.84 (0.60–1.17)	1	0.572
		GA/GG	1.74 (1.23–2.46)	1.14 (0.81–1.61)	0.76 (0.53–1.08)		2.05 (1.30–3.22)	1.29 (0.79–2.09)	1.14 (0.68–1.93)	
	rs9312661	AA	1.17 (0.85–1.61)	0.95 (0.69–1.30)	1	0.123	**2.26 (1.43–3.56)**	0.93 (0.58–1.48)	1	0.404
		GA/GG	1.54 (1.14–2.07)	1.09 (0.82–1.45)	0.88 (0.66–1.16)		**2.11 (1.38–3.23)**	1.15 (0.75–1.77)	1.32 (0.86–2.02)	
ARNTL	rs10766065	TT	1.66 (1.11–2.47)	0.99 (0.67–1.47)	1	0.434	2.46 (1.39–4.35)	0.72 (0.39–1.34)	1	0.113
		CT/CC	1.56 (1.12–2.17)	1.25 (0.91–1.73)	1.08 (0.79–1.49)		2.15 (1.32–3.51)	1.22 (0.75–1.99)	1.30 (0.79–2.11)	
	rs9633835	AA	1.48 (0.99–2.13)	1.14 (0.79–1.65)	1	0.953	1.11 (0.66–1.87)	0.68 (0.39–1.16)	1	0.070
		GA/GG	1.64 (1.19–2.27)	1.20 (0.88–1.68)	1.09 (0.80–1.48)		1.56 (0.99–2.48)	0.70 (0.44–1.10)	0.7 (0.44–1.12)	
PER2	rs2304672	GG	**1.49 (1.18–1.87)**	1.14 (0.92–1.42)	1	0.670	**1.85 (1.35–2.54)**	0.87 (0.64–1.19)	1	0.827
		CG/CC	1.59 (1.04–2.43)	0.94 (0.60–1.47)	1.02 (0.66–1.56)		1.28 (0.74–2.22)	0.76 (0.39–1.49)	0.68 (0.34–1.34)	
	rs3741892	GG	**1.60 (1.22–2.10)**	1.16 (0.90–1.51)	1	0.728	**1.90 (1.30–2.76)**	0.86 (0.59–1.26)	1	0.793
		CG/CC	**1.76 (1.30–2.38)**	1.38 (1.03–1.83)	1.29 (0.98–1.71)		1.70 (1.13–2.56)	0.93 (0.61–1.41)	0.98 (0.64–1.49)	
CRY1	rs11113192	GG	1.48 (1.12–1.96)	1.14 (0.87–1.49)	1	0.960	1.84 (1.25–2.70)	0.91 (0.61–1.34)	1	0.995
		CG/CC	1.37 (1.02–1.84)	1.00 (0.75–1.32)	0.91 (0.69–1.20)		1.89 (1.26–2.82)	0.91 (0.60–1.37)	1.03 (0.68–1.56)	
	rs2541891	CC	1.36 (0.96–1.94)	0.91 (0.64–1.28)	1	0.341	1.96 (1.20–3.20)	0.80 (0.48–1.32)	1	0.621
		GC/GG	1.55 (1.13–2.11)	1.23 (0.91–1.65)	0.99 (0.74–1.33)		1.96 (1.26–3.06)	1.05 (0.67–1.64)	1.11 (0.71–1.72)	
CRY2	rs7951225	AA	1.52 (1.10–2.08)	1.10 (0.80–1.51)	1	0.981	2.07 (1.32–3.24)	0.93 (0.58–1.49)	1	0.768
		TA/TT	1.63 (1.20–2.23)	1.23 (0.92–1.64)	1.09 (0.82–1.45)		1.96 (1.26–3.02)	1.01 (0.66–1.56)	1.15 (0.75–1.77)	

All odds ratios and 95% confidence intervals were calculated by performing multiple logistic regression. p-interaction: interaction between SNP and FC tertiles. Data in **bold** indicate statistically significant value after Bonferroni correction for multiple comparisons (corrected p-value: 0.05/45 = 0.001). [1] BMI ≥ 25 kg/m², odds ratio adjusted for age, sleep duration, energy intake, number of regular meals, alcohol intake, tobacco consumption, and moderate physical activity. [2] Waist circumference ≥85 cm for females, odds ratio adjusted for BMI and the same covariates as obesity.

In females, both genotypes of *CLOCK* rs9312661 in the VLFC showed an increased incidence of abdominal obesity compared with the reference group (AA genotype, OR: 2.26, 95% CI: 1.43–3.56, p = 0.0005; GA/GG genotype, OR: 2.11, 95% CI: 1.38–3.23, p = 0.0005). In addition, under the VLFC condition, *CRY1* rs3741892 had a significantly greater obesity risk than the reference regardless of genotype (GG genotype, OR: 1.60, 95% CI: 1.22–2.10, p = 0.0007; GA/GG genotype, OR: 1.76, 95% CI: 1.30–2.38, p = 0.0002). Intriguingly, the associations between macronutrient intake patterns and obesity risks were different depending on the genotypes of *CLOCK* rs11932595, *PER2* 2304672, and *CRY1* rs3741892. The major allele homozygous, AA genotype, of rs11932595 in the VLFC had a higher risk of abdominal obesity than the reference group (OR: 1.84, 95% CI: 1.32–2.56, p = 0.0003), but not in subjects carrying the minor G allele. Regarding *CRY1* rs3741892, which showed a higher obesity risk in both genotypes, the GG genotype, but not the CG/CC genotype, had a greater incidence of abdominal obesity (OR: 1.90, 95% CI: 1.30–2.76, p = 0.0008). Moreover, females with the GG genotype of *PER2* rs2304672 in the VLFC had significantly higher risks of obesity and abdominal obesity compared with the references (OR: 1.49, 95% CI:1.18–1.87, p = 0.0007; OR: 1.85, 95% CI 1.35–2.54, p = 0.0001 respectively), whereas no differences were detected in minor C allele carriers.

3.4. Potential Links between Genetic Variants and Gene Regulation

To explore the potential role of genetic variants on circadian gene regulation, we conducted an eQTL analysis at the SNP selection step. The four SNPs (rs11932595, rs9633835, rs2304672, and rs3741892), which had association with macronutrient intake patterns and obesity risk, contributed to gene expression in various tissues involved in metabolism (Appendix A). For instance, the genotypes of rs11932595 and rs9312661 influence *CLOCK* gene expression in the skeletal muscle, small intestine, colon, pancreas, and subcutaneous adipose tissue (Figure 3). Moreover, thyroidal *PER2* expression is impacted by rs2304672 genotypes, and the *CRY1* expression of the skeletal muscle is affected by rs3741892. Interestingly, the GG genotype of *PER2* rs2304672, which had a significantly increased risk of obesity in our results (Table 4), showed lower expression levels than C carriers (CC genotype: not found in the eQTL violin plot analysis, but a small portion of subjects were present in our data; n = 8 males and n = 12 females). These findings indicate that genetic variants might influence circadian gene expression levels in important metabolic tissues.

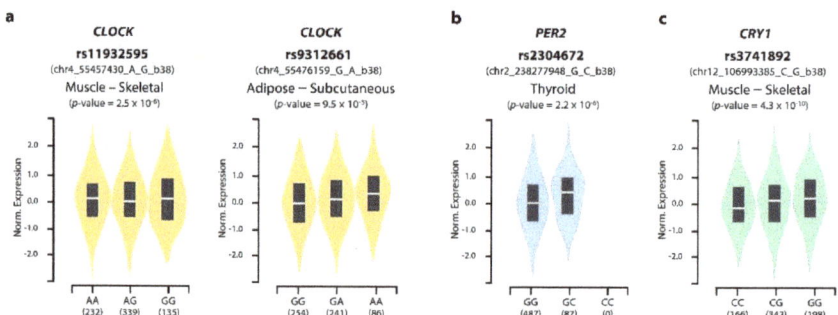

Figure 3. Relationship between genetic variants and circadian gene regulation. Effect of genetic variants on gene expression levels are shown by expression quantitative trait (eQTL) violin plot. The plot indicates the density distribution of samples in each genotype and number of subjects shown under each genotype. The white line in the box plot (black) shows the median value of the expression at each genotype. Association between rs11932595 and rs93126661 with *CLOCK* expression (**a**), Association between rs2304672 with *PER2* expression (**b**), and rs3741892 with *CRY1* expression (**c**). Data analysis was performed using GTEx Portal and included tissue-specific information provided by the website [54].

4. Discussion

In the present study, we explored macronutrient intake patterns in a Korean midlife population and observed associations between patterns and circadian clock gene variants and obesity. A categorization of the three patterns by the FC ratio revealed the high carbohydrate and relatively low-fat intake of subjects. The prevalence of obesity and abdominal obesity increased in the VLFC compared to the OFC in females. After stratification by the genotypes of nine SNPs, the obesity risk according to the patterns was different according to the genetic variants of *CLOCK*, *PER2*, and *CRY1*. In the VLFC pattern, the major allele homozygous genotype of rs11932595, rs3741892, and rs2304672 had greater risks of obesity and abdominal obesity than the reference group, whereas minor allele carriers had no difference in risk. These findings indicate that macronutrient intake patterns were associated with obesity susceptibility, and the associations were dependent on circadian clock genetic variants, particularly in females. To the best of our knowledge, this is the first study to investigate the roles of dietary macronutrient distribution and circadian clock genes in disease risk in the Korean population.

Dietary macronutrients induced alterations of circadian clock gene expression and phase shift in tissues [30,33–35]. The substitution of dietary components induced phase shifts of the hepatic circadian clock [35]. A high-fat diet altered the expression of circadian clock genes in the liver and adipose and, consequently, induced changes in the periods of circadian rhythms with advanced phase [30,32,33]. Mice fed a high-fat diet for 10 weeks revealed the reprogramming of the liver clock through the alternative oscillation of transcripts and metabolites in the liver [34]. The molecular mechanisms of reprogramming induced by high fat are the impairment of CLOCK:BMAL1 chromatin recruitment and a newly oscillating pattern of the peroxisome proliferator-activated receptor gamma (PPARγ), a nuclear receptor involved in glucose and lipid metabolism. The ketogenic diet, which consists of high fats and low carbohydrates, promotes BMAL1 chromatin recruitment in the liver and induces the tissue-specific oscillation of the peroxisome proliferator-activated receptor alpha (PPARα) and its target genes [36]. In a human study, the regulation of dietary fat and carbohydrate content altered the oscillations of peripheral clock genes and inflammatory genes [59]. A high-protein diet affected the expression of circadian genes and key gluconeogenic genes phosphoenolpyruvate carboxykinase (*PEPCK*) and glucose-6-phosphatase (*G6Pase*) in liver and kidney [37]. Therefore, interactions between dietary macronutrient distribution and circadian clock genes might influence downstream clock-controlled genes, leading to changes in metabolic outcomes. In this study, we identified macronutrient intake patterns in a Korean population and observed that the VLFC pattern was associated with increased risks of obesity and abdominal obesity. Moreover, this association was dependent on circadian genetic variants of *CLOCK*, *PER2*, and *CRY1*. Thus, these results suggest that the identification of patterns of dietary macronutrient distribution and understanding the effects of interactions between patterns and circadian genes are essential for the prevention of obesity.

To investigate the potential contribution of genetic variants to gene regulation, we selected nine SNPs by eQTL analysis. The eQTL from the GTEx portal uncovered genetic variants, including SNPs, that influenced differential levels of gene expression [53]. In the GTEx portal, tissue-specific gene expression and SNPs associations were investigated across all 49 human tissues. A combination of eQTL and SNP is useful for the comprehensive exploration of genetic effects on phenotypic variation and disease [60]. One study, which investigated disease-associated SNPs by applying an eQTL analysis, showed that several SNPs regulated gene expression levels in a tissue-specific manner, for example, the IRS1 gene in adipose tissue and influenced the risk of obesity and type 2 diabetes [61]. Rs1801260, a *CLOCK* polymorphism, has a role in the development of obesity, diabetes, and metabolic syndrome [12,18–20,23]. In a Korean population study, which used the same cohort data as our research but utilized a different genotype array chip, *CLOCK* rs1801260 affected the incidence of metabolic syndrome, and the association was more apparent after the stratification of monounsaturated fatty acid intake [22]. Moreover, the haplotype of three SNPs (rs1801260–rs11932595–rs4580704) influenced the risks of overweight and hyperglycemia. Considering the eQTL information of rs1801260 and rs11932595 was related to the differential expression of *CLOCK* in various tissues, these results imply that circadian genetic variants might regulate circadian genes as well as clock-controlled genes, resulting in different metabolic phenotypes. Having investigated the effects of genetic variants and macronutrient patterns on obesity risk, we found four significant SNPs. According to the eQTL analysis, the four SNPs influenced gene expression in various tissues (Appendix A). Genetic variants of *CLOCK*, *PER2*, and *CRY1* are associated with gene expression in muscle, adipose, and thyroid, which are known to regulate metabolism. In particular, the rs2304672 genotypes showed differential *PER2* expression levels, which were lower in the GG genotype compared with the GC genotype. *PER2* rs2304672 genetic variants were previously associated with psychiatric disorders including bipolar disorder, depression, and diurnal preference [62–64]. Two studies reported that the G allele of rs2304672 had morning preference [64,65], but no significance was found in a young Korean population [66]. In overweight/obese participants on a weight-reduction program, the G allele carriers of rs2304672 showed a lower waist to hip ratio values but had a greater probability of dropping out from the program with constant snacking and skipping breakfast than the CC genotype [21]. Moreover, the interactions between rs2304672 and plasma fatty acids on the modulation of lipoprotein-related biomarkers were reported [67]. Among metabolic syndrome patients with high plasma saturated fatty acid levels, the G allele carriers had higher plasma triglycerides, apolipoprotein C, and apolipoprotein B-48 concentrations than the CC genotype. Given that PER2 also interacts with nuclear receptors including PPARα and can regulate the expression of nuclear receptor target genes involved in lipid metabolism, *PER2* polymorphisms could contribute to metabolic disorder vulnerability [68]. In addition, rs2304672, which is located in the 5' untranslated region of the *PER2* gene, was suggested to alter the secondary structure of the transcript or change the folding of *PER2* mRNA, resulting in differential translation levels or functionality of proteins between the genotypes [64,67]. Although the mechanisms underlying disease susceptibility is not fully understood, these results support an important role of *PER2* genetic variants on obesity by regulating circadian gene expressions and functions. Further analysis is required to investigate the gene regulatory mechanisms of these SNPs.

We displayed distributions of Korean macronutrient intake patterns by the FC ratio stratification (Appendix C). The notable features in our study were a high proportion of carbohydrate intake and a positive correlation between protein and fat intake. The VLFC group, which had a low fat to carbohydrate ratio, had the highest carbohydrate intake and relatively low intake level of fat and protein. In contrast, the OFC group had a lower carbohydrate intake and increased fat and protein intake than the VLFC. Moreover, the OFC group had a balanced distribution with appropriate proportions of macronutrients that met the Korean AMDR.

The dietary intake proportion differed across populations. Western diets are characterized as having a high dietary level of saturated fats and refined carbohydrates and low levels of fiber. Previous studies have reported the effects of conventional dietary approach which applied a low-carbohydrate or low-fat diet to weight loss and improvement of obesity [38,69]. The types of intervention diets usually suggested for controlling weight can be categorized into three types: low-carbohydrate, low-fat, and moderate macronutrients [38]. Low-carbohydrate diets including Atkins and Zone diets contain 15~40% energy from carbohydrates, 30% energy from proteins, and 30~55% energy from fats. The low-fat diet is composed of 60~70% of energy from carbohydrates, 10~15% from proteins, and 10~20% from fats. In addition, a high-protein, low-fat diet had positive effects on body weight loss and metabolic benefits [69–72], providing 44%, 31%, and 25% of energy from carbohydrates, proteins, and fats, respectively. These results imply that previously utilized intervention diets are designed for western-style macronutrient distribution. For instance, there is a large difference in distribution between 'low-carbohydrate diets' or 'high-protein and low-fat' diets and Asian populations who have a much higher carbohydrate intake.

Although accumulating evidence supports the contribution of dietary macronutrient distribution to the development and prevention of metabolic diseases, the relationship between macronutrients and metabolic benefit is still controversial. Several research groups demonstrated that a low-carbohydrate diet is more effective at reducing weight, fat mass, and serum triglycerides and improving metabolic syndrome than a low-fat diet [73–77]. In contrast, other results showed both diets led to similar effects on weight control or clinical markers including glucose level, lipid profile, and blood pressure [40,74]. A meta-analysis study comparing 14 popular dietary programs found that most diets reduced weight and improved blood pressure at 6 months; however, the effects disappeared at 12 months [38]. One issue to consider is that previously conducted intervention diets modifying macronutrient distribution were usually based on energy restriction and have a short-term design. However, there were mouse studies with diets varying in protein to carbohydrate ratio, which examined the interactive effects of dietary macronutrient distribution and metabolic outcomes under *ad libitum* conditions [42,78]. Short-term 'high-protein and low-carbohydrate' diets decreased insulin sensitivity, impaired glucose tolerance, and increased triglycerides, resulting in metabolic dysregulation [78]. In contrast, 'low-protein and high-carbohydrate' diets prevented adiposity gain and improved metabolic health including insulin, glucose, and lipid levels, despite increased energy intake. As a result of chronic feeding over a lifetime in mice, 'high-protein and low-carbohydrate' diets reduced food intake and adiposity; however, they caused negative outcomes in metabolic health and shortened longevity [42]. Long-term 'low-protein and high-carbohydrate' diets increased food intake, body weight, and adiposity, but there were positive impacts on health and a longer lifespan, possibly through the regulation of mammalian target of rapamycin (mTORC1) activation [42].

Low-carbohydrate diets replaces carbohydrates with proteins or fats, a typical example is a ketogenic diet. The metabolic benefits of the low carbohydrate diets are inconsistent. Low-carbohydrate diets with increased fat or protein have been reported to be effective for weight loss and improving the lipid profile [39,75,76]. A meta-analysis comparing 'low-carbohydrate, high-fat' and 'high-carbohydrate, low-fat' diets found that the low-carbohydrate diet had a greater effect on weight loss than the high-carbohydrate diet, but no differences were observed for fat mass, glucose, and triglyceride levels, and blood pressure [41]. Results from prospective cohort studies, which investigated the effect of long-term dietary macronutrient distribution without calorie restriction, reported an association between low-carbohydrate intake and increased mortality [79–81]. Conversely, multinational and Asian studies have suggested that a high-carbohydrate intake contributed to increased mortality [82,83]. Interestingly, in a large prospective cohort study with a 25-year follow-up, midlife participants who had low (<40%) or high (>70%) energy from carbohydrate consumption were associated with increased mortality [84]. Moreover, those with a 50~55% carbohydrate intake showed the greatest lifespan, a level that might be considered moderate in the West but low in Asia. These conflicting results suggest the fact that the effects of macronutrient challenge in the short term, or energy restriction conditions might be different to those under long-term dietary intake and free-living individual conditions.

Although our study analyzed multiple variants of circadian core clock genes in Korean population cohort data, there were some limitations. The SNPs from the genomic data of the cohort did not cover the full list of variants, resulting in missing SNPs reported in previous studies. Therefore, the analysis of comprehensive genetic variant data including crucial variants will provide additional important SNPs. Secondly, our study analyzed local community-based cohort data because of the availability of genomic data. To confirm these findings, futures studies based on a national representative cohort study with a larger sample size are required. Third, even though we included the covariates (i.e., age, BMI, and energy intake) for adjustment in a statistical analysis process, the possibility of effects induced by potential confounding factors, such as residential area, socioeconomic position, and health-related behaviors, should be considered.

In conclusion, we investigated Korean macronutrient intake patterns and found associations between the patterns and circadian clock gene variants, and obesity risk. The VLFC pattern was related to higher incidences of obesity and abdominal obesity in females. After the genotype stratification of nine SNPs of circadian genes, the association between the FC ratio and obesity risk differed by the genetic variants of *CLOCK*, *PER2*, and *CRY1*. These findings suggest that the low dietary FC ratio influences obesity susceptibility and the association depends on circadian clock genetic variations. Our findings highlight an important role of the association of macronutrient distribution and circadian clock on obesity.

Author Contributions: Conceptualization, Y.J.P. and J.S.; investigation, J.S. and Y.H.; data curation, J.S.; writing—original draft preparation, J.S.; writing—review and editing, Y.J.P.; funding acquisition, Y.J.P. All authors have read and agreed to the published version of the manuscript.

Funding: This study was supported by Basic Science Research Programs through the National Research Foundation (NRF) funded by the Korean government (2021R1A2C2012578).

Institutional Review Board Statement: The study was conducted according to the guidelines of the Institutional Review Board of Ewha Womans University, Seoul, Korea (IRB approval number: ewha-202105-0003-01).

Informed Consent Statement: Written informed consent was waived by the Institutional Review Board due to all personal identifying information being removed from the dataset prior to analysis.

Data Availability Statement: The KoGES data are available on request from the National Research Institute of Health [47].

Acknowledgments: This study was conducted with bioresources from the National Biobank of Korea, the Korea Disease Control and Prevention Agency, and Korea (KBN-2021-035). J.S. was supported by NRF funded by the Ministry of Education (2020R1A6A3A13075729) and Hyundai Motor Chung Mong-Koo Foundation. Y.H. was supported by Brain Korea Four Project (Education Research Center for 4IR-Based Health Care).

Conflicts of Interest: The authors declare no conflict of interest.

Appendix A

Table A1. The expression quantitative trait loci information of SNPs.

SNP ID	Gene Symbol	Alleles	p-Value	Tissue
rs11932595	*CLOCK*	A/G	3×10^{-6}	Muscle–Skeletal
			5×10^{-7}	Cells–Cultured fibroblasts
rs9312661	*CLOCK*	A/G	2×10^{-25}	Thyroid
			2×10^{-17}	Skin–Sun Exposed (Lower leg)
			9×10^{-17}	Skin–Not Sun Exposed (Suprapubic)
			3×10^{-14}	Lung
			5×10^{-14}	Nerve–Tibial
			8×10^{-14}	Cells–Cultured fibroblasts
			7×10^{-13}	Spleen
			7×10^{-13}	Testis
			6×10^{-10}	Small Intestine–Terminal Ileum
			7×10^{-10}	Esophagus–Mucosa
			1×10^{-9}	Pancreas
			7×10^{-9}	Artery–Aorta
			2×10^{-7}	Colon–Transverse
			2×10^{-6}	Whole Blood
			1×10^{-5}	Breast–Mammary Tissue
			2×10^{-5}	Esophagus–Gastroesophageal Junction
			3×10^{-5}	Artery–Tibial
			1×10^{-4}	Adipose–Subcutaneous

Table A1. *Cont.*

SNP ID	Gene Symbol	Alleles	p-Value	Tissue
rs10766065	*ARNTL*	T/C	1×10^{-12}	Whole Blood
rs9633835	*ARNTL*	A/G	1×10^{-16}	Whole Blood
rs2304672	*PER2*	G/C	2×10^{-6}	Thyroid
rs3741892	*CRY1*	G/C	1×10^{-35}	Testis
			4×10^{-10}	Muscle–Skeletal
rs11113192	*CRY1*	G/C	1×10^{-6}	Testis
			6×10^{-5}	Esophagus–Gastroesophageal Junction
rs2541891	*CRY1*	C/G	1×10^{-4}	Testis
rs7951225	*CRY2*	A/T	3×10^{-12}	Whole Blood
			1×10^{-5}	Artery–Aorta
			1×10^{-5}	Artery–Tibial
			3×10^{-5}	Spleen

Expression quantitative loci (eQTL) information from GTEx database. Alleles are presented as major/minor allele.

Appendix B

Table A2. General characteristics of subjects.

Variables	Total (n = 5343)	Male (n = 2756)	Female (n = 2587)
General characteristics			
Age (year)	49.4 ± 7.3	48.9 ± 7.0	49.9 ± 7.6
BMI (kg/m^2)	24.7 ± 3.1	24.5 ± 2.9	24.8 ± 3.2
Sleep duration (h)	6.7 ± 1.3	6.7 ± 1.3	6.6 ± 1.4
Nutritional intake			
Energy (kcal/day)	1917.8 ± 550.6	1998.5 ± 527.5	1831.8 ± 561.8
Carbohydrate (g/day)	334.5 ± 92.2	342.7 ± 86.2	325.7 ± 97.3
Protein (g/day)	66.0 ± 23.9	69.6 ± 23.8	62.2 ± 23.4
Fat (g/day)	32.9 ± 17.2	36.4 ± 17.3	29.3 ± 16.3
% Energy from each macronutrient			
Protein	13.6 ± 2.2	13.8 ± 2.2	13.5 ± 2.2
Carbohydrate	70.3 ± 6.5	69.2 ± 6.2	71.6 ± 6.6
Fat	14.9 ± 5.0	15.9 ± 4.7	13.9 ± 5.1
Number of regular meal	2.8 ± 0.4	2.9 ± 0.3	2.8 ± 0.4
Alcohol intake (g/day)	10.8 ± 22.6	19.6 ± 28.4	1.5 ± 5.5
Tobacco consumption (pack/year)	9.2 ± 15.0	17.5 ± 16.9	0.3 ± 2.7
Moderate physical activity [1]	1956 (36.7)	1028 (37.3)	928 (35.87)

Data are presented as the mean ± standard deviation and number (percentage). [1] ≥30 min per day.

Appendix C

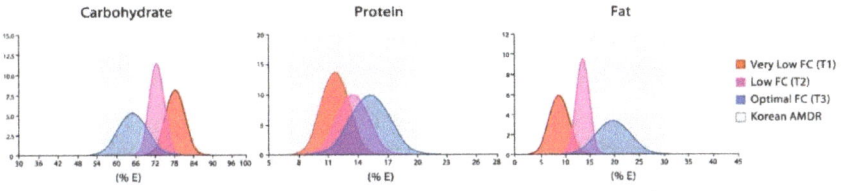

Figure A1. Macronutrient distribution according to FC group in females. Each macronutrient distribution of three FC groups was presented. The Very Low FC is represented in red; the Low FC and Optimal FC are represented in purple and blue, respectively. The gray background indicates Korean acceptable macronutrient distribution range (AMDR).

References

1. Takahashi, J.S.; Hong, H.-K.; Ko, C.H.; McDearmon, E.L. The genetics of mammalian circadian order and disorder: Implications for physiology and disease. *Nat. Rev. Genet.* **2008**, *9*, 764–775. [CrossRef] [PubMed]
2. Sato, F.; Kohsaka, A.; Bhawal, U.; Muragaki, Y. Potential roles of dec and bmal1 genes in interconnecting circadian clock and energy metabolism. *Int. J. Mol. Sci.* **2018**, *19*, 781. [CrossRef] [PubMed]
3. King, D.P.; Takahashi, J.S. Molecular genetics of circadian rhythms in mammals. *Annu. Rev. Neurosci.* **2000**, *23*, 713–742. [CrossRef] [PubMed]
4. Lee, C.; Etchegaray, J.-P.; Cagampang, F.R.; Loudon, A.S.; Reppert, S.M. Posttranslational mechanisms regulate the mammalian circadian clock. *Cell* **2001**, *107*, 855–867. [CrossRef]
5. Eckel-Mahan, K.; Sassone-Corsi, P. Metabolism and the circadian clock converge. *Physiol. Rev.* **2013**, *93*, 107–135. [CrossRef]
6. Rudic, R.D.; McNamara, P.; Curtis, A.-M.; Boston, R.C.; Panda, S.; Hogenesch, J.B.; FitzGerald, G.A. BMAL1 and CLOCK, two essential components of the circadian clock, are involved in glucose homeostasis. *PLoS Biol.* **2004**, *2*, e377. [CrossRef] [PubMed]
7. Shimba, S.; Ishii, N.; Ohta, Y.; Ohno, T.; Watabe, Y.; Hayashi, M.; Wada, T.; Aoyagi, T.; Tezuka, M. Brain and muscle Arnt-like protein-1 (BMAL1), a component of the molecular clock, regulates adipogenesis. *Proc. Natl. Acad. Sci. USA* **2005**, *102*, 12071–12076. [CrossRef] [PubMed]
8. Curtis, A.M.; Cheng, Y.; Kapoor, S.; Reilly, D.; Price, T.S.; FitzGerald, G.A. Circadian variation of blood pressure and the vascular response to asynchronous stress. *Proc. Natl. Acad. Sci. USA* **2007**, *104*, 3450–3455. [CrossRef] [PubMed]
9. Lamia, K.A.; Storch, K.-F.; Weitz, C.J. Physiological significance of a peripheral tissue circadian clock. *Proc. Natl. Acad. Sci. USA* **2008**, *105*, 15172–15177. [CrossRef] [PubMed]
10. Oishi, K.; Atsumi, G.-i.; Sugiyama, S.; Kodomari, I.; Kasamatsu, M.; Machida, K.; Ishida, N. Disrupted fat absorption attenuates obesity induced by a high-fat diet in Clock mutant mice. *FEBS Lett.* **2006**, *580*, 127–130. [CrossRef]
11. Turek, F.W.; Joshu, C.; Kohsaka, A.; Lin, E.; Ivanova, G.; McDearmon, E.; Laposky, A.; Losee-Olson, S.; Easton, A.; Jensen, D.R.; et al. Obesity and metabolic syndrome in circadian Clock mutant mice. *Science* **2005**, *308*, 1043–1045. [CrossRef] [PubMed]
12. Scott, E.; Carter, A.; Grant, P. Association between polymorphisms in the Clock gene, obesity and the metabolic syndrome in man. *Int. J. Obes.* **2008**, *32*, 658–662. [CrossRef] [PubMed]
13. Sookoian, S.; Gemma, C.; Gianotti, T.F.; Burgueño, A.; Castaño, G.; Pirola, C.J. Genetic variants of *Clock* transcription factor are associated with individual susceptibility to obesity. *Am. J. Clin. Nutr.* **2008**, *87*, 1606–1615. [CrossRef]
14. Woon, P.Y.; Kaisaki, P.J.; Bragança, J.; Bihoreau, M.-T.; Levy, J.C.; Farrall, M.; Gauguier, D. Aryl hydrocarbon receptor nuclear translocator-like (BMAL1) is associated with susceptibility to hypertension and type 2 diabetes. *Proc. Natl. Acad. Sci. USA* **2007**, *104*, 14412–14417. [CrossRef] [PubMed]
15. Kelly, M.A.; Rees, S.D.; Hydrie, M.Z.I.; Shera, A.S.; Bellary, S.; O'Hare, J.P.; Kumar, S.; Taheri, S.; Basit, A.; Barnett, A.H.; et al. Circadian gene variants and susceptibility to type 2 diabetes: A pilot study. *PLoS ONE* **2012**, *7*, e32670. [CrossRef] [PubMed]
16. Pappa, K.I.; Gazouli, M.; Anastasiou, E.; Iliodromiti, Z.; Antsaklis, A.; Anagnou, N.P. The major circadian pacemaker ARNT-like protein-1 (BMAL1) is associated with susceptibility to gestational diabetes mellitus. *Diabetes Res. Clin. Pract.* **2013**, *99*, 151–157. [CrossRef] [PubMed]
17. Škrlec, I.; Milić, J.; Steiner, R. The impact of the circadian genes clock and arntl on myocardial infarction. *J. Clin. Med.* **2020**, *9*, 484. [CrossRef] [PubMed]
18. Lo, M.-T.; Bandin, C.; Yang, H.-W.; Scheer, F.A.; Hu, K.; Garaulet, M. CLOCK 3111T/C genetic variant influences the daily rhythm of autonomic nervous function: Relevance to body weight control. *Int. J. Obes.* **2018**, *42*, 190. [CrossRef] [PubMed]
19. Garaulet, M.; Sánchez-Moreno, C.; Smith, C.E.; Lee, Y.-C.; Nicolás, F.; Ordovás, J.M. Ghrelin, sleep reduction and evening preference: Relationships to CLOCK 3111 T/C SNP and weight loss. *PLoS ONE* **2011**, *6*, e17435. [CrossRef] [PubMed]
20. Garaulet, M.; Lee, Y.-C.; Shen, J.; Parnell, L.D.; Arnett, D.K.; Tsai, M.Y.; Lai, C.-Q.; Ordovas, J.M. Genetic variants in human CLOCK associate with total energy intake and cytokine sleep factors in overweight subjects (GOLDN population). *Eur. J. Hum. Genet.* **2010**, *18*, 364–369. [CrossRef] [PubMed]
21. Garaulet, M.; Corbalán-Tutau, M.D.; Madrid, J.A.; Baraza, J.C.; Parnell, L.D.; Lee, Y.-C.; Ordovas, J.M. PERIOD2 variants are associated with abdominal obesity, psycho-behavioral factors, and attrition in the dietary treatment of obesity. *J. Am. Diet. Assoc.* **2010**, *110*, 917–921. [CrossRef] [PubMed]
22. Shin, D.; Lee, K.-W. CLOCK Gene Variation Is Associated with the Incidence of Metabolic Syndrome Modulated by Monounsaturated Fatty Acids. *J. Pers. Med.* **2021**, *11*, 412. [CrossRef]
23. Garcia-Rios, A.; Gomez-Delgado, F.J.; Garaulet, M.; Alcala-Diaz, J.F.; Delgado-Lista, F.J.; Marin, C.; Rangel-Zuñiga, O.A.; Rodriguez-Cantalejo, F.; Gomez-Luna, P.; Ordovas, J.M. Beneficial effect of CLOCK gene polymorphism rs1801260 in combination with low-fat diet on insulin metabolism in the patients with metabolic syndrome. *Chronobiol. Int.* **2014**, *31*, 401–408. [CrossRef]
24. Loria-Kohen, V.; Espinosa-Salinas, I.; Marcos-Pasero, H.; Lourenço-Nogueira, T.; Herranz, J.; Molina, S.; Reglero, G.; de Molina, A.R. Polymorphism in the CLOCK gene may influence the effect of fat intake reduction on weight loss. *Nutrition* **2016**, *32*, 453–460. [CrossRef]
25. Garaulet, M.; Lee, Y.-C.; Shen, J.; Parnell, L.D.; Arnett, D.K.; Tsai, M.Y.; Lai, C.-Q.; Ordovas, J.M. CLOCK genetic variation and metabolic syndrome risk: Modulation by monounsaturated fatty acids. *Am. J. Clin. Nutr.* **2009**, *90*, 1466–1475. [CrossRef]
26. Sahar, S.; Sassone-Corsi, P. Metabolism and cancer: The circadian clock connection. *Nat. Rev. Cancer* **2009**, *9*, 886. [CrossRef] [PubMed]

27. Yamazaki, S.; Numano, R.; Abe, M.; Hida, A.; Takahashi, R.-i.; Ueda, M.; Block, G.D.; Sakaki, Y.; Menaker, M.; Tei, H. Resetting central and peripheral circadian oscillators in transgenic rats. *Science* **2000**, *288*, 682–685. [CrossRef] [PubMed]
28. Oike, H.; Oishi, K.; Kobori, M. Nutrients, clock genes, and chrononutrition. *Curr. Nutr. Rep.* **2014**, *3*, 204–212. [CrossRef] [PubMed]
29. Oosterman, J.E.; Kalsbeek, A.; la Fleur, S.E.; Belsham, D.D. Impact of nutrients on circadian rhythmicity. *Am. J. Physiol. Regul. Integr. Comp. Physiol.* **2015**, *308*, R337–R350. [CrossRef] [PubMed]
30. Kohsaka, A.; Laposky, A.D.; Ramsey, K.M.; Estrada, C.; Joshu, C.; Kobayashi, Y.; Turek, F.W.; Bass, J. High-fat diet disrupts behavioral and molecular circadian rhythms in mice. *Cell Metab.* **2007**, *6*, 414–421. [CrossRef]
31. Kuroda, H.; Tahara, Y.; Saito, K.; Ohnishi, N.; Kubo, Y.; Seo, Y.; Otsuka, M.; Fuse, Y.; Ohura, Y.; Hirao, A.; et al. Meal frequency patterns determine the phase of mouse peripheral circadian clocks. *Sci. Rep.* **2012**, *2*, 711. [CrossRef]
32. Ribas-Latre, A.; Santos, R.B.; Fekry, B.; Tamim, Y.M.; Shivshankar, S.; Mohamed, A.M.; Baumgartner, C.; Kwok, C.; Gebhardt, C.; Rivera, A.; et al. Cellular and physiological circadian mechanisms drive diurnal cell proliferation and expansion of white adipose tissue. *Nat. Commun.* **2021**, *12*, 3482. [CrossRef] [PubMed]
33. Pendergast, J.S.; Branecky, K.L.; Yang, W.; Ellacott, K.L.; Niswender, K.D.; Yamazaki, S. High-fat diet acutely affects circadian organisation and eating behavior. *Eur. J. Neurosci.* **2013**, *37*, 1350–1356. [CrossRef] [PubMed]
34. Eckel-Mahan, K.L.; Patel, V.R.; De Mateo, S.; Orozco-Solis, R.; Ceglia, N.J.; Sahar, S.; Dilag-Penilla, S.A.; Dyar, K.A.; Baldi, P.; Sassone-Corsi, P. Reprogramming of the circadian clock by nutritional challenge. *Cell* **2013**, *155*, 1464–1478. [CrossRef] [PubMed]
35. Hirao, A.; Tahara, Y.; Kimura, I.; Shibata, S. A balanced diet is necessary for proper entrainment signals of the mouse liver clock. *PLoS ONE* **2009**, *4*, e6909. [CrossRef] [PubMed]
36. Tognini, P.; Murakami, M.; Liu, Y.; Eckel-Mahan, K.L.; Newman, J.C.; Verdin, E.; Baldi, P.; Sassone-Corsi, P. Distinct circadian signatures in liver and gut clocks revealed by ketogenic diet. *Cell Metab.* **2017**, *26*, 523–538.e5. [CrossRef]
37. Oishi, K.; Uchida, D.; Itoh, N. Low-carbohydrate, high-protein diet affects rhythmic expression of gluconeogenic regulatory and circadian clock genes in mouse peripheral tissues. *Chronobiol. Int.* **2012**, *29*, 799–809. [CrossRef] [PubMed]
38. Ge, L.; Sadeghirad, B.; Ball, G.D.; da Costa, B.R.; Hitchcock, C.L.; Svendrovski, A.; Kiflen, R.; Quadri, K.; Kwon, H.Y.; Karamouzian, M.; et al. Comparison of dietary macronutrient patterns of 14 popular named dietary programmes for weight and cardiovascular risk factor reduction in adults: Systematic review and network meta-analysis of randomised trials. *BMJ* **2020**, *369*, m696. [CrossRef]
39. Foster, G.D.; Wyatt, H.R.; Hill, J.O.; McGuckin, B.G.; Brill, C.; Mohammed, B.S.; Szapary, P.O.; Rader, D.J.; Edman, J.S.; Klein, S. A randomized trial of a low-carbohydrate diet for obesity. *N. Engl. J. Med.* **2003**, *348*, 2082–2090. [CrossRef] [PubMed]
40. Gardner, C.D.; Trepanowski, J.F.; Del Gobbo, L.C.; Hauser, M.E.; Rigdon, J.; Ioannidis, J.P.; Desai, M.; King, A.C. Effect of low-fat vs low-carbohydrate diet on 12-month weight loss in overweight adults and the association with genotype pattern or insulin secretion: The DIETFITS randomized clinical trial. *JAMA* **2018**, *319*, 667–679. [CrossRef]
41. Yang, Q.; Lang, X.; Li, W.; Liang, Y. The effects of low-fat, high-carbohydrate diets vs. low-carbohydrate, high-fat diets on weight, blood pressure, serum liquids and blood glucose: A systematic review and meta-analysis. *Eur. J. Clin. Nutr.* **2022**, *76*, 16–27. [CrossRef]
42. Solon-Biet, S.M.; McMahon, A.C.; Ballard, J.W.O.; Ruohonen, K.; Wu, L.E.; Cogger, V.C.; Warren, A.; Huang, X.; Pichaud, N.; Melvin, R.G.; et al. The ratio of macronutrients, not caloric intake, dictates cardiometabolic health, aging, and longevity in ad libitum-fed mice. *Cell Metab.* **2014**, *19*, 418–430. [CrossRef] [PubMed]
43. Hatori, M.; Vollmers, C.; Zarrinpar, A.; DiTacchio, L.; Bushong, E.A.; Gill, S.; Leblanc, M.; Chaix, A.; Joens, M.; Fitzpatrick, J.A.; et al. Time-restricted feeding without reducing caloric intake prevents metabolic diseases in mice fed a high-fat diet. *Cell Metab.* **2012**, *15*, 848–860. [CrossRef] [PubMed]
44. Chaix, A.; Zarrinpar, A.; Miu, P.; Panda, S. Time-restricted feeding is a preventative and therapeutic intervention against diverse nutritional challenges. *Cell Metab.* **2014**, *20*, 991–1005. [CrossRef] [PubMed]
45. McHill, A.W.; Czeisler, C.A.; Phillips, A.J.; Keating, L.; Barger, L.K.; Garaulet, M.; Scheer, F.A.; Klerman, E.B. Caloric and macronutrient intake differ with circadian phase and between lean and overweight young adults. *Nutrients* **2019**, *11*, 587. [CrossRef]
46. Xiao, Q.; Garaulet, M.; Scheer, F.A. Meal timing and obesity: Interactions with macronutrient intake and chronotype. *Int. J. Obes.* **2019**, *43*, 1701–1711. [CrossRef]
47. Kim, Y.; Han, B.-G.; The KoGES Group. Cohort profile: The Korean genome and epidemiology study (KoGES) consortium. *Int. J. Epidemiol.* **2017**, *46*, 1350. [CrossRef]
48. Jang, S.-N.; Kawachi, I.; Chang, J.; Boo, K.; Shin, H.-G.; Lee, H.; Cho, S.-i. Marital status, gender, and depression: Analysis of the baseline survey of the Korean Longitudinal Study of Ageing (KLoSA). *Soc. Sci. Med.* **2009**, *69*, 1608–1615. [CrossRef]
49. Consortium, G.P. An integrated map of genetic variation from 1092 human genomes. *Nature* **2012**, *491*, 56. [CrossRef]
50. Cho, Y.S.; Go, M.J.; Kim, Y.J.; Heo, J.Y.; Oh, J.H.; Ban, H.-J.; Yoon, D.; Lee, M.H.; Kim, D.-J.; Park, M.; et al. A large-scale genome-wide association study of Asian populations uncovers genetic factors influencing eight quantitative traits. *Nat. Genet.* **2009**, *41*, 527–534. [CrossRef]
51. Purcell, S.; Neale, B.; Todd-Brown, K.; Thomas, L.; Ferreira, M.A.; Bender, D.; Maller, J.; Sklar, P.; De Bakker, P.I.; Daly, M.J.; et al. PLINK: A tool set for whole-genome association and population-based linkage analyses. *Am. J. Hum. Genet.* **2007**, *81*, 559–575. [CrossRef] [PubMed]

52. Barrett, J.C.; Fry, B.; Maller, J.; Daly, M.J. Haploview: Analysis and visualization of LD and haplotype maps. *Bioinformatics* **2004**, *21*, 263–265. [CrossRef] [PubMed]
53. Lonsdale, J.; Thomas, J.; Salvatore, M.; Phillips, R.; Lo, E.; Shad, S.; Hasz, R.; Walters, G.; Garcia, F.; Young, N.; et al. The genotype-tissue expression (GTEx) project. *Nat. Genet.* **2013**, *45*, 580–585. [CrossRef] [PubMed]
54. The Genotype-Tissue Expression Project (GTEx). Available online: https://www.gtexportal.org (accessed on 20 April 2021).
55. Ahn, Y.; Kwon, E.; Shim, J.; Park, M.; Joo, Y.; Kimm, K.; Park, C.; Kim, D. Validation and reproducibility of food frequency questionnaire for Korean genome epidemiologic study. *Eur. J. Clin. Nutr.* **2007**, *61*, 1435–1441. [CrossRef]
56. World Health Organization. *The Asia-Pacific Perspective: Redefining Obesity and Its Treatment*; Health Communications Australia Pty Limited: Balmain, NSW, Australia, 2000.
57. Lee, S.; Park, H.S.; Kim, S.M.; Kwon, H.S.; Kim, D.Y.; Kim, D.J.; Cho, G.J.; Han, J.H.; Kim, S.R.; Park, C.Y.; et al. Cut-off points of waist circumference for defining abdominal obesity in the Korean population. *Korean J. Obes.* **2006**, *15*, 1–9.
58. The Korean Nutrition Society. *Dietary Reference Intakes for Koreans*; Ministry of Health and Welfare: Sejong, Korea, 2020; p. 9.
59. Pivovarova, O.; Jürchott, K.; Rudovich, N.; Hornemann, S.; Ye, L.; Möckel, S.; Murahovschi, V.; Kessler, K.; Seltmann, A.-C.; Maser-Gluth, C.; et al. Changes of dietary fat and carbohydrate content alter central and peripheral clock in humans. *J. Clin. Endocrinol. Metab.* **2015**, *100*, 2291–2302. [CrossRef]
60. Stranger, B.E.; Forrest, M.S.; Dunning, M.; Ingle, C.E.; Beazley, C.; Thorne, N.; Redon, R.; Bird, C.P.; De Grassi, A.; Lee, C.; et al. Relative impact of nucleotide and copy number variation on gene expression phenotypes. *Science* **2007**, *315*, 848–853. [CrossRef]
61. Fadason, T.; Ekblad, C.; Ingram, J.R.; Schierding, W.S.; O'Sullivan, J.M. Physical interactions and expression quantitative traits loci identify regulatory connections for obesity and type 2 diabetes associated SNPs. *Front. Genet.* **2017**, *8*, 150. [CrossRef]
62. Lavebratt, C.; Sjöholm, L.K.; Partonen, T.; Schalling, M.; Forsell, Y. PER2 variation is associated with depression vulnerability. *Am. J. Med. Genet. Part B Neuropsychiatr. Genet.* **2010**, *153B*, 570–581. [CrossRef]
63. Forbes, E.E.; Dahl, R.E.; Almeida, J.R.; Ferrell, R.E.; Nimgaonkar, V.L.; Mansour, H.; Sciarrillo, S.R.; Holm, S.M.; Rodriguez, E.E.; Phillips, M.L. PER2 rs2304672 polymorphism moderates circadian-relevant reward circuitry activity in adolescents. *Biol. Psychiatry* **2012**, *71*, 451–457. [CrossRef]
64. Carpen, J.D.; Archer, S.N.; Skene, D.J.; Smits, M.; von Schantz, M. A single-nucleotide polymorphism in the 5′-untranslated region of the hPER2 gene is associated with diurnal preference. *J. Sleep Res.* **2005**, *14*, 293–297. [CrossRef]
65. Satoh, K.; Mishima, K.; Inoue, Y.; Ebisawa, T.; Shimizu, T. Two pedigrees of familial advanced sleep phase syndrome in Japan. *Sleep* **2003**, *26*, 416–417. [CrossRef]
66. Lee, H.-J.; Kim, L.; Kang, S.-G.; Yoon, H.-K.; Choi, J.-E.; Park, Y.-M.; Kim, S.J.; Kripke, D.F. PER2 variation is associated with diurnal preference in a Korean young population. *Behav. Genet.* **2011**, *41*, 273–277. [CrossRef] [PubMed]
67. Garcia-Rios, A.; Perez-Martinez, P.; Delgado-Lista, J.; Phillips, C.M.; Gjelstad, I.M.; Wright, J.W.; Karlström, B.; Kieć-Wilk, B.; van Hees, A.; Helal, O. A Period 2 genetic variant interacts with plasma SFA to modify plasma lipid concentrations in adults with metabolic syndrome. *J. Nutr.* **2012**, *142*, 1213–1218. [CrossRef] [PubMed]
68. Schmutz, I.; Ripperger, J.A.; Baeriswyl-Aebischer, S.; Albrecht, U. The mammalian clock component PERIOD2 coordinates circadian output by interaction with nuclear receptors. *Genes Dev.* **2010**, *24*, 345–357. [CrossRef]
69. Martinez, J.A.; Navas-Carretero, S.; Saris, W.H.; Astrup, A. Personalized weight loss strategies—The role of macronutrient distribution. *Nat. Rev. Endocrinol.* **2014**, *10*, 749–760. [CrossRef]
70. Farnsworth, E.; Luscombe, N.D.; Noakes, M.; Wittert, G.; Argyiou, E.; Clifton, P.M. Effect of a high-protein, energy-restricted diet on body composition, glycemic control, and lipid concentrations in overweight and obese hyperinsulinemic men and women. *Am. J. Clin. Nutr.* **2003**, *78*, 31–39. [CrossRef] [PubMed]
71. Wycherley, T.P.; Moran, L.J.; Clifton, P.M.; Noakes, M.; Brinkworth, G.D. Effects of energy-restricted high-protein, low-fat compared with standard-protein, low-fat diets: A meta-analysis of randomized controlled trials. *Am. J. Clin. Nutr.* **2012**, *96*, 1281–1298. [CrossRef]
72. Noakes, M.; Keogh, J.B.; Foster, P.R.; Clifton, P.M. Effect of an energy-restricted, high-protein, low-fat diet relative to a conventional high-carbohydrate, low-fat diet on weight loss, body composition, nutritional status, and markers of cardiovascular health in obese women. *Am. J. Clin. Nutr.* **2005**, *81*, 1298–1306. [CrossRef]
73. Gardner, C.D.; Kiazand, A.; Alhassan, S.; Kim, S.; Stafford, R.S.; Balise, R.R.; Kraemer, H.C.; King, A.C. Comparison of the Atkins, Zone, Ornish, and LEARN diets for change in weight and related risk factors among overweight premenopausal women: The A TO Z Weight Loss Study: A randomized trial. *JAMA* **2007**, *297*, 969–977. [CrossRef]
74. Brehm, B.J.; Seeley, R.J.; Daniels, S.R.; D'Alessio, D.A. A randomized trial comparing a very low carbohydrate diet and a calorie-restricted low fat diet on body weight and cardiovascular risk factors in healthy women. *J. Clin. Endocrinol. Metab.* **2003**, *88*, 1617–1623. [CrossRef]
75. Bazzano, L.A.; Hu, T.; Reynolds, K.; Yao, L.; Bunol, C.; Liu, Y.; Chen, C.-S.; Klag, M.J.; Whelton, P.K.; He, J. Effects of low-carbohydrate and low-fat diets: A randomized trial. *Ann. Intern. Med.* **2014**, *161*, 309–318. [CrossRef]
76. Volek, J.S.; Phinney, S.D.; Forsythe, C.E.; Quann, E.E.; Wood, R.J.; Puglisi, M.J.; Kraemer, W.J.; Bibus, D.M.; Fernandez, M.L.; Feinman, R.D. Carbohydrate restriction has a more favorable impact on the metabolic syndrome than a low fat diet. *Lipids* **2009**, *44*, 297–309. [CrossRef] [PubMed]

77. Volek, J.S.; Sharman, M.J.; Gómez, A.L.; Judelson, D.A.; Rubin, M.R.; Watson, G.; Sokmen, B.; Silvestre, R.; French, D.N.; Kraemer, W.J. Comparison of energy-restricted very low-carbohydrate and low-fat diets on weight loss and body composition in overweight men and women. *Nutr. Metab.* **2004**, *1*, 13. [CrossRef] [PubMed]
78. Solon-Biet, S.M.; Mitchell, S.J.; Coogan, S.C.; Cogger, V.C.; Gokarn, R.; McMahon, A.C.; Raubenheimer, D.; de Cabo, R.; Simpson, S.J.; Le Couteur, D.G. Dietary protein to carbohydrate ratio and caloric restriction: Comparing metabolic outcomes in mice. *Cell Rep.* **2015**, *11*, 1529–1534. [CrossRef] [PubMed]
79. Fung, T.T.; van Dam, R.M.; Hankinson, S.E.; Stampfer, M.; Willett, W.C.; Hu, F.B. Low-carbohydrate diets and all-cause and cause-specific mortality: Two cohort studies. *Ann. Intern. Med.* **2010**, *153*, 289–298. [CrossRef]
80. Trichopoulou, A.; Psaltopoulou, T.; Orfanos, P.; Hsieh, C.; Trichopoulos, D. Low-carbohydrate–high-protein diet and long-term survival in a general population cohort. *Eur. J. Clin. Nutr.* **2007**, *61*, 575–581. [CrossRef] [PubMed]
81. Noto, H.; Goto, A.; Tsujimoto, T.; Noda, M. Low-carbohydrate diets and all-cause mortality: A systematic review and meta-analysis of observational studies. *PLoS ONE* **2013**, *8*, e55030. [CrossRef]
82. Nakamura, Y.; Okuda, N.; Okamura, T.; Kadota, A.; Miyagawa, N.; Hayakawa, T.; Kita, Y.; Fujiyoshi, A.; Nagai, M.; Takashima, N.; et al. Low-carbohydrate diets and cardiovascular and total mortality in Japanese: A 29-year follow-up of NIPPON DATA80. *Br. J. Nutr.* **2014**, *112*, 916–924. [CrossRef]
83. Dehghan, M.; Mente, A.; Zhang, X.; Swaminathan, S.; Li, W.; Mohan, V.; Iqbal, R.; Kumar, R.; Wentzel-Viljoen, E.; Rosengren, A.; et al. Associations of fats and carbohydrate intake with cardiovascular disease and mortality in 18 countries from five continents (PURE): A prospective cohort study. *Lancet* **2017**, *390*, 2050–2062. [CrossRef]
84. Seidelmann, S.B.; Claggett, B.; Cheng, S.; Henglin, M.; Shah, A.; Steffen, L.M.; Folsom, A.R.; Rimm, E.B.; Willett, W.C.; Solomon, S.D. Dietary carbohydrate intake and mortality: A prospective cohort study and meta-analysis. *Lancet Public Health* **2018**, *3*, e419–e428. [CrossRef]

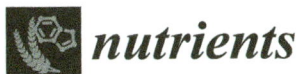

Article

FTO and ADRB2 Genetic Polymorphisms Are Risk Factors for Earlier Excessive Gestational Weight Gain in Pregnant Women with Pregestational Diabetes Mellitus: Results of a Randomized Nutrigenetic Trial

Karina dos Santos [1], Eliane Lopes Rosado [1], Ana Carolina Proença da Fonseca [2], Gabriella Pinto Belfort [1], Letícia Barbosa Gabriel da Silva [1], Marcelo Ribeiro-Alves [3], Verônica Marques Zembrzuski [2], J. Alfredo Martínez [4] and Cláudia Saunders [1,*]

1. Programa de Pós-Graduação em Nutrição, Instituto de Nutrição Josué de Castro, Universidade Federal do Rio de Janeiro, Avenida Carlos Chagas Filho, 373-Bloco J 2° andar, Cidade Universitária, Rio de Janeiro 21941-902, Brazil; karsantos@gmail.com (K.d.S.); elianerosado@nutricao.ufrj.br (E.L.R.); belfortgabriella@hotmail.com (G.P.B.); leticiabgs.nut04@gmail.com (L.B.G.d.S.)
2. Laboratório de Genética Humana, Instituto Oswaldo Cruz, Fundação Oswaldo Cruz, Pavilhão Leônidas Deane, Avenida Brasil 4365, Rio de Janeiro 21040-360, Brazil; ana_carol_pf@hotmail.com (A.C.P.d.F.); vezembrzuski@gmail.com (V.M.Z.)
3. Instituto Nacional de Infectologia Evandro Chagas, Fundação Oswaldo Cruz, Avenida Brasil 4365, Rio de Janeiro 21040-360, Brazil; mribalves@gmail.com
4. Precision Nutrition and Cardiometabolic Health Program, IMDEA Food Institute, Crta. de Canto Blanco, n 8, E-28049 Madrid, Spain; jalfredo.martinez@imdea.org

* Correspondence: claudiasaunders@nutricao.ufrj.br

Abstract: Excessive gestational weight gain (GWG) is associated with increased risk of maternal and neonatal complications. We investigated obesity-related polymorphisms in the FTO gene (rs9939609, rs17817449) and ADRB2 (rs1042713, rs1042714) as candidate risk factors concerning excessive GWG in pregnant women with pregestational diabetes. This nutrigenetic trial, conducted in Brazil, randomly assigned 70 pregnant women to one of the groups: traditional diet ($n = 41$) or DASH diet ($n = 29$). Excessive GWG was the total weight gain above the upper limit of the recommendation, according to the Institute of Medicine guidelines. Genotyping was performed using real-time PCR. Time-to-event analysis was performed to investigate risk factors for progression to excessive GWG. Regardless the type of diet, AT carriers of rs9939609 (FTO) and AA carriers of rs1042713 (ADRB2) had higher risk of earlier exceeding GWG compared to TT (aHR 2.44; CI 95% 1.03–5.78; $p = 0.04$) and GG (aHR 3.91; CI 95% 1.12–13.70; $p = 0.03$) genotypes, respectively, as the AG carriers for FTO haplotype rs9939609:rs17817449 compared to TT carriers (aHR 1.79; CI 95% 1.04–3.06; $p = 0.02$).

Keywords: gestational weight gain; ADRB2; FTO; DASH diet; diabetes mellitus; nutrigenetics

1. Introduction

Excessive gestational weight gain (GWG) affects half of pregnancies worldwide [1] and nearly 40% of pregnancies in Brazil [2]. In women with pregestational diabetes mellitus (DM), excessive GWG is associated with a higher risk of preterm delivery, cesarean section, large-for-gestational-age newborn, macrosomia, neonatal distress, and neonatal malformations [3,4]. In addition to increasing the immediate risk of perinatal complications, excessive GWG is associated with short- and long-term metabolic consequences for mothers and children and probably plays a key role in the metabolic programming of chronic diseases in the offspring [5].

The GWG recommendations [6,7] are based on the pre-pregnancy body mass index (BMI), but genetics, dietetics, and environmental factors appear to be involved in significant interindividual variation in weight gain during pregnancy [8,9]. The fat mass and obesity-associated (FTO) gene is located on chromosome 16, and common polymorphisms in the first intron are strongly associated with obesity. FTO encodes a protein with demethylase function and is highly expressed in the hypothalamus, particularly in the arcuate nucleus, suggesting that this gene plays an essential role in energy balance and body weight control [10].

The polymorphisms rs9939609 (T/A) and rs17817449 (T/G) in FTO are associated with body weight, BMI, and extreme obesity in the Brazilian population [11]. The A allele of the polymorphism rs9939609 is associated with higher GWG in North America [12,13] and Spanish women [14] but not with excessive GWG in Brazilian women [15]. Despite the association of rs17817449 (GG) with higher maternal BMI in pregnant Iraqi women [16], its relationship with GWG has not yet been explored in the literature.

The adrenoceptor beta 2 (ADRB2) gene is located on chromosome 5, and some polymorphisms in this gene have been consistently associated with a predisposition to obesity due to its expression in adipose tissue and its role in lipolysis and energy balance [17]. Two common polymorphisms in ADRB2 are the most studied, rs1042713 (G/A) and rs1042714 (C/G), although the results are quite divergent, with only rs1042714 (CG/GG) associated with obesity in a meta-analysis [18]. The relationship between ADRB2 polymorphisms and GWG has not yet been explored.

Interventions that focus on a healthy diet have been found to be effective in optimizing GWG [5] and should start as early as possible, even during the periconceptional period [19]. The adherence to an "Western" dietary pattern—characterized by unhealthy and energy-dense foods with high intake of red meat, fries, dipping sauces, salty snacks, and alcoholic drinks—was associated with increased GWG, especially among obese women, in a cohort of women from Southern Europe [19].

Pregnant women with DM especially benefit from nutritional guidance to prevent excessive GWG and related adverse outcomes, which are more common in high-risk pregnancies [20]. The Dietary Approach to Stop Hypertension (DASH) diet encourages the consumption of fruits, vegetables, fat-free/low-fat dairy, whole grains, nuts, and legumes as well as limits the intake of saturated fat, cholesterol, refined sugar, sodium, red, and processed meats [21]. The DASH diet was originally proposed to control hypertension; however, in recent years, it has been recommended for pregnant women with DM, obesity, and hypertension to reduce the risk of obstetric and perinatal complications [22,23].

However, the effects of diet on body physiology vary greatly among individuals, which may be partially explained by nutrigenetic interactions. The association between FTO and ADRB2 genetic polymorphisms and obesity phenotypes appears to be modified by diet composition [24–26]. Personalized nutrition may benefit individuals genetically predisposed to have a higher BMI using a dietary pattern that minimizes risk [27]. Studies are needed to elucidate the association between genetic variants, diet, and GWG, especially for high-risk pregnancies, such as in mothers with pregestational DM.

The aim of this study was to investigate the FTO genetic polymorphisms (rs9939609, rs17817449) and the ADRB2 genetic polymorphisms (rs1042713, rs1042714) as candidate genetic risk factors for excessive GWG in pregnant women with pregestational DM using two different types of diets, a traditional diet and the DASH diet, as well as to ascertain nutrigenetic interactions associated to the genetic make-up.

2. Materials and Methods

2.1. Subjects

The participants were pregnant women who were enrolled in the DASDIA (DASh diet for pregnant women with DIAbetes) randomized controlled clinical trial carried out at the Maternity School of the Federal University of Rio de Janeiro, Rio de Janeiro, Brazil, with the aim of evaluating the effect of the DASH diet on perinatal outcomes in pregnant women with pregestational DM (2016–2020, Brazilian Clinical Trials Registry RBR-4tbgv6). Eighty-seven pregnant women participated in the DASDIA trial, of whom 70 were included in the present study because valid data were available for performing the nutrigenetic analyses.

The participants were pregnant women with pregestational DM; 18 years or older; less than 28 weeks pregnant at the time of inclusion in the study; single fetus; no alcohol, tobacco, or drug use; no sexually transmitted disease (e.g., syphilis, genital herpes, HPV); no psychiatric diseases (e.g., anxiety, depression, eating disorders); and no DM complications (e.g., diabetic nephropathy or retinopathy). Pregnant women with treated and controlled hypothyroidism (TSH 0.1–2.5 mUI/L in the first trimester or 0.3–3.0 mUI/L in the second trimester, using levothyroxine) or chronic hypertension (systolic blood pressure <160 mmHg and diastolic blood pressure <110, using methyldopa, without SHG) were included. The eligible participants were randomly assigned to one of two parallel study groups, traditional diet or DASH diet, using a computer-generated list of random numbers prepared by the head investigator (even numbers to DASH diet group and odd numbers to traditional diet group). The participants were blinded to allocation.

The research was approved by the Ethics Committee of the Maternity School of Federal University of Rio de Janeiro (CAAE–46913115.0.0000.5275; July/2015).

2.2. Pregestational Diabetes Diagnosis and Treatment

Women with type 1 or 2 DM were included in this study, with a pre-pregnancy diagnosis or diagnosed during pregnancy, after presenting with a fasting glucose level ≥126 mg/dL [20]. Women with gestational DM were excluded from the study. Following the institutional protocol, all participants were treated with insulin therapy, which was prescribed by physicians according to individual needs.

2.3. Diet Groups and Nutritional Guidance

The participants were randomly assigned to one of two groups of nutritional guidance, a traditional diet or the DASH diet. Women in both groups received individual nutritional guidance from a registered dietitian from the date of inclusion in the study until the last prenatal appointment in six scheduled visits. The time of intervention was defined as the time between inclusion in the study and childbirth.

Both traditional and DASH diets were designed to contain 45–55% carbohydrates, 15–20% protein, and 25–30% total fat. However, the DASH diet was richer in fruits, vegetables, whole grains, and low-fat dairy products and included a serving of nuts per day. The original North American version of the DASH diet was translated and adapted for the DASDIA trial, considering the characteristics of Brazilian pregnant women with DM, as detailed elsewhere [28]. The traditional diet was a healthy diet currently prescribed for all pregnant women with DM-attending prenatal care at the maternity hospital.

The main differences in the composition of the traditional and DASH diets based on the 2100 kcal meal plan are provided in Table 1.

Table 1. Daily composition of the diets used in the study.

	Traditional Diet	DASH Diet
Saturated fatty acids *	9.7% E	7.2% E
Monounsaturated fatty acids *	8.5% E	9.2% E
Polyunsaturated fatty acids *	2.8% E	5.6% E
Fiber	42 g	55 g
Calcium	1500 mg	2280 mg
Magnesium	315 mg	496 mg
Potassium	4081 mg	4418 mg
Sodium	2400 mg	2400 mg

* Expressed as percentual of daily energy intake (% E). Data are presented for a daily energy intake of 2100 kcal, as an example.

The daily energy intake was calculated individually in order to formulate recommendations according to age, physical activity, pre-pregnancy BMI, and recommended GWG for each woman in both groups. All participants received a meal plan with a list of equivalents based on the traditional or DASH diet, which was explained in detail and revised at each appointment with the registered dietitian, with reinforcement of the nutritional orientations for both diets until the last visit [28].

Adherence to the diets was assessed using a 24-h dietary recall and by applying a tool with four evaluation items, which was scored from 0 to 4 points according to (1) quantity of food consumed—portions; (2) food groups consumed—variety; (3) consumed meals—number and time; and (4) gestational weight gain—adequate when no more than 20% less or above the recommended amount [29]. The adherence score was stratified into low-to-moderate adherence (<2 points) and high adherence (≥ 2 points). For the present analyses, we considered the adherence score obtained at the visit closest to childbirth to reflect the longest possible time of exposure to the intervention.

To improve adherence, participants in the traditional diet group received a bottle of extra virgin olive oil (500 mL) at the first visit, a can of powdered semi-skimmed milk (300 mg), and a pack of oats (250 mg) at each subsequent visit, while the participants in the DASH diet group received a bottle of extra virgin olive oil (500 mL) at the first visit, a can of powdered skimmed milk (280 mg), and a pack of nuts (150 mg) and seeds (200 mg) at each subsequent visit.

2.4. Outcome

The main outcome was excessive GWG (kg). The recommended GWG was defined according to the Institute of Medicine guidelines [6,7] considering the pre-pregnancy BMI: underweight, 12.5 to 18 kg; normal weight, 11.5 to 16 kg; overweight, 7 to 11.5 kg; and obesity, 5 to 9 kg. Excessive GWG was the total weight gain of pregnancy exceeding the maximum amount recommended by IOM [6,7] according to pre-pregnancy BMI: GWG > 18 kg, >16 kg, >11.5 kg, and >9 kg for underweight, normal weight, overweight, and obese women, respectively. The time until excessive GWG was estimated by linear interpolation, assuming a linearly increasing weight gain between different measurements.

To calculate the pre-pregnancy BMI, height was measured during the first prenatal visit, and weight was measured at each prenatal visit by nursing technicians and registered in the medical record. Pre-pregnancy weight was the self-reported weight of a woman near conception [30]. The pre-pregnancy BMI was calculated as (pre-pregnancy weight/height^2) and was classified as underweight (BMI < 18.5 kg/m^2), normal weight (BMI 18.5–24.9 kg/m^2), overweight (BMI 25.0–29.9 kg/m^2), or obesity (BMI $\geq$ 30.0 kg/m^2) [31].

The last pregnancy weight was measured on admission for childbirth. GWG was calculated as (weight at admission for childbirth−pre-pregnancy weight), representing the total weight gain during pregnancy.

2.5. Genotyping

We collected saliva samples from each pregnant woman participating in the study, and genomic DNA was isolated from buccal epithelial cells using the Aidar and Line (2007) protocol [32]. FTO (rs9939609 and rs17817449) and ADRB2 (rs1042713 and rs1042714) polymorphisms were genotyped by real-time PCR using TaqMan® assays (Thermo Fisher Scientific, Carlsbad, CA, USA). Reactions were performed in 10-µL volumes containing DNA (2 µL), Universal Master Mix (5 µL), TaqMan Genotyping Assay specific for each polymorphism (0.25 µL), and MiliQ (2.75 µL). Amplification was carried out in a StepOne® Plus Real-Time PCR System (ThermoFisher) according to the manufacturer's recommendations for the number of cycles and temperatures. Negative and positive controls were included in the plate.

2.6. Co-Variates

Data, such as age (years), DM type (1 or 2), education level (elementary, middle, or high school), marital status (married/single), employment (yes/no), per capita income (total family income divided by the number of persons living in the same house, in USD), housing conditions (adequate when all had regular garbage collection, tap water, and sewerage system), pre-existing chronic diseases (hypothyroidism or chronic hypertension), and parity (number of previous childbirths) were obtained from medical records and were complemented in a personal interview with the researchers using structured questionnaires. Physical activity was assessed at baseline using the short form of the International Physical Activity Questionnaire (active, irregularly active, and sedentary) [33].

Skin color (white/black/brown/yellow) and years living with DM were self-reported. Energy intake (kcal) at baseline was obtained using a 24-h dietary recall from which the reported portions of food were converted into grams to quantify the energy content using food composition tables [34,35]. Gestational age (weeks) was calculated using the first ultrasonography performed in prenatal care, which was obtained at the time of inclusion in the study (all <28 weeks of pregnancy).

2.7. Statistical Analyses

Data are presented as medians and interquartile ranges (IQR) for numeric variables, and absolute (n) and relative frequencies (%) for categorical variables. The normality of the continuous variables was assessed using histograms, kurtosis, and asymmetry measures. Mann–Whitney U and Kruskal–Wallis tests were used to compare continuous numerical variables, and chi-square or Fisher's exact tests were used for categorical variables. Genotype and allele frequencies of each variant were determined by direct counting, and deviations from Hardy–Weinberg equilibrium (HWE) were evaluated using chi-square tests.

Paired linkage disequilibrium (LD) patterns were determined for each gene using r^2 statistics (r^2 cutoff ≥ 0.8). Haplotype frequencies or allelic phase determination were estimated by expectation maximization (EM algorithm), and estimation uncertainty was included in the statistical models applied for association analyses in the form of weights. The homozygous/heterozygous genotypes and lower frequency alleles (minor allele frequency, MAF) in our population, or those containing them, were compared with the higher frequency alleles or genotypes containing higher frequency alleles (reference). Haplotype analyses used the most common haplotype in our population as a reference.

The incidences of excessive GWG were analyzed based on the events and years of persons at risk based on the follow-up time from the most likely date of conception to the most probable date of the outcome. Incidences and 95% confidence intervals (95% CIs) were estimated according to asymptotic standard errors calculated from a gamma distribution. Pregnant women who did not present with the outcome were considered from the most likely date of conception and censored on the day of delivery.

The results of the time-to-event analyses were presented in the form of hazard ratios (HRs) with 95% CIs, and the risks of progression to the events described above were estimated using Cox proportional hazard models. The assumption of risk proportionality was tested using correlation analyses and χ^2 tests based on Schoenfeld scaled residuals and transformed survival times. The effects of the genetic characteristics of interest were corrected for phenotypic characteristics with at least one suggested association (p-value ≤ 0.1) with the outcome of interest and the marginal effects presented in the form of aHR. Pregestational BMI was not included in the adjusted model because of its potential mediating effect between genotype and outcome. Each polymorphism was evaluated using the additive, dominant, and recessive models.

Statistical analyses were performed using R software (Version 4.1.1) and its "genetics" and "survival" packages. Power analysis and sample size estimates were performed using the R code available on the Power and Sample Size platform (http://powerandsamplesize.com/Calculators/Test-Time-To-Event-Data/Cox-PH-2-Sided-Equality) accessed on 18 January 2022. Considering the overall prevalence of the event of 50%, the frequency of minor allele carriers of 35%, a mean hazard ratio of 2, and alpha = 0.05, the minimum sample size for Cox proportional models estimated for power (1-eta) of 0.8 was 144. Nonetheless, we had a limited sample size (n = 70) that reached 56.35% statistical power for this analysis.

3. Results

Of the 249 pregnant women with pregestational DM assessed for eligibility, 87 were included in the DASDIA clinical trial, and 70 were included in the present study because there were sufficient data for the analyses: 41 in the traditional diet group and 29 in the DASH diet group (Figure 1).

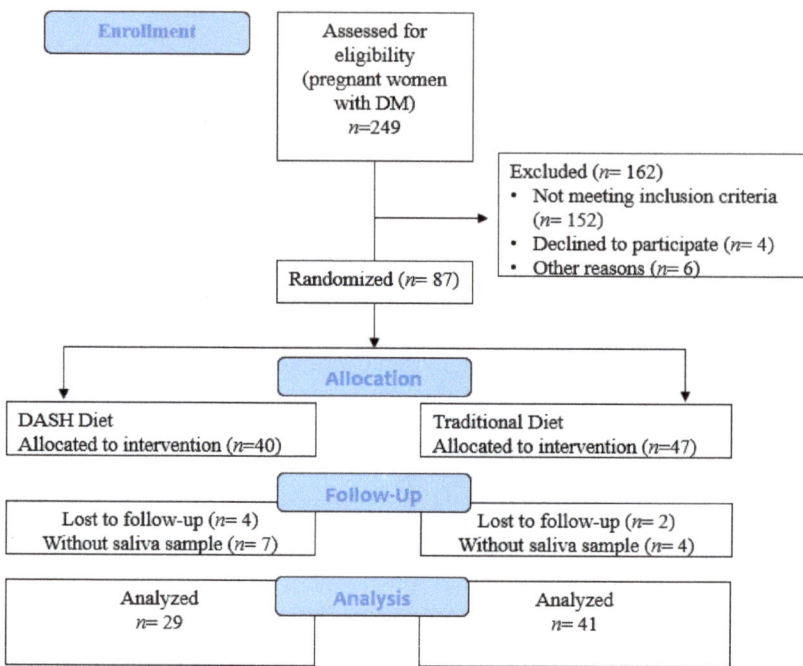

Figure 1. Flowchart of the study (Rio de Janeiro/Brazil, 2016–2020).

The median age was 32 years (IQR 25.7–36.0), and the gestational age at randomization was 15 weeks (IQR 11.1–20.1). DM type 1 was 51.4% (n = 36) of the cases. The distribution of the variables was homogeneous among the diet groups (Table 2).

Table 2. General characteristics of the participants at baseline (Rio de Janeiro/Brazil, 2016–2020).

	Overall n = 70	Trad. Diet n = 41	DASH Diet n = 29	p-Value *
Age (years)	32 (25.7–36.0)	31 (25.0–35.0)	34 (28.0–37.0)	0.28
Gestational age (weeks)	15.0 (11.1–20.1)	14.4 (11.6–21.6)	16.0 (10.1–18.6)	0.66
DM type n (%)				
DM1	36 (51.4)	21 (51.2)	15 (51.7)	0.97
DM2	34 (48.6)	20 (48.8)	14 (48.3)	
Years living with DM	8 (2.0–13.5)	6 (1.9–12.5)	9 (2.0–14.5)	0.36
Skin color n (%)				
Brown	27 (38.6)	15 (36.6)	12 (41.4)	
White	22 (31.4)	12 (29.3)	10 (34.5)	
Black	16 (22.9)	11 (26.8)	5 (17.2)	0.59
Yellow	1 (1.4)	0 (0)	1 (3.4)	
Unknown	4 (5.7)	3 (7.3)	1 (3.4)	

Table 2. Cont.

	Overall n = 70	Trad. Diet n = 41	DASH Diet n = 29	p-Value *
Marital status n (%)				
Married	56 (80.0)	33 (80.5)	23 (79.3)	
Single	12 (17.1)	6 (14.6)	6 (20.7)	0.57
Missing	2 (2.9)	2 (4.9)	0 (0)	
Education level n (%)				
Elementary/middle school	46 (65.7)	26 (63.4)	20 (69.0)	
High school	23 (32.9)	14 (34.2)	9 (31.0)	0.73
Missing	1 (1.4)	1 (2.4)	0 (0)	
Employment n (%)				
Yes	42 (60.0)	26 (63.4)	16 (55.2)	
No	27 (38.6)	14 (34.1)	13 (44.8)	0.41
Missing	1 (1.4)	1 (2.4)	0 (0)	
per capita income (USD †)	151.51 (103.04–227.27)	154.54 (113.33–228.78)	136.36 (91.67–221.04)	0.59
Housing conditions				
Adequate	64 (91.4)	37 (90.2)	27 (93.1)	1.00
Inadequate	3 (4.3)	2 (4.9)	1 (3.5)	
Missing	3 (4.3)	2 (4.9)	1 (3.5)	
Parity n (%)	1 (0–1.25)	1 (0–1.5)	1 (0–1.5)	0.92
Preexisting chronic disease n (%)				
None	48 (68.4)	31 (75.6)	17 (58.6)	
Hypertension	9 (12.9)	4 (9.8)	5 (17.2)	0.06
Hypothyroidism	8 (11.4)	2 (4.9)	6 (20.7)	
Both	1 (1.4)	0 (0)	1 (3.4)	
Missing	4 (5.7)	4 (9.8)	0 (0)	
Pre-pregnancy BMI (kg/m^2)	27.85 (24.4–32.3)	27.10 (24.3–31.9)	28.60 (25.7–33.3)	0.16
Pre-pregnany BMI n (%)				
Normal weight	20 (28.6)	14 (34.1)	6 (20.7)	
Overweight	25 (35.7)	14 (34.1)	11 (37.9)	0.45
Obesity	25 (35.7)	13 (31.7)	12 (41.4)	
Energy intake (kcal)	1808.3 (1578.7–2228.6)	1823.8 (1528.9–2362.2)	1780.7 (1644.5–1968.8)	0.68
Physical Activity n (%)				
Active	30 (42.9)	15 (36.6)	15 (51.7)	
Irregularly active	27 (38.6)	17 (41.5)	10 (34.5)	0.51
Sedentary	7 (10.0)	5 (12.1)	2 (6.9)	
Missing	6 (8.6)	4 (9.8)	2 (6.9)	

Data presented as median (interquartile range) or as absolute and relative frequencies n (%). † Estimated for exchange rate of 1 real (BRL) = USD 5.5. * Mann–Whitney U test or Kruskal–Wallis test to compare medians and chi-square test or Fisher exact test to compare frequencies.

The genotypic frequencies of rs9939609–FTO were TT 40%, AT 48.6%, and AA 11.4%, while for rs17817449–FTO, the values were TT 45.7%, GT 44.3%, and GG 10%, without differences among diet groups ($p = 0.48$ and $p = 0.73$, respectively; Table 3). The MAFs for rs9939609 (A) were 35.7%, while it was 32.1% for rs17817449 (G).

The genotypic frequencies of rs1042713–ADRB2 were GG 35.7%, AG 52.9%, and AA 11.4%, while for rs1042714–ADRB2, the values were CC 50%, CG 44.3%, and GG 5.7%, without differences among diet groups ($p = 0.35$ and $p = 0.28$, respectively; Table 3). The MAFs for rs1042713 (A) were 37.9% and 27.9% for rs1042714 (G). The genotypes of all evaluated polymorphisms were in HWE ($p > 0.05$).

Table 3. Genetic background of the participants concerning FTO and ADRB2 polymorphisms (Rio de Janeiro/Brazil, 2016–2020).

	Overall n = 70	Traditional Diet n = 41	DASH Diet n = 29	p-Value *
FTO rs9939609 n (%)				
T Allele	90 (64.3)			
A Allele	50 (35.7)			
TT	28 (40.0)	17 (41.5)	11 (37.9)	
AT	34 (48.6)	21 (51.2)	13 (44.8)	0.48
AA	8 (11.4)	3 (7.3)	5 (17.2)	
FTO rs17817449 n (%)				
T Allele	95 (67.9)			
G Allele	45 (32.1)			
TT	32 (45.7)	19 (46.3)	13 (44.8)	
GT	31 (44.3)	19 (46.3)	12 (41.4)	0.73
GG	7 (10.0)	3 (7.3)	4 (13.8)	
ADRB2 rs1042713 n (%)				
G Allele	87 (62.1)			
A Allele	53 (37.9)			
GG	25 (35.7)	12 (29.3)	13 (44.8)	
AG	37 (52.9)	23 (56.1)	14 (48.3)	0.35
AA	8 (11.4)	6 (14.6)	2 (6.9)	
ADRB2 rs1042714 n (%)				
C Allele	101 (72.1)			
G Allele	39 (27.9)			
CC	35 (50.0)	20 (48.3)	15 (51.7)	
CG	31 (44.3)	17 (41.5)	14 (48.3)	0.28
GG	4 (5.7)	4 (9.8)	0 (0)	

FTO, fat mass and obesity-associated gene; ADRB2, adrenoceptor beta 2 gene. Data presented as absolute and relative frequencies n (%). Genotypes were in Hardy–Weinberg equilibrium. * Chi-square test or Fisher's exact test to compare frequencies.

The median time of intervention was 22.50 weeks (IQR 15.50–26.04). Most pregnant women attended six scheduled appointments (n = 38, 54.3%) or at least five of them (n = 16, 22.9%). Almost 40% of the participants had the highest adherence scores in both groups (39.5% in the traditional diet group and 40.7% in the DASH diet group).

In the overall sample (n = 70), 28.6% of the women had a normal pre-pregnancy BMI, 35.7% were overweight, and 35.7% were obese. None of the pregnant women were underweight pre-pregnancy. The median GWG was 13.7 kg (IQR 11.5–17.5), 11.8 kg (IQR 7.5–16.4), and 11.0 (IQR 5.9–14.1) for normal-weight, overweight, and obese women, respectively, without differences between diet groups (Supplementary Table S1). We found no statistically significant interaction between diet and genotype on GWG but a marginal effect for the AA genotype of rs9939609–FTO and GG genotype of rs17817449–FTO ($p = 0.05$ and $p = 0.08$, respectively) on higher GWG comparing to another genotypes, only in the traditional diet group (Supplementary Figure S1).

Thirty-seven pregnant women (52.9%) presented with excessive GWG, and the median gestational age of exceeding GWG was 31.6 weeks (IQR 26.6–35.0). Compared to the traditional diet, the DASH diet did not modify the risk of progression to excessive GWG (aHR 1.32, CI 95% 0.62–2.79; $p = 0.46$) in our sample. Instead, the time of living with DM $\geq$ 8 years (aHR 1.99, CI 95% 1.01–3.93; $p = 0.04$), pre-pregnancy overweight (aHR 3.15, CI 95% 1.23–8.09; $p = 0.02$) or obesity (aHR 2.87, CI 95% 1.11–7.42; $p = 0.03$) status, previous hypothyroidism (aHR 4.37, CI 95% 1.62–11.77; $p = 0.00$), and yellow color of the skin (aHR 74.40; CI 95% 4.25–1302.72; $p = 0.00$, not shown in the table) were risk factors for earlier GWG. In contrast, age $\geq$ 32 years was a protective factor (aHR 0.41, CI 95% 0.21–0.80; $p = 0.01$) (Table 4).

Table 4. Cox proportional hazard models or time-to-event analyses (from conception to excessive gestational weight gain) of diet groups and general characteristics of the participants (Rio de Janeiro/Brazil, 2016–2020).

Characteristics	Outcome	pY	Crude Incidence/ 100 pY (CI 95%)	HR (CI 95%)	p-Value	aHR * (CI 95%)	p-Value
Overall	37	44.4	83.29 (58.65–114.81)	-	-	-	-
Diet							
Traditional diet	18	26.0	69.12 (40.97–109.25)	Reference	-	Reference	-
DASH diet	19	18.4	103.36 (62.23–161.41)	1.66 (0.87–3.17)	0.12	1.32 (0.62–2.79)	0.46
Type of DM							
DM1	17	23.2	73.36 (42.73–117.46)	Reference	-	Reference	-
DM2	20	21.2	94.12 (57.49–145.37)	1.39 (0.728–2.657)	0.32	0.92 (0.38–2.22)	0.86
Years living with DM (years)							
<8	18	25.3	71.25 (42.23–112.61)	Reference	-	Reference	-
≥8	19	18.4	103.10 (62.07–161.00)	1.62 (0.85–3.09)	0.14	1.99 (1.01–3.93)	0.04
Age (years)							
<32	21	23.0	91.20 (56.46–139.41)	Reference	-	Reference	-
≥32	16	21.4	74.78 (42.74–121.44)	0.80 (0.41–1.53)	0.49	0.41 (0.21–0.80)	0.01
Color of the skin							
Brown	14	17.2	81.17 (44.37–136.18)	Reference	-	Reference	-
White	10	14.0	71.30 (34.19–131.11)	0.838 (0.372–1.888)	0.67	0.681 (0.293–1.586)	0.37
Black	10	10.2	98.29 (47.13–180.76)	1.404 (0.622–3.171)	0.41	1.132 (0.458–2.8)	0.79
Marital Status							
Married	30	36.9	81.30 (54.86–116.07)	Reference	-	Reference	-
Single	7	6.8	102.84 (41.35–211.90)	1.44 (0.63–3.29)	0.38	1.92 (0.79–4.68)	0.15
Employment							
Yes	20	26.9	74.18 (45.31–114.56)	Reference	-	Reference	-
No	17	16.7	101.54 (59.15–162.58)	1.40 (0.74–2.68)	0.30	1.45 (0.76–2.79)	0.26
Housing Conditions							
Adequate	35	41.1	85.10 (59.27–118.35)	Reference	-	Reference	-
Inadequate	2	1.1	183.54 (22.23–663.01)	4.49 (1.04–19.43)	0.04	4.25 (0.84–21.59)	0.08
Pre-pregnancy BMI							
Normal weight	6	13.5	44.43 (16.31–96.71)	Reference	-	Reference	-
Overweight	16	15.6	102.54 (58.61–166.52)	3.15 (1.23–8.09)	0.02	3.15 (1.23–8.09)	0.02
Obesity	15	15.3	97.94 (54.82–161.53)	2.87 (1.11–7.42)	0.03	2.87 (1.11–7.42)	0.03

Table 4. Cont.

Characteristics	Outcome	pY	Crude Incidence/ 100 pY (CI 95%)	HR (CI 95%)	p-Value	aHR * (CI 95%)	p-Value
Chronic disease							
None	24	31.1	70.74 (44.33–107.10)	Reference	-	Reference	-
Chronic hypertension	5	5.6	89.26 (28.98–208.30)	1.53 (0.58–4.04)	0.39	1.33 (0.48–3.70)	0.59
Hypothyroidism	7	4.9	141.02 (56.70–290.56)	2.66 (1.13–6.30)	0.02	4.37 (1.62–11.77)	0.00
Both	1	0.7	141.02 (3.57–785.72)	1.64 (0.22–12.19)	0.63	1.21 (0.15–9.98)	0.86

pY, person-years; CI, confidence interval; DASH, Dietary Approach to stop Hypertension; DM, diabetes mellitus; BMI, body mass index. * Adjusted HR for skin color, previous chronic diseases, and housing conditions.

Adjusting for the main confounders, the A allele carriers (AT/AA) had a higher risk of earlier exceeding GWG (aHR 2.55; CI 95% 1.14–5.69; p = 0.02) than the rs9939609 TT genotype in the FTO gene, which was also found in the comparison of AT vs. TT genotypes (aHR 2.44; CI 95% 1.03–5.78; p = 0.04) (Table 5).

Table 5. Cox proportional hazard models or time-to-event analyses (from conception to excessive gestational weight gain) stratified by the FTO polymorphisms rs9939609 and rs17817449 (Rio de Janeiro/Brazil, 2016–2020).

Genotypes		Outcome	pY	Crude Incidence/ 100 pY (CI 95%)	HR (CI 95%)	p	aHR * (CI 95%)	p
Overall		37	44.4	83.29 (58.65–114.31)	-	-	-	-
rs9939609								
Additive Model	TT	12	18.6	64.33 (33.24–112.38)	Reference	-	Reference	-
	AT	19	20.6	92.06 (55.43–143.77)	1.56 (0.76–3.21)	0.23	2.44 (1.03–5.78)	0.04
	AA	6	5.1	116.94 (42.92–254.53)	2.08 (0.78–5.55)	0.14	2.83 (0.93–8.62);	0.07
Dominant Model	TT	12	18.6	64.33 (33.24–112.38)	Reference	-	Reference	-
	AT/AA	25	25.8	97.02 (62.78–143.21)	1.66 (0.83–3.30);	0.15	2.55 (1.14–5.69)	0.02
Recessive Model	AA	6	5.1	116.94 (42.92–254.53)	Reference	-	Reference	-
	AT/TT	31	39.3	78.9 (53.61–111.99)	0.62 (0.26–1.48)	0.28	0.54 (0.20–1.49)	0.24
rs17817449								
Additive Model	TT	15	21.0	71.42 (39.97–117.80)	Reference	-	Reference	-
	GT	17	18.8	90.55 (52.75–144.98)	1.30 (0.65–2.61)	0.46	1.66 (0.75–3.65)	0.21
	GG	5	4.6	107.62 (34.94–251.14)	1.54 (0.56–4.25)	0.40	2.18 (0.65–7.33)	0.21
Dominant Model	TT	15	21.0	71.42 (39.97–117.8)	Reference	-	Reference	-
	GT/GG	22	23.4	93.94 (58.87–142.22)	1.35 (0.70–2.60)	0.37	1.74 (0.82–3.70)	0.15
Recessive Model	GG	5	4.6	107.62 (34.94–251.14)	Reference	-	Reference	-
	GT/TT	32	39.8	80.45 (55.03–113.57)	0.74 (0.29–1.90)	0.53	0.60 (0.20–1.83)	0.37

pY, person-years; CI, confidence interval; FTO, fat mass and obesity-associated gene. * Adjusted HR for skin color, previous chronic diseases, and housing conditions.

The A allele carriers for rs1042713 in the ADRB2 gene had a higher risk of earlier exceeding GWG than the GG genotype (aHR 2.37; CI 95% 1.01–5.52; p = 0.04), being almost four times higher for the AA carriers (aHR 3.91; CI 95% 1.12–13.70; p = 0.03). We found that the genotypes for rs17817449 (FTO) and rs1042714 (ADRB2) had no effect on the risk of excess GWG in our sample (Table 6).

Table 6. Cox proportional hazard models or time-to-event analyses (from conception to excessive gestational weight gain) stratified by the ADRB2 polymorphisms rs1042713 and rs1042714 (Rio de Janeiro/Brazil, 2016–2020).

Genotypes		Outcome	pY	Crude Incidence/ 100 pY (CI 95%)	HR (CI 95%)	p	aHR * (CI 95%)	p
Overall		37	44.4	83.29 (58.65–114.31)	-	-	-	-
rs1042713								
Additive Model	GG	10	16.3	61.44 (29.46–112.99)	Reference	-	Reference	-
	AG	22	23.6	93.36 (58.51–141.35)	1.72 (0.81–3.64)	0.16	2.14 (0.89–5.14)	0.09
	AA	5	4.6	109.16 (35.44–254.74)	2.05 (0.70–6.02)	0.19	3.91 (1.12–13.70)	0.03
Dominant Model	GG	10		61.44 (29.46–112.99)	Reference	-	Reference	-
	AG/AA	27		95.93 (63.22–139.57)	1.772 (0.856–3.667)	0.12	2.37 (1.01–5.52)	0.04
Recessive Model	AA	5	4.6	109.16 (35.44–254.74)	Reference	-	Reference	-
	AG/GG	32	39.8	80.32 (54.94–113.38)	0.69 (0.27–1.77)	0.44	0.41 (0.14–1.21)	0.11
rs1042714								
Additive Model	CC	20	21.2	94.11 (57.49–145.35)	Reference	-	Reference	-
	CG	15	20.4	73.41 (41.09–121.08)	0.71 (0.36–1.39)	0.32	0.78 (0.37–1.63)	0.51
	GG	2	2.7	73.05 (8.85–263.88)	0.65 (0.15–2.80)	0.57	0.29 (0.04–1.91)	0.20
Dominant Model	CC	20	21.2	94.11 (57.49–145.35)	Reference	-	Reference	-
	CG/GG	17	23.2	73.37 (42.74–117.47)	0.70 (0.37–1.34)	0.29	0.70 (0.34–1.44)	0.33
Recessive Model	GG	2	2.7	73.05 (8.85–263.88)	Reference	-	Reference	-
	CG/CC	35	41.7	83.96 (58.48–116.77)	1.30 (0.31–5.40)	0.72	3.20 (0.48–21.53)	0.23

pY, person-years; CI, confidence interval; ADRB2, adrenoceptor beta 2 gene. * Adjusted HR for skin color, previous chronic diseases, and housing conditions.

Although rs17817449 alone was not associated with the outcome, in the haplotype analysis of rs9939609:rs17817449 (TT/AG/AT), we found a higher risk for earlier excessive GWG among AG carriers: the A allele for rs9939609 and the G allele for rs17817449 (aHR 1.79; CI 95% 1.04–3.06; $p = 0.02$). We found no association between haplotype analysis of the ADRB2 gene in our sample (Table 7).

Table 7. Cox proportional hazard models or time-to-event analyses (from conception to excessive gestational weight gain) of the haplotypes ADRB2 rs1042713:rs1042714 and FTO rs9939609:rs17817449 (Rio de Janeiro/Brazil, 2016–2020).

Haplotypes	Outcome	pY	Crude Incidence/ 100 pY (CI 95%)	HR (CI 95%)	p-Value	aHR * (CI 95%)	p-Value
ADRB2 rs1042713:rs1042714							
AC	32	32.7	97.78 (66.88–138.04)	Reference	-	Reference	-
GC	23	30.2	76.13 (48.26–114.24)	0.74 (0.43–1.26)	0.26	0.63 (0.36–1.12)	0.12
GG	19	25.9	73.33 (44.15–114.52)	0.67 (0.38–1.19)	0.17	0.59 (0.32–1.09)	0.09
FTO rs9939609:rs17817449							
TT	43	57.2	75.17 (54.40–101.26)	Reference	-	Reference	-
AG	27	27.3	98.81 (65.12–143.77)	1.37 (0.85–2.22)	0.18	1.79 (1.04–3.06)	0.02
AT	4	3.6	111.87 (30.48–286.42)	2.03 (0.73–5.67)	0.26	1.40 (0.46–4.28)	0.49

pY, person-years; CI, confidence interval; FTO, fat mass and obesity-associated gene; ADRB2, adrenoceptor beta 2 gene. * Adjusted HR for skin color, previous chronic diseases, and housing conditions.

4. Discussion

In a sample of 70 Brazilian pregnant women with pregestational DM, we found that the A allele carriers for rs9939609 (FTO gene) and rs1042713 (ADRB2 gene) had more than twice the risk of earlier exceeding GWG compared to TT and GG genotypes, respectively. The haplotype rs9939609:rs17817449 (AG) was also a risk factor, increasing 1.8 times in terms of the progression to excessive GWG. Time of living with DM of ≥8 years, pre-pregnancy overweight or obesity, and previous hypothyroidism were risk factors for earlier excessive GWG. However, age ≥ 32 years old was a protective factor. We found no effect of the DASH diet on the risk for progression to excessive GWG, but our results of non-association need to be interpreted with caution because of our limited statistical power.

The allele frequencies in our sample were close to the frequencies in global databases (www.ncbi.nlm.nih.gov/snp (accessed on 18 January 2022)). Common polymorphisms (>5% allele frequency) are expected to be shared across different geographical regions and populations [36]. However, the Brazilian population is highly admixed and underrepresented in genomic studies as a potential source of new phenotype-associated genetic variants [37].

The A allele for the rs9939609 polymorphism in the FTO gene was previously associated with higher BMI before and after pregnancy [38,39] but not with excessive GWG [15] in Brazilian women. Studies from the USA [12,13] and Spain [14] found a higher risk of having higher GWG among A-allele carriers, contradicting the results from Turkey [40] and Mexico [41], both without association. The other evaluated polymorphisms (FTO rs17817449, ADRB2 rs1042713, and rs1042714) have not been previously investigated for GWG. The haplotype rs9939609:rs17817449 (AT) was found to increase the risk of obesity in the Brazilian adult population [11], but we identified the role of AG in the risk of progression to GWG.

The effect of the DASH diet on weight gain during pregnancy is controversial. Van Horn et al. (2018) noted that overweight and obese pregnant women (*n* = 280, EUA) gained less weight and had less excessive GWG using the DASH diet than by using a control diet [42], whereas Fulay et al. (2018) reported that high adherence to the DASH diet was associated with more weight gain during pregnancy in obese women (*n* = 1760, EUA) [43].

Genetics may partially explain the interindividual variation in body weight in response to nutritional intervention [44]; thus, it was hypothesized that the FTO and ADRB2 polymorphisms could modify the effect of diet on GWG. We found a marginal association of the FTO polymorphisms on the GWG according to the type of diet: women with the AA genotype for rs9939609 and women with the GG genotype for rs17817449 had higher GWG in the traditional diet group. This result could represent some benefit of the DASH diet on limiting GWG for women with these genotypes, but it was not confirmed in the analysis adjusted for the main confounders, as we found no effect of diet on the risk for progression to excessive GWG in our sample.

Martins et al. (2018) reported that the A allele for rs9939609 was associated with an increase in the total energy intake and increase in the percentage of energy from ultra-processed foods during pregnancy in a cohort of Brazilian women [45]. In our study, we calculated the individualized meal plan for all participants in both groups, considering the appropriate GWG, and we found similar high adherence to diet in the groups (40%). Indeed, the evaluation of dietary intake in details deserves further analyses to clarify if the genetic polymorphisms affect the GWG by dietary characteristics other than the dietary pattern (traditional or DASH), such as the level of food processing, for example.

Pregestational overweight and obesity were risk factors for progression to excessive GWG in our sample. This result agrees with the study by Brandão et al. (2021), which involved a large cohort of healthy Brazilian women and found that excessive GWG was observed in 30.1%, 30.7%, 56.4%, and 46.2% of underweight, normal weight, overweight, and obese women, respectively [2]. According to the IOM guidelines, GWG recommendations decrease when BMI increases. Thus, obese women should gain less weight than overweight and normal weight women, but the guidelines do not provide specific recommendations for women with pregestational DM [6].

In this context, Siegel et al. (2015) found no difference between BMI classes to gain less, within, or above the IOM recommendations in a sample of women with pregestational DM but noticed a higher risk for macrosomia (aOR 4.02; CI 95% 1.16–13.9) and large-for-gestational-age infants (aOR 3.08; CI 95% 1.13–8.39) in women who gained excessive weight compared to women who gained weight within the recommended amounts, even after adjusting for pregestational BMI [46]. The results from the study by Egan et al. (2014) were similar, reporting that excessive GWG in women with pregestational DM was a risk factor for macrosomia (aOR 3.58; CI 95% 1.77–7.24) and large-for-gestational-age infants (aOR 3.97; CI 95% 1.85–8.53), but they found more women with overweight or obesity presenting with excessive GWG than non-excessive GWG (44% vs. 27% for overweight and 37% vs. 25% for obesity; $p < 0.01$) [3].

We found that the number of years living with DM was a risk factor for progression to excessive GWG, but older age (≥ 32 years) was a protective factor, which appears controversial. The studies by Egan (2014) and Siegel (2015) did not find any association between age and excessive GWG [3,46], but in a cohort of 8184 healthy Brazilian women, the GWG decreased as the age increased [2].

A longer time of living with DM is expected in women with type 1 DM, who usually have lower pregestational BMI compared to those with type 2 DM [47]. Given our results for the effect of pregestational BMI on excessive GWG, it seems contradictory. However, the type of DM was not a risk factor for earlier excessive GWG in our sample. Therefore, we suggest that longer years of living with DM may impact the metabolic and behavioral factors influencing GWG not covered in the present study.

Only one participant had yellow skin. This woman was overweight before pregnancy and had the highest GWG in our sample (28.2 kg). Therefore, even though we had found the yellow color of the skin to be a risk factor for progression to excessive GWG, we considered that it cannot be properly interpreted or discussed, as it was an isolated case with a very wide confidence interval. Three women who had excessive GWG in our sample reported the color of the skin as unknown.

A meta-analysis comparing the prevalence of excessive GWG among racial/ethnic groups found that White women were more likely to exceed the IOM guidelines than their Asian and Hispanic counterparts, but White and Black women had a similar prevalence of excessive GWG [48]. Differences in the GWG regarding the color of the skin are often related to socioeconomic discrepancies [48]. We found a marginal effect of inadequate housing conditions on the risk of earlier excessive GWG, but it was not statistically significant.

Of the nine women with hypothyroidism included in our sample, eight had excessive GWG, with a risk more than four times higher than that of women without hypothyroidism (aHR 4.37, CI 95% 1.62–11.77; $p = 0.00$). Collares et al. (2017) found that higher maternal TSH and lower free T4 levels in early pregnancy were associated with a higher GWG [49]. Hypothyroidism is a common endocrine disorder that occurs during pregnancy [50]. In our sample, all women diagnosed with hypothyroidism were treated with oral repositioning of the T4 hormone and had adequate hormone levels at the time of inclusion in the study; however, monitoring adherence to treatment and hormone levels during pregnancy was outside the scope of this study.

Identifying risk factors for earlier exceeding GWG and implementing a dietary intervention to mitigate it may help decrease the related adverse outcomes. The sooner the excess weight is present, the more that the metabolic effects can harm the mother and fetus [51]. Of particular interest for pregnant women with DM is that an increase in maternal fat mass during early pregnancy can increase insulin resistance and thus worsen glycemic control [52]. As excess GWG does influence offspring obesity over the short- and long-term [53], faster fist and second trimester GWG but not third trimester was associated with higher mid-childhood adiposity in a cohort of 979 mother–child pairs from whom children were evaluated between 6.6 and 10.9 years of age [54].

Our study is novel in terms of several relevant characteristics. First, we investigated candidate genetic risk factors for progression to excessive GWG, and we did not find previous studies with this objective. Second, we investigated the influence of obesity-related polymorphisms in Brazilian women with pregestational diabetes since studies enrolling Brazilian pregnant women in this field are scarce and were not designed for women with DM. Additionally, women were administered two distinct types of diets, and we noticed that it had no effect on the risk of progression to excessive GWG in our sample.

However, this study had some limitations. First, we had a limited sample size to include in these analyses because the clinical trial was originally designed to analyze the effect of the two types of diets on perinatal outcomes without making use of the nutrigenetics approach. Given the increasing evidence regarding the effects of genetic characteristics and gene-diet interactions on BMI and obesity predisposition, we considered that it should gain more attention in the field of maternal and child nutrition. Therefore, we believe that this study will contribute to paving this way.

Furthermore, we had to make adaptations to maintain the study when the COVID-19 pandemic began in 2020. We used telemedicine to complete the follow-up of six women (8.6% of the sample) who were already enrolled in the study at the beginning of the pandemic quarantine. The same study protocol was used for the present visits. Prenatal visits to the physicians were maintained at the local level of the study, maintaining the measurements of weight at each visit. We also asked the participants to send a photograph of the prenatal card containing this information using a popular free smartphone application. Once the pandemic quarantine began, we did not include more participants in the study.

5. Conclusions

In this study, we investigated obesity-related polymorphisms in FTO and ADRB2 genes as candidate genetic risk factors for excessive GWG in pregnant women with pregestational DM using traditional or DASH diets.

Regardless the type of diet, the AT carriers of rs9939609 (FTO gene) had more than twice the risk of earlier exceeding GWG compared to the TT genotype, and the AA carriers of rs1042713 (ADRB2 gene) had almost four times higher risk than the GG carriers. The frequencies of these genotypes in our study population were 48.6% and 11.4%, respectively.

We found no effect of the genotypes of rs17817449 (FTO gene) and rs1042714 (ADRB2 gene) on the risk of progression to excessive GWG; however, the AG carriers for FTO haplotype rs9939609:rs17817449 had almost twice the risk of earlier exceeding GWG compared to TT carriers. Non-genetic characteristics associated with the risk of progression to GWG were time living with DM ≥ 8 years, pre-pregnancy overweight or obesity, and previous hypothyroidism. In contrast, age ≥ 32 years old was a protective factor.

Identifying women at a higher risk for exceeding GWG earlier may help improve nutritional interventions to mitigate this risk. The next step in advancing personalized nutrition is to understand which diet patterns may protect these women against excessive GWG and to investigate other genes and potential gene-diet-environment interactions with effects on GWG.

Supplementary Materials: The following supporting information can be downloaded at: https://www.mdpi.com/article/10.3390/nu14051050/s1, Table S1: Comparison of gestational weight gain (kg) between diet groups according to pregestational BMI (Rio de Janeiro/Brazil, 2016–2020); Figure S1: Gestational weight gain according to genotypes and dietary patterns.

Author Contributions: Conceptualization, K.d.S., E.L.R. and C.S.; data curation, K.d.S., G.P.B. and L.B.G.d.S.; formal analysis, K.d.S and M.R.-A.; funding acquisition, E.L.R. and C.S.; investigation, K.d.S., A.C.P.d.F., G.P.B., L.B.G.d.S. and V.M.Z.; project administration, C.S.; writing—original draft, K.d.S.; writing—review and editing, E.L.R., J.A.M., and C.S. All authors have read and agreed to the published version of the manuscript.

Funding: This research received financial support from the Conselho Nacional de Desenvolvimento Científico e Tecnológico–CNPq (National Council for Scientific and Technological Development, grant number: 409032/2016-6), the Fundação Carlos Chagas Filho de Amparo à Pesquisa do Estado do Rio de Janeiro—FAPERJ (Carlos Chagas Filho Foundation to Research in the State of Rio de Janeiro, grant numbers: E-26/202.972/2016-6 and E-26/201.193/2021), and the Coordenação de Aperfeiçoamento de Pessoal de Nível Superior–CAPES–Brasil (Coordination for the Improvement of Higher Education Personnel). This study was financed in part by the Coordenação de Aperfeiçoamento de Pessoal de Nível Superior-Brasil (CAPES)—Finance Code 001.

Institutional Review Board Statement: The study was conducted in accordance with the Declaration of Helsinki and approved by the Ethics Committee of Maternidade Escola da UFRJ (CAAE–46913115.0.0000.5275; 15 July 2015). The study was registered in the Brazilian Registry of Clinical Trials (RBR-4tbgv6).

Informed Consent Statement: Informed consent was obtained from all subjects involved in the study.

Acknowledgments: Lenita Zajdenverg, Marcus Miranda, Karina Bilda de Castro Rezende, Rita Bornia, Joffre Amin Jr., and Jorge Rezende Filho for their support during the study.

Conflicts of Interest: The authors declare no conflict of interest. The funders had no role in the design of the study; in the collection, analyses, or interpretation of data; in the writing of the manuscript, or in the decision to publish the results.

References

1. Goldstein, R.F.; Abell, S.K.; Ranasinha, S.; Misso, M.; Boyle, J.A.; Black, M.H.; Li, N.; Hu, G.; Corrado, F.; Rode, L.; et al. Association of gestational weight gain with maternal and infant outcomes: A systematic review and meta-analysis. *J. Am. Med. Assoc.* **2017**, *317*, 2207–2225. [CrossRef]
2. Brandão, T.; de Carvalho Padilha, P.; de Barros, D.C.; Dos Santos, K.; Nogueira da Gama, S.G.; Leal, M.D.C.; da Silva Araújo, R.G.P.; Esteves Pereira, A.P.; Saunders, C. Gestational weight gain adequacy for favourable obstetric and neonatal outcomes: A nationwide hospital-based cohort gestational weight gain for favourable obstetric and neonatal outcomes. *Clin. Nutr. ESPEN* **2021**, *45*, 374–380. [CrossRef]
3. Egan, A.M.; Dennedy, M.C.; Al-Ramli, W.; Heerey, A.; Avalos, G.; Dunne, F. ATLANTIC-DIP: Excessive gestational weight gain and pregnancy outcomes in women with gestational or pregestational diabetes mellitus. *J. Clin. Endocrinol. Metab.* **2014**, *99*, 212–219. [CrossRef] [PubMed]
4. Gualdani, E.; Di Cianni, G.; Seghieri, M.; Francesconi, P.; Seghieri, G. Pregnancy outcomes and maternal characteristics in women with pregestational and gestational diabetes: A retrospective study on 206,917 singleton live births. *Acta Diabetol.* **2021**, *58*, 1169–1176. [CrossRef] [PubMed]
5. McDowell, M.; Cain, M.A.; Brumley, J. Excessive Gestational Weight Gain. *J. Midwifery Women's Heal.* **2018**, *64*, 46–54. [CrossRef]
6. Institute of Medicine. *Weight Gain during Pregnancy: Reexamining the Guidelines*; The National Academies Press: Washington, DC, USA, 2009.
7. Institute of Medicine. *Implementing Guidelines on Weight Gain and Pregnancy*; The National Academies Press: Washington, DC, USA, 2013.
8. Warrington, N.M.; Richmond, R.; Fenstra, B.; Myhre, R.; Gaillard, R.; Paternoster, L.; Wang, C.A.; Beaumont, R.N.; Das, S.; Murcia, M.; et al. Maternal and fetal genetic contribution to gestational weight gain. *Int. J. Obes.* **2018**, *42*, 775–784. [CrossRef] [PubMed]
9. Maugeri, A.; Magnano San Lio, R.; La Rosa, M.C.; Giunta, G.; Panella, M.; Cianci, A.; Caruso, M.A.T.; Agodi, A.; Barchitta, M. The Relationship between Telomere Length and Gestational Weight Gain: Findings from the Mamma & Bambino Cohort. *Biomedicines* **2021**, *10*, 67. [CrossRef]
10. Loos, R.J.; Yeo, G.S. The bigger picture of FTO: The first GWAS-identified obesity gene. *Nat. Rev. Endocrinol.* **2014**, *10*, 51–61. [CrossRef]
11. Fonseca, A.C.P.D.; Marchesini, B.; Zembrzuski, V.M.; Voigt, D.D.; Ramos, V.G.; Carneiro, J.R.I.; Nogueira Neto, J.F.; Cabello, G.M.K.; Cabello, P.H. Genetic variants in the fat mass and obesity-associated (FTO) gene confer risk for extreme obesity and modulate adiposity in a Brazilian population. *Genet Mol. Biol.* **2020**, *43*, e20180264. [CrossRef]
12. Groth, S.W.; LaLonde, A.; Wu, T.; Fernandez, I.D. Obesity candidate genes, gestational weight gain, and body weight changes in pregnant women. *Nutrition* **2018**, *48*, 61–66. [CrossRef]
13. Groth, S.W.; Morrison-Beedy, D. GNB3 and FTO Polymorphisms and Pregnancy Weight Gain in Black Women. *Biol. Res. Nurs.* **2014**, *17*, 405–412. [CrossRef] [PubMed]
14. Gesteiro, E.; Sánchez-Muniz, F.J.; Ortega-Azorín, C.; Guillén, M.; Corella, D.; Bastida, S. Maternal and neonatal FTO rs9939609 polymorphism affect insulin sensitivity markers and lipoprotein profile at birth in appropriate-for-gestational-age term neonates. *J. Physiol. Biochem.* **2016**, *72*, 169–181. [CrossRef] [PubMed]
15. Martins, M.C.; Trujillo, J.; Farias, D.R.; Struchiner, C.J.; Kac, G. Association of the FTO (rs9939609) and MC4R (rs17782313) gene polymorphisms with maternal body weight during pregnancy. *Nutrition* **2016**, *32*, 1223–1230. [CrossRef]

16. Al-Ogaidi, S.O.; Abdulsattar, S.; Al-dulaimi, M. FTO rs17817449 Gene Polymorphism as a Predictor for Maternal Obesity in Iraqi Pregnant Women. *Indian J. Public Heal. Res. Dev.* **2019**, *10*, 678–683. [CrossRef]
17. Steemburgo, T.; Azevedo, M.J.; Martínez, J.A. Interação entre gene e nutriente e sua associação à obesidade e ao diabetes melito [Gene-nutrient interaction and its association with obesity and diabetes mellitus]. *Arq. Bras. de Endocrinol. Metabol.* **2009**, *53*, 497–508. (In Portuguese) [CrossRef]
18. Zhang, H.; Wu, J.; Yu, L. Association of Gln27Glu and Arg16Gly polymorphisms in Beta2-adrenergic receptor gene with obesity susceptibility: A meta-analysis. *PLoS ONE* **2014**, *9*, e100489. [CrossRef]
19. Maugeri, A.; Barchitta, M.; Favara, G.; La Rosa, M.C.; La Mastra, C.; Magnano San Lio, R.; Agodi, A. Maternal Dietary Patterns Are Associated with Pre-Pregnancy Body Mass Index and Gestational Weight Gain: Results from the "Mamma & Bambino". Cohort. *Nutr.* **2019**, *11*, 1308. [CrossRef]
20. American Diabetes Association. 14. Management of Diabetes in Pregnancy: Standards of Medical Care in Diabetes—2021. *Diabetes Care* **2020**, *44*, S200–S210. [CrossRef]
21. Svetkey, L.P.; Sacks, F.M.; Obarzanek, E.; Vollmer, W.M.; Appel, L.J.; Lin, P.H.; Karanja, N.M.; Harsha, D.W.; Bray, G.A.; Aickin, M.; et al. The DASH Diet, Sodium Intake and Blood Pressure Trial (DASH-sodium): Rationale and design. DASH-Sodium Collaborative Research Group. *J. Am. Diet. Assoc.* **1999**, *99*, S96–S104. [CrossRef]
22. Asemi, Z.; Tabassi, Z.; Samimi, M.; Fahiminejad, T.; Esmaillzadeh, A. Favourable effects of the Dietary Approaches to Stop Hypertension diet on glucose tolerance and lipid profiles in gestational diabetes: A randomised clinical trial. *Br. J. Nutr.* **2012**, *109*, 2024–2030. [CrossRef]
23. Li, S.; Gan, Y.; Chen, M.; Wang, M.; Wang, X.; Santos, H.O.; Okunade, K.; Kathirgamathamby, V. Effects of the Dietary Approaches to Stop Hypertension (DASH) on Pregnancy/Neonatal Outcomes and Maternal Glycemic Control: A Systematic Review and Meta-analysis of Randomized Clinical Trials. *Complement. Ther. Med.* **2020**, *54*, 102551. [CrossRef]
24. Hosseini-Esfahani, F.; Koochakpoor, G.; Daneshpour, M.S.; Sedaghati-Khayat, B.; Mirmiran, P.; Azizi, F. Mediterranean Dietary Pattern Adherence Modify the Association between FTO Genetic Variations and Obesity Phenotypes. *Nutrients* **2017**, *9*, 1064. [CrossRef]
25. Hosseini-Esfahani, F.; Koochakpoor, G.; Mirmiran, P.; Daneshpour, M.S.; Azizi, F. Dietary patterns modify the association between fat mass and obesity-associated genetic variants and changes in obesity phenotypes. *Br. J. Nutr.* **2019**, *121*, 1247–1254. [CrossRef]
26. Martínez, J.A.; Corbalán, M.S.; Sánchez-Villegas, A.; Forga, L.; Marti, A.; Martínez-González, M.A. Obesity risk is associated with carbohydrate intake in women carrying the Gln27Glu beta2-adrenoceptor polymorphism. *J. Nutr.* **2003**, *133*, 2549–2554. [CrossRef] [PubMed]
27. Ferguson, L.R.; De Caterina, R.; Görman, U.; Allayee, H.; Kohlmeier, M.; Prasad, C.; Choi, M.S.; Curi, R.; de Luis, D.A.; Gil, Á.; et al. Guide and Position of the International Society of Nutrigenetics/Nutrigenomics on Personalised Nutrition: Part 1-Fields of Precision Nutrition. *J. Nutr. Nutr.* **2016**, *9*, 12–27. [CrossRef]
28. Saunders, C.; Moreira, T.M.; Belfort, G.P.; da Silva, C.F.M.; dos Santos, K.; da Silva, L.B.G.; Scancetti, L.B.; Fagherazzi, S.; Pereira, A.F.; Rosado, E.L.; et al. Procedimentos metodológicos para elaboração de plano alimentar adaptado baseado na dieta DASH para gestantes com diabetes mellitus. *BJD* **2021**, *7*, 116769–116788. [CrossRef]
29. Della Líbera, B.; Ribeiro Baião, M.; de Souza Santos, M.M.; Padilha, P.; Dutra Alves, P.; Saunders, C. Adherence of pregnant women to dietary counseling and adequacy of total gestational weight gain. *Nutr. Hosp.* **2011**, *26*, 79–85.
30. Carrilho, T.R.B.; Rasmussen, K.; Farias, D.R.; Freitas Costa, N.C.; Araújo Batalha, M.; Reichenheim, M.E.; Ohuma, E.O.; Hutcheon, J.A.; Kac, G.; Brazilian Maternal and Child Nutrition Consortium. Agreement between self-reported pre-pregnancy weight and measured first-trimester weight in Brazilian women. *BMC Pregnancy Childbirth* **2020**, *20*, 734. [CrossRef]
31. World Health Organization (WHO). *Physical Status: The Use and Interpretation of Anthropometry*; Report of a WHO Expert Committee; WHO: Geneva, Switzerland, 1995; Volume 452, pp. 1–542.
32. Aidar, M.; Line, S.R.P. A simple and cost-effective protocol for DNA isolation from buccal epithelial cells. *Braz. Dent. J.* **2007**, *18*, 148–152. [CrossRef]
33. Matsudo, S.; Araújo, T.; Matsudo, V.; Andrade, D.; Andrade, E.; Oliveira, L.C.; Braggion, G. Questionário Internacional de Atividade Física (IPAQ): Estudo de validade e reprodutibilidade no Brasil. *RBAFS* **2001**, *6*, 5–18.
34. Núcleo de Estudos e Pesquisas em Alimentação (NEPA). Tabela Brasileira de Composição de Alimentos (TACO/NEPA-Unicamp). Available online: http://www.nepa.unicamp.br/taco/tabela.php?ativo=tabela (accessed on 25 February 2022).
35. United States Department of Agriculture. USDA National Nutrient Database for Standard Reference. Available online: https://fdc.nal.usda.gov/ (accessed on 25 February 2022).
36. Biddanda, A.; Rice, D.P.; Novembre, J. A variant-centric perspective on geographic patterns of human allele frequency variation. *Elife* **2020**, *9*, e60107. [CrossRef] [PubMed]
37. Scliar, M.O.; Sant'Anna, H.P.; Santolalla, M.L.; Leal, T.P.; Araújo, N.M.; Alvim, I.; Borda, V.; Magalhães, W.C.S.; Gouveia, M.H.; Lyra, R.; et al. Admixture/fine-mapping in Brazilians reveals a West African associated potential regulatory variant (rs114066381) with a strong female-specific effect on body mass and fat mass indexes. *Int. J. Obes.* **2021**, *45*, 1017–1029. [CrossRef] [PubMed]
38. Kroll, C.; Farias, D.R.; Carrilho, T.R.B.; Kac, G.; Mastroeni, M.F. Association of ADIPOQ-rs2241766 and FTO-rs9939609 genetic variants with body mass index trajectory in women of reproductive age over 6 years of follow-up: The PREDI study. *Eur. J. Clin. Nutr.* **2021**, *76*, 159–172. [CrossRef] [PubMed]

39. Kroll, C.; de França, P.H.C.; Mastroeni, M.F. Association between FTO gene polymorphism and excess body weight in women from before to after pregnancy: A cohort study. *Am. J. Hum. Biol.* **2018**, *30*, e23164. [CrossRef]
40. Beysel, S.; Eyerci, N.; Ulubay, M.; Caliskan, M.; Kizilgul, M.; Hafızoğlu, M.; Cakal, E. Maternal genetic contribution to pre-pregnancy obesity, gestational weight gain, and gestational diabetes mellitus. *Diabetol. Metab. Syndr.* **2019**, *11*, 37. [CrossRef] [PubMed]
41. Saucedo, R.; Valencia, J.; Gutierrez, C.; Basurto, L.; Hernandez, M.; Puello, E.; Rico, G.; Vega, G.; Zarate, A. Gene variants in the FTO gene are associated with adiponectin and TNF-alpha levels in gestational diabetes mellitus. *Diabetol. Metab. Syndr.* **2017**, *9*, 32. [CrossRef]
42. Van Horn, L.; Peaceman, A.; Kwasny, M.; Vincent, E.; Fought, A.; Josefson, J.; Spring, B.; Neff, L.M.; Gernhofer, N. Dietary Approaches to Stop Hypertension Diet and Activity to Limit Gestational Weight: Maternal Offspring Metabolics Family Intervention Trial, a Technology Enhanced Randomized Trial. *Am. J. Prev. Med.* **2018**, *55*, 603–614. [CrossRef]
43. Fulay, A.P.; Rifas-Shiman, S.L.; Oken, E.; Perng, W. Associations of the dietary approaches to stop hypertension (DASH) diet with pregnancy complications in Project Viva. *Eur. J. Clin. Nutr.* **2018**, *72*, 1385–1395. [CrossRef]
44. Camp, K.M.; Trujillo, E. Position of the Academy of Nutrition and Dietetics: Nutritional genomics. *J. Acad. Nutr. Diet.* **2014**, *114*, 299–312. [CrossRef]
45. Martins, M.C.; Trujillo, J.; Freitas-Vilela, A.A.; Farias, D.R.; Rosado, E.L.; Struchiner, C.J.; Kac, G. Associations between obesity candidate gene polymorphisms (fat mass and obesity-associated (FTO), melanocortin-4 receptor (MC4R), leptin (LEP) and leptin receptor (LEPR)) and dietary intake in pregnant women. *Br. J. Nutr.* **2018**, *120*, 454–463. [CrossRef]
46. Siegel, A.M.; Tita, A.; Biggio, J.R.; Harper, L.M. Evaluating gestational weight gain recommendations in pregestational diabetes. *Am. J. Obstet. Gynecol.* **2015**, *213*, 563.e1–563.e5. [CrossRef] [PubMed]
47. Alessi, J.; Wiegand, D.M.; Hirakata, V.N.; Oppermann, M.L.R.; Reichelt, A.J. Temporal changes in characteristics and outcomes among pregnant women with pre-gestational diabetes. *Int. J. Gynecol. Obstet.* **2018**, *143*, 59–65. [CrossRef] [PubMed]
48. Denize, K.M.; Acharya, N.; Prince, S.A.; da Silva, D.F.; Harvey, A.L.J.; Ferraro, Z.M.; Adamo, K.B. Addressing cultural, racial and ethnic discrepancies in guideline discordant gestational weight gain: A systematic review and meta-analysis. *PeerJ* **2018**, *6*, e5407. [CrossRef] [PubMed]
49. Collares, F.M.; Korevaar, T.I.M.; Hofman, A.; Steegers, E.A.P.; Peeters, R.P.; Jaddoe, V.W.V.; Gaillard, R. Maternal thyroid function, prepregnancy obesity and gestational weight gain-The Generation R Study: A prospective cohort study. *Clin. Endocrinol.* **2017**, *87*, 799–806. [CrossRef] [PubMed]
50. Alexander, E.K.; Pearce, E.N.; Brent, G.A.; Brown, R.S.; Chen, H.; Dosiou, C.; Grobman, W.A.; Laurberg, P.; Lazarus, J.H.; Mandel, S.J.; et al. 2017 Guidelines of the American Thyroid Association for the Diagnosis and Management of Thyroid Disease During Pregnancy and the Postpartum. *Thyroid* **2017**, *27*, 315–389. [CrossRef]
51. Cheney, K.; Berkemeier, S.; Sim, K.A.; Gordon, A.; Black, K. Prevalence and predictors of early gestational weight gain associated with obesity risk in a diverse Australian antenatal population: A cross-sectional study. *BMC Pregnancy Childbirth* **2017**, *17*, 296. [CrossRef] [PubMed]
52. Herring, S.J.; Oken, E.; Rifas-Shiman, S.L.; Rich-Edwards, J.W.; Stuebe, A.M.; Kleinman, K.P.; Gillman, M.W. Weight gain in pregnancy and risk of maternal hyperglycemia. *Am. J. Obstet. Gynecol.* **2009**, *201*, 61.e1–61.e7. [CrossRef]
53. Mamun, A.A.; Mannan, M.; Doi, S.A. Gestational weight gain in relation to offspring obesity over the life course: A systematic review and bias-adjusted meta-analysis. *Obes. Rev.* **2013**, *15*, 338–347. [CrossRef]
54. Hivert, M.F.; Rifas-Shiman, S.L.; Gillman, M.W.; Oken, E. Greater early and mid-pregnancy gestational weight gains are associated with excess adiposity in mid-childhood. *Obesity* **2016**, *24*, 1546–1553. [CrossRef]

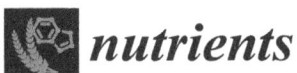

Article

Genetic Variants in Folate and Cobalamin Metabolism-Related Genes in Pregnant Women of a Homogeneous Spanish Population: The Need for Revisiting the Current Vitamin Supplementation Strategies

Gemma Rodriguez-Carnero [1,2,†], Paula M. Lorenzo [1,3,†], Ana Canton-Blanco [1,2], Leire Mendizabal [4], Maddi Arregi [4], Mirella Zulueta [4], Laureano Simon [4], Manuel Macia-Cortiñas [5], Felipe F. Casanueva [3,6] and Ana B. Crujeiras [1,3,*]

1. Epigenomics in Endocrinology and Nutrition Group, Epigenomics Unit, Instituto de Investigacion Sanitaria de Santiago de Compostela (IDIS), Complejo Hospitalario Universitario de Santiago de Compostela (CHUS/SERGAS), 15706 Santiago de Compostela, Spain; maria.gemma.rodriguez.carnero@sergas.es (G.R.-C.); paula.marino.lorenzo@sergas.es (P.M.L.); ana.canton.blanco@sergas.es (A.C.-B.)
2. Endocrinology and Nutrition Division, Complejo Hospitalario Universitario de Santiago de Compostela (CHUS/SERGAS), 15706 Santiago de Compostela, Spain
3. CIBER Fisiopatologia de la Obesidad y Nutricion (CIBERobn), 28029 Madrid, Spain; felipe.casanueva@usc.es
4. Patia Europe, 20009 San Sebastian, Spain; lmendizabal@patiadiabetes.com (L.M.); marregui@patiadiabetes.com (M.A.); mzulueta@patiadiabetes.com (M.Z.); lsimon@patiadiabetes.com (L.S.)
5. Gynecology and Obstetrics Division, Complejo Hospitalario Universitario de Santiago de Compostela (CHUS/SERGAS), 15706 Santiago de Compostela, Spain; manuel.macia.cortinas@sergas.es
6. Molecular and Cellular Endocrinology Group, Instituto de Investigacion Sanitaria de Santiago de Compostela (IDIS), Complejo Hospitalario Universitario de Santiago de Compostela (CHUS/SERGAS), Santiago de Compostela University (USC), 15706 Santiago de Compostela, Spain
* Correspondence: ana.belen.crujeiras.martinez@sergas.es or anabelencrujeiras@hotmail.com; Tel.: +34-981955710
† These authors contributed equally to this work.

Abstract: Polymorphisms of genes involved in the metabolism and transport of folate and cobalamin could play relevant roles in pregnancy outcomes. This study assessed the prevalence of genetic polymorphisms of folate and cobalamin metabolism-related genes such as MTHFR, MTR, CUBN, and SLC19A1 in pregnant women of a homogeneous Spanish population according to conception, pregnancy, delivery, and newborns complications. This study was conducted on 149 nulliparous women with singleton pregnancies. Sociodemographic and obstetrics variables were recorded, and all patients were genotyped in the MTHFR, MTR, CUBN, and SLC10A1 polymorphisms. The distribution of genotypes detected in this cohort was similar to the population distribution reported in Europe, highlighting that more than 50% of women were carriers of risk alleles of the studied genes. In women with the MTHFR risk allele, there was a statistically significant higher frequency of assisted fertilisation and a higher frequency of preeclampsia and preterm birth. Moreover, CUBN (rs1801222) polymorphism carriers showed a statistically significantly lower frequency of complications during delivery. In conclusion, the prevalence of genetic variants related to folic acid and vitamin B12 metabolic genes in pregnant women is related to mother and neonatal outcomes. Knowing the prevalence of these polymorphisms may lead to a personalised prescription of vitamin intake.

Keywords: vitamin B9; vitamin B12; pregnancy; newborn; polymorphism; one-carbon metabolism; MTHFR; MTR; CUBN; SLC10A1

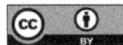

1. Introduction

Pregnancy is a critical period during which a mother's nutrition and lifestyle have a decisive influence on maternal and child outcomes. Multiple factors can affect pregnancy health, including maternal sociodemographic characteristics, environmental exposures, maternal nutrition, age, obesity, lifestyle, and socioeconomic status, as well as genetic background and gene–environment interactions [1–3].

The maternal diet and nutritional stores provide nutrients for the developing embryo and foetus [4–8]. Among nutrients, folic acid (vitamin B9) and cobalamin (vitamin B12) stand out for their role in foetal growth and prevention of neural tube defects, through their role as essential co-factors in the one-carbon metabolism pathway [9–11]. Moreover, deficiencies in these vitamins were also associated with important impacts on the health of mothers such as preeclampsia [12], gestational diabetes [13], or maternal neurocognitive symptoms [14]. Considering this issue, supplementation with folic acid was particularly recommended by the World Health Organisation (WHO) in order to prevent pregnancy outcomes [15]. However, maternal vitamin levels depend on dietary and supplement intake but also are influenced by genetic polymorphisms in the gene coding for enzymes involved in vitamin metabolism and transport, which may lead to changes in their catalytic activity. Functional polymorphisms of genes encoding enzymes involved in one-carbon metabolism can cause disturbances in B9 and B12 vitamin status due to a reduction in enzyme activity [16–19]. Polymorphisms of genes involved in the metabolism and transport of these vitamins were associated with disturbances in the health of mother and child [20].

In this regard, determining genetic variants in folate and cobalamin metabolism-related genes in pregnant women can lead to personalised treatment with higher amounts of folic acid and cobalamin for the sake of improving pregnancy and neonatal health outcomes. Therefore, the aim of the present study was to assess the prevalence of the common target genetic polymorphisms of folate and cobalamin metabolism-related genes in the literature such as methylenetetrahydrofolate reductase (*MTHFR*), methionine synthase (*MTR*), cubilin (*CUBN*), and *SLC19A1* (commonly known as reduced folate carrier (RFC1)) in pregnant women of a homogeneous Spanish population according to conception, pregnancy, delivery, and newborn complications.

2. Patients and Methods

2.1. Study Population and Design

This study was conducted on 149 nulliparous women with singleton pregnancies. Pregnant women were recruited in the Endocrinology and Obstetrics departments of the "Complejo Hospitalario Universitario de Santiago de Compostela (CHUS)" in Santiago de Compostela, Galicia (northeastern Spain) from September 2018 to February 2020. Women were recruited between 24 and 28 weeks of pregnancy and then followed up throughout the pregnancy to delivery. The inclusion criteria were an age of 16 years old or older, singleton pregnancy, lack of any chronic disease or being under medical treatment, absence of any language barrier, and correct monitoring of pregnancy and delivery in our centre.

2.2. Sociodemographic and Obstetrics Variables

At the time of recruitment, the following data were collected: age; ethnicity; maternal lifestyles (tobacco smoking, alcohol consumption, or drug abuse) during the pregnancy; singleton or multiple pregnancies; previous miscarriages, abortions, or ectopic pregnancies; use of assisted reproductive technologies and medical history (hypertension, diabetes); maternal height; and self-reported pre-pregnancy weight and weight at week 36 (or last weight in the case of preterm delivery) of pregnancy, which allowed for calculation of weight gain during pregnancy and body mass index pre-pregnancy.

2.3. Vitamin B12 and Folic Acid Supplementation Use

Information on vitamin supplementation was obtained by reviewing electronic medical records and asking pregnant women from recruitment to delivery. Information on supplement intake included brand name, dosage per day, and the start and end dates of consumption. This information was used to determine supplemental vitamin B12 and folate doses per day for each woman.

2.4. Maternal and Neonatal Outcomes and Definitions

Participants were followed prospectively from recruitment until delivery. Maternal and neonatal outcomes were collected from electronic medical records.

Maternal outcomes such as gestational diabetes mellitus (GDM), gestational hypertension (GHT), and preeclampsia were obtained. GDM was defined as diabetes diagnosed in the second or third trimester of pregnancy that was not clearly overt diabetes prior to gestation and was diagnosed according to our Hospital's protocol and the one-step approach [21]. GHT was defined as blood pressure $\geq 140/90$ mmHg arising after 20-week gestation, without any other feature of the multisystem disorder that resolves within 3 months postpartum [22]. PE was defined as GHT with ≥ 1 proteinuria/abnormal renal or liver function tests or platelet count/symptoms and signs consistent with end-organ damage of preeclampsia [22].

Gestational age and anthropometric measurements (weight, height, head circumference, and chest circumference) at birth were obtained from electronic medical records. Weight index was calculated as the ratio of birth weight (grams) to height (cm^3). Size for gestational age was estimated based on Carrascosa et al. (2004) [23], using neonatal gestational age at delivery, anthropometric measurements (AM: weight, height, and head circumference), and sex. Newborns were categorised into three groups: small for gestational age (SGA) (AM less than 10th percentile for gestational age); appropriate for gestational age (AGA) (AM 10th to 90th percentile for gestational age, which was the reference group); and large for gestational age (LGA) (AM greater than 90th percentile for gestational age). For birth weight, newborns were considered to be LGA if their birth weight was >2.0 standard deviation (SD) or over the 90th percentile for sex and gestational age, and SGA infants were considered to have a birth weight that was <-2.0 SD or under the 10th percentile for sex and gestational age. Normal birth weight was considered for values between -2.0 and $+2.0$ SD for sex and gestational age (between the 10th and 90th percentile). Low birth weight (LBW) was defined as birth weight less than 2500 g. Macrosomia was defined as neonates whose birth weight was equal to or greater than 4000 g.

Other obstetric complications such as miscarriage, stillbirth, and neonatal death were also collected. Delivery data were obtained, with special attention to the type of delivery (spontaneous onset of labour, induced labour, instrumental delivery, and route of delivery), preterm delivery, perinatal complications, admission to intensive care unit, and hospital stay. Spontaneous preterm birth (PTB) was spontaneous preterm labour or preterm premature rupture of the membranes, resulting in birth at <37-week gestation. Uncomplicated pregnancy was defined as a pregnancy in which no antenatal medical or obstetric complication had been diagnosed, resulting in the delivery of an appropriately grown, healthy baby at ≥ 37 weeks of gestation.

2.5. Sample Collection

Participants were asked to refrain from eating, drinking, brushing teeth, and using mouthwash for at least 30 min prior to sample collection for which a buccal swab of the Puritan Medical Products PurFlock Ultra® (25-3606-U, Guilford, NC, USA) was used. Genomic DNA was extracted from the buccal swab using a MagMax DNA Multi-Sample Ultra Kit (Applied biosystems by Thermo Fisher Scientific, Waltham, MA, USA).

2.6. Genotyping

Genotyping was performed via IPLEX MassARRAY PCR using the Agena platform (Agena Bioscience, San Diego, CA, USA). IPLEX MassARRAY PCR and extension primers were designed from sequences containing each target SNP and 150 upstream and downstream bases with Assay Designer 4.0.0.2 (Agena Bioscience, San Diego, CA, USA) using the default settings. Single base extension reactions were performed on the PCR reactions with the iPLEX Gold Kit (Agena Bioscience) and 0.8 µL of the custom UEP pool. PCR reactions were dispensed onto SpectroChipArrays with a Nanodispenser (Agena Bioscience). An Agena Bioscience Compact MassArray Spectrometer was used to perform MALDI–TOF mass spectrometry according to the iPLEX Gold Application Guide. The Typer 4 software package (Agena Bioscience) was used to analyse the resulting spectra, and the composition of the target bases was determined from the mass of each extended oligo. These panels were designed in collaboration with PATIA, and genotyping was performed using the Agena platform located at the Epigenetics and Genotyping laboratory, Central Unit for Research in Medicine (UCIM), Faculty of Medicine, University of Valencia, Valencia, Spain.

2.7. Statistics Analysis

For the statistical analysis, 136 of the 149 patients were included, for whom genetic data were available. Different statistical tests were applied to examine the association between polymorphism in CUBN, MTHFR, MTR, and SLC19A1 and maternal and infant phenotypes and delivery complications. Maternal complications included preeclampsia, hypertension, and a family history of type 2 diabetes. Delivery complications included caesarean birth and induced birth. Neonatal phenotypes included macrosomia, admission to the intensive care unit, and PTB. The SNP information was decoded to numerical type depending on the presence of a reference or an alternative nucleotide of each sample. p values were computed using the chi-square test to determine whether the prevalence of genotype risk groups varied significantly depending on the phenotype or complication. $p \leq 0.05$ was considered statistically significant. All of the aforementioned statistical analyses were performed using R software (version 3.2.0).

3. Results

3.1. Baseline Characteristics

Table 1 describes the characteristics of participants in this study (n = 149), including vitamin supplementation in the first trimester and neonatal and maternal outcomes. The mean age was 34.7 ± 5.2 years old, and the mean pregestational BMI was 26.4 ± 5.50 kg/m^2; the average weight gain at final of pregnancy was 11.6 ± 5.84 kg. Spontaneous gestation was observed with a higher frequency than assisted. Delivery was spontaneous in the majority of patients. Regarding maternal complications during gestation, 62.4% had GDM, 2.0% GHT, and 3.4% preeclampsia. Regarding neonatal outcomes, the mean birth weight was 3.18 ± 0.57 kg, 7.4% were PTB, and 8.8% were admitted to intensive care.

Table 1. Characteristics of the participants in this study.

Variables	Data
N	149
Maternal age (years)	34.7 ± 5.2
Pregestational BMI (kg/m^2)	26.4 ± 5.50
GDM (%)	62.4
Socioeconomic status (% active)	80.4
Type of gestation (%)	
Spontaneous	83.9
Assisted	15.1
Weight gain (kg)	11.6 ± 5.84
Type of delivery (%)	
Vaginal	70.5
Caesarean	29.5
Induced	17.7
Spontaneous	82.3
Hospital stay (days)	3.18 ± 1.37
GHT (%)	2.0
Preeclampsia (%)	3.4

Table 1. Cont.

Variables	Data
Vitamin and mineral supplementation (%)	
Vitamin complex	81.2
Iodine and folic acid	13.4
Folic acid	5.4
Iron	55.0
Gestational week (wks)	39.2 ± 1.9
Baby weight at birth (kg)	3.18 ± 0.57
PTB (%)	7.4
Neonatal ICU income (%)	8.8
Baby sex (% women)	48.3
SGA (%)	3.4
AGA (%)	89.9
LGA (%)	6.7
Low birth weight (%)	9.4
Macrosomia (%)	6.7

Data show mean ± standard deviation or frequency (%). N, number; BMI, body mass index; GDM, gestational diabetes mellitus; GHT, gestational hypertension; PTB, preterm birth; ICU, intensive care unit; SGA, small for gestational age; AGA, appropriate for gestational age; LGA, large for gestational age.

All women received folic acid supplementation in the first trimester of pregnancy; 81.2% received a multivitamin complex that included folic acid, iodine, and B12; 13.4% received folic acid plus iodine; and 5.4% just folic acid. In addition to the supplementation with folic acid or multivitamin complex, 55.0% of women were prescribed iron supplementation.

3.2. Distribution of SNP Genotypes of Genes Related to Folate and Cobalamin Metabolism and Transport in the Study Population

The distribution of genotypes detected in women from the CHUS cohort was similar to the population distribution reported in Europe (Figure 1). It is important to highlight that 61% of the women analysed in this study carried risk alleles in the MTHFR gene, approximately 72% of women in this study carried risk alleles in the SCL19A1 gene, and risk alleles were detected in the CUBN gene in 47% of these women, while the majority of this population carried the reference allele for the MTR gene (99%).

3.3. Association between SNP Genotypes and Pregnancy Outcomes

The association between maternal SNP and neonatal and maternal outcomes is shown in Table 2. Although only 1% of women were risk genotype carriers of *MTR*, and 75% of women in this study carried risk alleles in the *SCL19A1* gene, statistically significant associations were not found between the polymorphisms analysed of these genes, nor in *CUBN* and maternal or neonatal outcomes.

In women with the *MTHFR* risk allele, there was a statistically significant higher frequency of assisted fertilization (lower frequency of spontaneous gestation). In addition, there was a higher frequency of preeclampsia and PTB in women with variation in the genotype of *MTHFR*.

When the cohort was analysed according to complications in the mother's health, neonate's health, or delivery, no association was found between genotypes and complications except for *CUBN* (rs1801222), which showed a lower frequency of complications during delivery associated with the risk allele (white bars, $p = 0.024$; Figure 2).

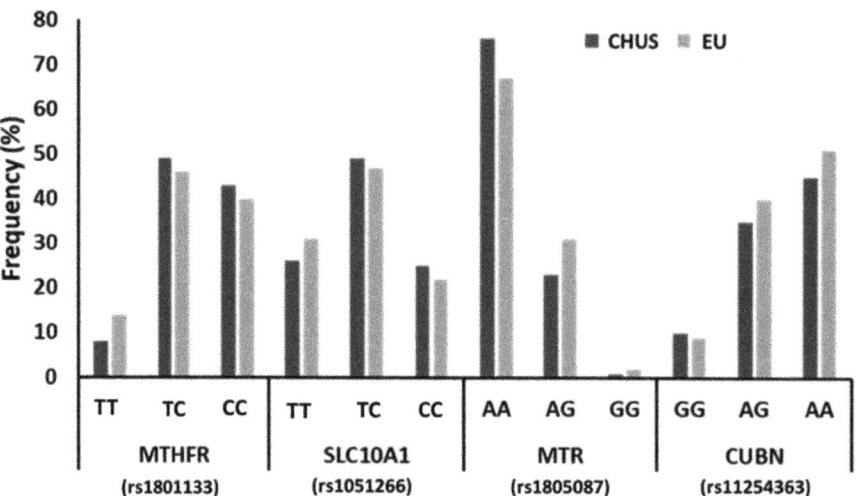

Figure 1. Prevalence of SNP genotypes of genes related to folate and cobalamin metabolism and transport in the study population (CHUS), compared with European population (EU). AA, adenine-adenine genotype; AG, adenine-guanine genotype; GG, guanine-guanine genotype; TT, thymine-thymine genotype; TG, thymine-guanine genotype; CC, cytosine-cytosine genotype; TC, thymine-cytosine genotype; MTHFR, methylenetetrahydrofolate reductase; SLC10A1, reduced folate carrier (RFC1); MTR, methionine synthase; CUBN, cubilin.

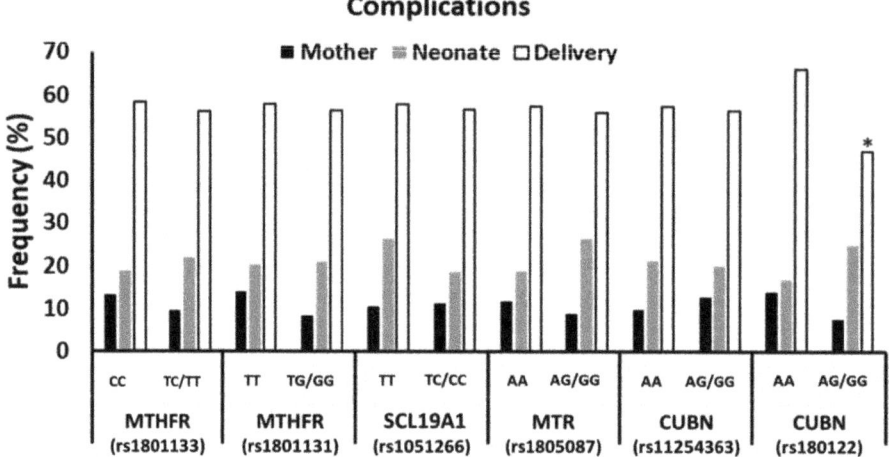

Figure 2. Association between complications in health of the mother, that of the neonate, or during delivery and SNP genotypes of genes related to folate and cobalamin metabolism and transport in the study population. (*) indicates statistically significant differences in delivery complications (white bars) between both groups of genotypes (AA vs. AG/GG). AA, adenine-adenine genotype; AG, adenine-guanine genotype; GG, guanine-guanine genotype; TT, thymine-thymine genotype; TG, thymine-guanine genotype; CC, cytosine-cytosine geno-type; TC, thymine-cytosine genotype; MTHFR, methylenetetrahydrofolate reductase; SLC10A1, reduced folate carrier (RFC1); MTR, methionine synthase; CUBN, cubilin.

Table 2. Association between pregnancy outcomes and SNP genotypes of genes related to folate and cobalamin metabolism and transport in the study population.

Prevalence (%)	SCL19A1 (rs1051266)			CUBN (rs11254363)			CUBN (rs1801222)			MTR (rs1805087)			MTHFR (rs1801133)			MTHFR (rs1801131)		
	TT	TC/CC	p Value	AA	AG/GG	p Value	AA	AG/GG	p Value	AA	AG/GG	p Value	CC	TC/TT	p Value	TT	TG/GG	p Value
Samples	28.15	71.85		59.26	40.74		52.59	47.41		74.81	25.19		39.26	60.74		47.41	52.59	
Spontaneous gestation	84.21	78.35	0.429	80.00	80.00	1.000	84.51	75.00	0.177	79.21	82.35	0.689	73.58	84.15	0.155	87.50	73.24	0.035
Assisted fertilization	7.89	18.56	0.075	15.00	16.36	0.836	11.27	20.31	0.158	16.83	11.76	0.460	20.75	12.20	0.208	9.38	21.13	0.055
Vaginal delivery	47.37	43.30	0.673	43.75	45.45	0.846	38.03	51.56	0.116	43.56	47.06	0.726	45.28	43.90	0.876	45.31	43.66	0.849
Vaginal-instrumental delivery	28.95	20.62	0.334	27.50	16.36	0.120	25.35	20.31	0.492	22.77	23.53	0.929	24.53	21.95	0.735	23.44	22.54	0.903
Caesarean	23.68	32.99	0.276	26.25	36.36	0.221	36.62	23.44	0.095	31.68	26.47	0.563	28.30	31.71	0.676	28.13	32.39	0.594
Induced delivery	18.42	15.46	0.693	16.25	16.36	0.986	19.72	12.50	0.261	15.84	17.65	0.815	18.87	14.63	0.535	20.31	12.68	0.243
Spontaneous delivery	81.58	83.51	0.798	83.75	81.82	0.777	80.28	85.94	0.390	82.18	85.29	0.672	79.25	85.37	0.380	79.69	85.92	0.350
Preeclampsia	2.63	4.12	0.698	3.75	3.64	0.977	2.82	4.69	0.625	2.97	5.88	0.567	0.00	6.10	0.000	4.69	2.82	0.625
Preterm birth	7.89	7.22	0.902	10.00	3.64	0.139	4.23	10.94	0.155	6.93	8.82	0.748	1.89	10.98	0.013	6.25	8.45	0.646
Neonatal ICU income	10.53	8.25	0.706	10.00	7.27	0.594	7.04	10.94	0.454	6.93	14.71	0.261	11.32	7.32	0.466	7.81	9.86	0.692

ICU, intensive care unit. AA, adenine-adenine genotype; AG, adenine-guanine genotype; GG, guanine-guanine genotype; TT, thymine-thymine genotype; TC, thymine-cytosine genotype; CC, cytosine-cytosine genotype; TG, thymine-guanine genotype; MTHFR, methylenetetrahydrofolate reductase; SLC10A1, reduced folate carrier (RFC1); MTR, methionine synthase; CUBN, cubilin. Numbers in bold show statistically significant differences.

4. Discussion

The present study was carried out on pregnant women from northwestern Spain, which showed diversity in the prevalence of one-carbon metabolism risk polymorphisms. Importantly, among the evaluated SNPs, those related to *MTHFR* were associated with a lower frequency of spontaneous gestation and higher frenquecy of preeclampsia, and PTB, while the *CUBN* polymorphism was associated with a lower frequency of complications during delivery. Detection of risk alleles in women may lead to personalised medicine with targeted treatment based on increased vitamin intake that can improve success in conception and maternal and foetal outcomes.

Different genetic variants have been related to vitamin deficiency. The population prevalence of most of the polymorphisms associated with altered vitamin levels is unknown. The most widely studied polymorphism of one-carbon metabolism is the *MTHFR* genotype 677 C > T (rs1801133), which is responsible for the synthesis of the *MTHFR* enzyme and whose activity is decreased in TT homozygosis (by 60%) and in CT heterozygosis (by 30%) with respect to the CC genotype [24]. The prevalence of the TT SNP, the highest risk genotype, represented between 14.2% and 19.9% [25,26] of the cases described in studies carried out in Europe. More recently, Aguilar-Lacasaña et al. (2021) showed a higher prevalence (38%) in pregnant women in southern Spain [27]. In the current study, the prevalence in pregnant women carriers of TT SNP was 57%. This alteration has great relevance because individuals with TT have lower levels of folic acid than those with CC and CT [28–30].

Several studies have shown that the homozygous TT genotype has a lower response to folic acid treatment than those with the homozygous CC genotype, suggesting that the TT genotype requires higher folic acid intake [31]. The impact of these genetic alterations on folic acid levels and their effect on different diseases [31,32] such as breast, lung, or colorectal cancer [33] is widely known. Specifically, in pregnant women, the homozygous TT genotype has been associated with an increased risk of neural tube defects [34–37], reinforcing the idea of the well-known link between folic acid deficiency during pregnancy and the risk of neural tube defects in the newborn.

In our study, all women received supplements with folic acid or folic acid and B12. In this regard, Colson et al. (2017) [38] showed that a dose of 400 mcg daily of folic acid would be sufficient to overcome the deficits resulting from these polymorphisms. However, a recent study by Aguilar-Lacasaña et al. (2021) [27] showed that, although their population had received a correct folic acid intake during gestation, the prevalence of SGA and LGA was higher in pregnant women with T or TT in relation to the hetero or homo polymorphism CC, suggesting that there must be other factors that influence these results.

In addition, different studies have shown that women with the *MTHFR* 677 TT genotype are predisposed to elevated homocysteine levels when folic acid intake is inadequate [39], endothelial damage, arterial constriction, and thrombosis [40,41], all of which can lead to placental hypoperfusion resulting in worse neonatal outcomes with PTB and LBW [42]. In our study, women with the *MTHFR* risk alleles had a higher frequency of PTB, even though they all received adequate folic acid, but no higher frequency of LBW was observed. In addition, this higher frequency of premature newborns is concomitant with a higher frequency of LBW, which is a frequent neonatal complication [43,44] that has a direct implication in adolescence and adulthood, with a higher prevalence of chronic diseases such as obesity, diabetes, metabolic syndrome, or cardiovascular pathology [45].

Elevated homocysteine levels, derived from the incorrect functioning of the *MTHFR* enzyme, have also been related to an increased risk of spontaneous abortions [46]. In our series, women with the *MTHFR* risk allele had a lower frequency of spontaneous pregnancy, i.e., a greater need for assisted fertilization, which may reflect a difficulty in gestation derived from the incorrect functioning of the one-carbon metabolism pathway. The *MTHFR* risk allele in our population was associated with a lower frequency of spontaneous pregnancy, which is known to have a negative impact on health care costs and maternal mental health.

In our series, women with risk alleles of *MTHFR* had a higher frequency of preeclampsia than those without. Preeclampsia is characterised by hypertension accompanied by proteinuria in pregnant women over 20 weeks of gestation. This disease can affect both the foetus and the mother and, in extreme situations, can compromise the life of both [47–49]. A meta-analysis report by Wang et al. (2013) [50] showed a significant association between the *MTHFR* T allele and pre-eclampsia among Caucasians and people of Asian descent but not among people of African descent. However, a recent study carried out in Lagos, southwestern Nigeria, has shown an occurrence of preeclampsia was significantly associated with the presence of the T allele of *MTHFR* (OR = 1.855; $p < 0.05$) [51].

As for the cubilin gene (*CUBN*), the intrinsic factor-vitamin B12 receptor, we found that the allelic distribution of SNP rs1801222 was significantly different depending on complications during delivery—namely, a higher frequency of delivery complications was found among carriers of the wild-type allele. This suggests that carrying this genetic variant could reduce the risk of delivery complications. In this regard, previous studies have observed a significant increase in the risk of congenital heart disease for carriers of the wild-type allele of the *CUBN* SNP rs11254363 [52]. Cubilin favours the absorption of intrinsic factor-vitamin B12 complex in the intestinal mucosa. Polymorphisms in the cubilin gene were associated with variability in the binding and transport of vitamin B12. In this regard, it was demonstrated in a meta-analysis that participants homozygous for the rs1801222 G allele had higher plasmatic B12 levels [53]. Adequate maternal vitamin B12 status is associated with advantageous maternal and child health outcomes [54]. Therefore, the low frequency of delivery complications observed in G carriers in the current study could be related to higher plasmatic B12 levels in these participants. As far as we know, this is the first study that found a different distribution of *CUBN* SNPs in women with delivery complications, such as caesarean section and induced or instrumental delivery.

Other relevant polymorphisms involved in the one-carbon metabolism are *MTR* and *SLC19A1*. *MTR* encoded an enzyme involved in the synthesis of methionine through homocysteine methylation with the presence of vitamin B12 (Vit. B12) as a co-factor, and SNPs in this gene were associated with risk during pregnancy [55]. SLC19A1 gene encodes a typical transporter with 12 transmembrane domains involved in the active transport of 5-methyltetrahydrofolate from plasma to the cytosol and regulation of intracellular folate concentration. It may limit the absorption of folic acid by the developing foetus, thus affecting the growth of the foetus [56]. In the current study, we did not observe an association between the studies SPNs of these genes and pregnancy or newborn complications.

The present study has several limitations such as a small sample size and short follow-up time. Moreover, all women included in this study were prescribed folic acid and vitamin B12 supplementation during pregnancy which possibly mask the association between one-carbon polymorphisms and pregnancy or newborn complications. Among the mother complications, a higher prevalence of GDM than the general population was found in this cohort. This is because pregnant women between 24 and 28 weeks of gestation who attended both the endocrinology and obstetrics departments were invited to participate in the study, and, in particular, the pregnant women who attended the endocrinology department mainly visited for metabolic problems, mostly GDM. Another limitation of this study could be that there are no metabolic data to assess the consequences of polymorphisms on the metabolism of single carbons, which limits the analysis of the significance of the associations. However, this may be the beginning of future studies with larger sample sizes and longer follow-up times that include both pregnant women as well as women with gestational desire to know the implication of these polymorphisms and their possible approach in the preconception stage.

5. Conclusions

In conclusion, our data show a high prevalence of genetic variants related to folic acid and vitamin B12 metabolic genes in pregnant women that may justify the difference in maternal and neonatal outcomes. This study warrants the need to perform further studies to elucidate whether knowing the prevalence of these polymorphisms on an individual basis and its association with the mother and newborn health may lead to personalised medicine with a nutritional assessment of vitamin intake.

Author Contributions: Conceptualisation, A.B.C.; data curation, G.R.-C., P.M.L. and A.C.-B.; formal analysis, G.R.-C., P.M.L., A.B.C., M.A., M.Z. and L.M.; investigation, F.F.C. and A.B.C.; methodology, A.B.C., L.M., L.S., M.M.-C. and F.F.C.; supervision, A.B.C.; writing—original draft preparation, G.R.-C., P.M.L. and A.B.C.; writing—review and editing, G.R.-C., P.M.L. and A.B.C. All authors have read and agreed to the published version of the manuscript.

Funding: The research work of the authors is supported by Fundación Paideia Galiza and Fundación de la Sociedad Gallega de Endocrinología, Nutrición y Metabolismo (SGENM), as well as Xunta de Galicia-Gain (IN607B2020/09) and Centro de Investigación Biomedica en Red fisiopatología de la obesidad y nutricion (CIBERobn), the Miguel Servet Project (CP17/0008) and research projects (PI20/00650; PI20/00628), under the initiative of Instituto de Salud Carlos III (ISCIII) and co-financed by the European Regional Development Fund (FEDER). PML is funded by a predoctoral grant from Xunta de Galicia (IN606-2020/013). ABC is a Miguel Servet researcher (ISCIII; CP17/0008).

Institutional Review Board Statement: The study was conducted according to the guidelines of the Declaration of Helsinki and approved by the Autonomic Committee of Clinical Research Ethics of Galicia, Spain (protocol code 2017/622). The participants did not receive economic profit.

Informed Consent Statement: Informed consent was obtained from all subjects involved in the study.

Data Availability Statement: Data are available upon reasonable request from the corresponding author.

Acknowledgments: The authors thank all participants in this study and the research group involved in the project, as well as the individuals who performed the fieldwork, such as the Laboratory Technician Jesus Iglesias and Data Manager Maribel Rendo.

Conflicts of Interest: The authors declare no conflict of interest.

References

1. Sengpiel, V.; Bacelis, J.; Myhre, R.; Myking, S.; Devold Pay, A.S.; Haugen, M.; Brantsæter, A.-L.; Meltzer, H.M.; Nilsen, R.M.; Magnus, P.; et al. Folic acid supplementation, dietary folate intake during pregnancy and risk for spontaneous preterm delivery: A prospective observational cohort study. *BMC Pregnancy Childbirth* **2014**, *14*, 375. [CrossRef] [PubMed]
2. Alves-Santos, N.H.; Cocate, P.G.; Benaim, C.; Farias, D.R.; Emmett, P.M.; Kac, G. Prepregnancy Dietary Patterns and Their Association with Perinatal Outcomes: A Prospective Cohort Study. *J. Acad. Nutr. Diet.* **2019**, *119*, 1439–1451. [CrossRef] [PubMed]
3. Bulloch, R.E.; Wall, C.R.; McCowan, L.M.E.; Taylor, R.S.; Roberts, C.T.; Thompson, J.M.D. The Effect of Interactions between Folic Acid Supplementation and One Carbon Metabolism Gene Variants on Small-for-Gestational-Age Births in the Screening for Pregnancy Endpoints (SCOPE) Cohort Study. *Nutrients* **2020**, *12*, 1677. [CrossRef] [PubMed]
4. de Bildt, A.; Oosterling, I.J.; van Lang, N.D.J.; Sytema, S.; Minderaa, R.B.; van Engeland, H.; Roos, S.; Buitelaar, J.K.; van der Gaag, R.-J.; de Jonge, M.V. Standardized ADOS scores: Measuring severity of autism spectrum disorders in a Dutch sample. *J. Autism Dev. Disord.* **2011**, *41*, 311–319. [CrossRef] [PubMed]
5. Furness, D.; Fenech, M.; Dekker, G.; Khong, T.Y.; Roberts, C.; Hague, W. Folate, vitamin B12, vitamin B6 and homocysteine: Impact on pregnancy outcome. *Matern. Child Nutr.* **2013**, *9*, 155–166. [CrossRef] [PubMed]
6. Furness, D.L.F.; Dekker, G.A.; Roberts, C.T. DNA damage and health in pregnancy. *J. Reprod. Immunol.* **2011**, *89*, 153–162. [CrossRef]
7. Maloney, C.A.; Rees, W.D. Gene-nutrient interactions during fetal development. *Reproduction* **2005**, *130*, 401–410. [CrossRef]
8. Redman, C.W.G.; Sargent, I.L. Immunology of pre-eclampsia. *Am. J. Reprod. Immunol.* **2010**, *63*, 534–543. [CrossRef]
9. Imbard, A.; Benoist, J.-F.; Blom, H.J. Neural tube defects, folic acid and methylation. *Int. J. Environ. Res. Public Health* **2013**, *10*, 4352–4389. [CrossRef]
10. van Gool, J.D.; Hirche, H.; Lax, H.; De Schaepdrijver, L. Folic acid and primary prevention of neural tube defects: A review. *Reprod. Toxicol.* **2018**, *80*, 73–84. [CrossRef]
11. Wahbeh, F.; Manyama, M. The role of Vitamin B12 and genetic risk factors in the etiology of neural tube defects: A systematic review. *Int. J. Dev. Neurosci.* **2021**, *81*, 386–406. [CrossRef] [PubMed]
12. Mardali, F.; Fatahi, S.; Alinaghizadeh, M.; Kord Varkaneh, H.; Sohouli, M.H.; Shidfar, F.; Găman, M.-A. Association between abnormal maternal serum levels of vitamin B12 and preeclampsia: A systematic review and meta-analysis. *Nutr. Rev.* **2021**, *79*, 518–528. [CrossRef]

13. Saravanan, P.; Sukumar, N.; Adaikalakoteswari, A.; Goljan, I.; Venkataraman, H.; Gopinath, A.; Bagias, C.; Yajnik, C.S.; Stallard, N.; Ghebremichael-Weldeselassie, Y.; et al. Association of maternal vitamin B12 and folate levels in early pregnancy with gestational diabetes: A prospective UK cohort study (PRiDE study). *Diabetologia* **2021**, *64*, 2170–2182. [CrossRef] [PubMed]
14. Ramadan, E.F.; Grisdale, M.; Morais, M. Maternal Vitamin B12 Levels During Pregnancy and Their Effects on Maternal Neurocognitive Symptoms: A Systematic Review. *J. Obstet. Gynaecol. Can.* **2022**, *44*, 390–394.e3. [CrossRef] [PubMed]
15. WHO; FAO. Vitamin B12. In *Vitamin and Mineral Requirements in Human Nutrition*, 2nd ed.; World Health Organization: Rome, Italy, 2004; pp. 279–302.
16. Zinck, J.W.; de Groh, M.; MacFarlane, A.J. Genetic modifiers of folate, vitamin B-12, and homocysteine status in a cross-sectional study of the Canadian population. *Am. J. Clin. Nutr.* **2015**, *101*, 1295–1304. [CrossRef]
17. Solanky, N.; Requena Jimenez, A.; D'Souza, S.W.; Sibley, C.P.; Glazier, J.D. Expression of folate transporters in human placenta and implications for homocysteine metabolism. *Placenta* **2010**, *31*, 134–143. [CrossRef] [PubMed]
18. Talaulikar, V.S.; Arulkumaran, S. Folic acid in obstetric practice: A review. *Obstet. Gynecol. Surv.* **2011**, *66*, 240–247. [CrossRef]
19. Nazki, F.H.; Sameer, A.S.; Ganaie, B.A. Folate: Metabolism, genes, polymorphisms and the associated diseases. *Gene* **2014**, *533*, 11–20. [CrossRef]
20. McNulty, H.; Ward, M.; Hoey, L.; Hughes, C.F.; Pentieva, K. Addressing optimal folate and related B-vitamin status through the lifecycle: Health impacts and challenges. *Proc. Nutr. Soc.* **2019**, *78*, 449–462. [CrossRef]
21. American Diabetes Association. Classification and Diagnosis of Diabetes: Standards of Medical Care in Diabetes-2018. *Diabetes Care* **2018**, *41*, S13–S27. [CrossRef]
22. Garovic, V.D.; Dechend, R.; Easterling, T.; Karumanchi, S.A.; McMurtry Baird, S.; Magee, L.A.; Rana, S.; Vermunt, J.V.; August, P.; American Heart Association Council on Hypertension; et al. Hypertension in Pregnancy: Diagnosis, Blood Pressure Goals, and Pharmacotherapy: A Scientific Statement From the American Heart Association. *Hypertension* **2022**, *79*, e21–e41. [CrossRef] [PubMed]
23. Carrascosa, A.; Yeste, D.; Copil, A.; Almar, J.; Salcedo, S.; Gussinyé, M. Anthropometric growth patterns of preterm and full-term newborns (24–42 weeks' gestational age) at the Hospital Materno-Infantil Vall d'Hebron (Barcelona)(1997–2002). *An. Pediatr.* **2004**, *60*, 406–416.
24. Torres-Sánchez, L.; López-Carrillo, L.; Blanco-Muñoz, J.; Chen, J. Maternal dietary intake of folate, vitamin B12 and MTHFR 677C>T genotype: Their impact on newborn's anthropometric parameters. *Genes Nutr.* **2014**, *9*, 429. [CrossRef] [PubMed]
25. Guéant-Rodriguez, R.-M.; Guéant, J.-L.; Debard, R.; Thirion, S.; Hong, L.X.; Bronowicki, J.-P.; Namour, F.; Chabi, N.W.; Sanni, A.; Anello, G.; et al. Prevalence of methylenetetrahydrofolate reductase 677T and 1298C alleles and folate status: A comparative study in Mexican, West African, and European populations. *Am. J. Clin. Nutr.* **2006**, *83*, 701–707. [CrossRef]
26. Wilcken, B.; Bamforth, F.; Li, Z.; Zhu, H.; Ritvanen, A.; Renlund, M.; Stoll, C.; Alembik, Y.; Dott, B.; Czeizel, A.E.; et al. Geographical and ethnic variation of the 677C>T allele of 5,10 methylenetetrahydrofolate reductase (MTHFR): Findings from over 7000 newborns from 16 areas world wide. *J. Med. Genet.* **2003**, *40*, 619–625. [CrossRef] [PubMed]
27. Aguilar-Lacasaña, S.; López-Flores, I.; González-Alzaga, B.; Giménez-Asensio, M.J.; Carmona, F.D.; Hernández, A.F.; López Gallego, M.F.; Romero-Molina, D.; Lacasaña, M. Methylenetetrahydrofolate Reductase (MTHFR) Gene Polymorphism and Infant's Anthropometry at Birth. *Nutrients* **2021**, *13*, 831. [CrossRef]
28. Bueno, O.; Molloy, A.M.; Fernandez-Ballart, J.D.; García-Minguillán, C.J.; Ceruelo, S.; Ríos, L.; Ueland, P.M.; Meyer, K.; Murphy, M.M. Common Polymorphisms That Affect Folate Transport or Metabolism Modify the Effect of the MTHFR 677C > T Polymorphism on Folate Status. *J. Nutr.* **2016**, *146*, 1–8. [CrossRef]
29. de Batlle, J.; Matejcic, M.; Chajes, V.; Moreno-Macias, H.; Amadou, A.; Slimani, N.; Cox, D.G.; Clavel-Chapelon, F.; Fagherazzi, G.; Romieu, I. Determinants of folate and vitamin B12 plasma levels in the French E3N-EPIC cohort. *Eur. J. Nutr.* **2018**, *57*, 751–760. [CrossRef]
30. Shane, B.; Pangilinan, F.; Mills, J.L.; Fan, R.; Gong, T.; Cropp, C.D.; Kim, Y.; Ueland, P.M.; Bailey-Wilson, J.E.; Wilson, A.F.; et al. The 677C→T variant of MTHFR is the major genetic modifier of biomarkers of folate status in a young, healthy Irish population. *Am. J. Clin. Nutr.* **2018**, *108*, 1334–1341. [CrossRef]
31. Hiraoka, M.; Kagawa, Y. Genetic polymorphisms and folate status. *Congenit. Anom.* **2017**, *57*, 142–149. [CrossRef]
32. Molloy, A.M. Genetic aspects of folate metabolism. *Subcell. Biochem.* **2012**, *56*, 105–130. [PubMed]
33. Lee, S.-A. Gene-diet interaction on cancer risk in epidemiological studies. *J. Prev. Med. Public Health* **2009**, *42*, 360–370. [CrossRef] [PubMed]
34. Shin, J.-A.; Kim, Y.-J.; Park, H.; Kim, H.-K.; Lee, H.-Y. Localization of folate metabolic enzymes, methionine synthase and 5,10-methylenetetrahydrofolate reductase in human placenta. *Gynecol. Obstet. Investig.* **2014**, *78*, 259–265. [CrossRef]
35. Moulik, N.R.; Kumar, A.; Agrawal, S. Folic acid, one-carbon metabolism & childhood cancer. *Indian J. Med. Res.* **2017**, *146*, 163–174.
36. Field, M.S.; Stover, P.J. Safety of folic acid. *Ann. N. Y. Acad. Sci.* **2018**, *1414*, 59–71. [CrossRef] [PubMed]
37. Yila, T.A.; Sasaki, S.; Miyashita, C.; Braimoh, T.S.; Kashino, I.; Kobayashi, S.; Okada, E.; Baba, T.; Yoshioka, E.; Minakami, H.; et al. Effects of maternal 5,10-methylenetetrahydrofolate reductase C677T and A1298C Polymorphisms and tobacco smoking on infant birth weight in a Japanese population. *J. Epidemiol.* **2012**, *22*, 91–102. [CrossRef]
38. Colson, N.J.; Naug, H.L.; Nikbakht, E.; Zhang, P.; McCormack, J. The impact of MTHFR 677 C/T genotypes on folate status markers: A meta-analysis of folic acid intervention studies. *Eur. J. Nutr.* **2017**, *56*, 247–260. [CrossRef]

39. Shelnutt, K.P.; Kauwell, G.P.A.; Gregory, J.F.; Maneval, D.R.; Quinlivan, E.P.; Theriaque, D.W.; Henderson, G.N.; Bailey, L.B. Methylenetetrahydrofolate reductase 677C–>T polymorphism affects DNA methylation in response to controlled folate intake in young women. *J. Nutr. Biochem.* **2004**, *15*, 554–560. [CrossRef]
40. Kupferminc, M.J.; Eldor, A.; Steinman, N.; Many, A.; Bar-Am, A.; Jaffa, A.; Fait, G.; Lessing, J.B. Increased frequency of genetic thrombophilia in women with complications of pregnancy. *N. Engl. J. Med.* **1999**, *340*, 9–13. [CrossRef]
41. Chen, H.; Yang, X.; Lu, M. Methylenetetrahydrofolate reductase gene polymorphisms and recurrent pregnancy loss in China: A systematic review and meta-analysis. *Arch. Gynecol. Obstet.* **2016**, *293*, 283–290. [CrossRef]
42. Valdez, L.L.; Quintero, A.; Garcia, E.; Olivares, N.; Celis, A.; Rivas, F.; Rivas, F. Thrombophilic polymorphisms in preterm delivery. *Blood Cells. Mol. Dis.* **2004**, *33*, 51–56. [CrossRef] [PubMed]
43. Sapkota, A.; Chelikowsky, A.P.; Nachman, K.E.; Cohen, A.J.; Ritz, B. Exposure to particulate matter and adverse birth outcomes: A comprehensive review and meta-analysis. *Air Qual. Atmos. Health* **2012**, *5*, 369–381. [CrossRef]
44. Martínez-Martínez, R.E.; Moreno-Castillo, D.F.; Loyola-Rodríguez, J.P.; Sánchez-Medrano, A.G.; Miguel-Hernández, J.H.S.; Olvera-Delgado, J.H.; Domínguez-Pérez, R.A. Association between periodontitis, periodontopathogens and preterm birth: Is it real? *Arch. Gynecol. Obstet.* **2016**, *294*, 47–54. [CrossRef] [PubMed]
45. Jiang, M.; Qiu, J.; Zhou, M.; He, X.; Cui, H.; Lerro, C.; Lv, L.; Lin, X.; Zhang, C.; Zhang, H.; et al. Exposure to cooking fuels and birth weight in Lanzhou, China: A birth cohort study. *BMC Public Health* **2015**, *15*, 712. [CrossRef]
46. Dai, C.; Fei, Y.; Li, J.; Shi, Y.; Yang, X. A Novel Review of Homocysteine and Pregnancy Complications. *Biomed Res. Int.* **2021**, *2021*, 6652231.
47. Rigotti, A. Absorption, transport, and tissue delivery of vitamin E. *Mol. Aspects Med.* **2007**, *28*, 423–436. [CrossRef]
48. Zhao, Y.; Lee, M.-J.; Cheung, C.; Ju, J.-H.; Chen, Y.-K.; Liu, B.; Hu, L.-Q.; Yang, C.S. Analysis of multiple metabolites of tocopherols and tocotrienols in mice and humans. *J. Agric. Food Chem.* **2010**, *58*, 4844–4852. [CrossRef]
49. Niforou, A.; Konstantinidou, V.; Naska, A. Genetic Variants Shaping Inter-individual Differences in Response to Dietary Intakes-A Narrative Review of the Case of Vitamins. *Front. Nutr.* **2020**, *7*, 558598. [CrossRef]
50. Wang, X.; Wu, H.; Qiu, X. Methylenetetrahydrofolate reductase (MTHFR) gene C677T polymorphism and risk of preeclampsia: An updated meta-analysis based on 51 studies. *Arch. Med. Res.* **2013**, *44*, 159–168. [CrossRef]
51. Osunkalu, V.O.; Taiwo, I.A.; Makwe, C.C.; Quao, R.A. Methylene tetrahydrofolate reductase and methionine synthase gene polymorphisms as genetic determinants of pre-eclampsia. *Pregnancy Hypertens.* **2020**, *20*, 7–13. [CrossRef]
52. Wang, J.; Zhao, J.-Y.; Wang, F.; Peng, Q.-Q.; Hou, J.; Sun, S.-N.; Gui, Y.-H.; Duan, W.-Y.; Qiao, B.; Wang, H.-Y. A genetic variant in vitamin B12 metabolic genes that reduces the risk of congenital heart disease in Han Chinese populations. *PLoS ONE* **2014**, *9*, e88332.
53. Hazra, A.; Kraft, P.; Lazarus, R.; Chen, C.; Chanock, S.J.; Jacques, P.; Selhub, J.; Hunter, D.J. Genome-wide significant predictors of metabolites in the one-carbon metabolism pathway. *Hum. Mol. Genet.* **2009**, *18*, 4677–4687. [CrossRef] [PubMed]
54. Behere, R.V.; Deshmukh, A.S.; Otiv, S.; Gupte, M.D.; Yajnik, C.S. Maternal Vitamin B12 Status During Pregnancy and Its Association With Outcomes of Pregnancy and Health of the Offspring: A Systematic Review and Implications for Policy in India. *Front. Endocrinol.* **2021**, *12*, 619176. [CrossRef] [PubMed]
55. Coppedè, F.; Bosco, P.; Lorenzoni, V.; Migheli, F.; Barone, C.; Antonucci, I.; Stuppia, L.; Romano, C.; Migliore, L. The MTR 2756A>G polymorphism and maternal risk of birth of a child with Down syndrome: A case-control study and a meta-analysis. *Mol. Biol. Rep.* **2013**, *40*, 6913–6925. [CrossRef] [PubMed]
56. Yi, K.; Ma, Y.-H.; Wang, W.; Zhang, X.; Gao, J.; He, S.-E.; Xu, X.-M.; Ji, M.; Guo, W.-F.; You, T. The roles of reduced folate carrier-1 (RFC1) A80G (rs1051266) polymorphism in congenital heart disease: A meta-analysis. *Med. Sci. Monit.* **2021**, *27*, e929911. [CrossRef]

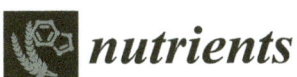

Article

Sex-Dependent Mediation of Leptin in the Association of Perilipin Polymorphisms with BMI and Plasma Lipid Levels in Children

Claudia Vales-Villamarín [1], Jairo Lumpuy-Castillo [2], Teresa Gavela-Pérez [3], Olaya de Dios [1], Iris Pérez-Nadador [1], Leandro Soriano-Guillén [3] and Carmen Garcés [1,*]

1 Lipid Research Laboratory, IIS-Fundación Jiménez Díaz, 28040 Madrid, Spain; claudia.vales@quironsalud.es (C.V.-V.); olaya.dios@quironsalud.es (O.d.D.); iris.perezn@quironsalud.es (I.P.-N.)
2 Laboratory of Diabetes and Vascular Pathology, IIS-Fundación Jiménez Díaz, UAM, 28040 Madrid, Spain; jairo.lumpuy@estudiante.uam.es
3 Department of Pediatrics, IIS-FJD, 28040 Madrid, Spain; TGavela@fjd.es (T.G.-P.); LSoriano@fjd.es (L.S.-G.)
* Correspondence: cgarces@fjd.es; Tel.: +34-91-5404892

Abstract: Variations in the perilipin (*PLIN*) gene have been suggested to be associated with obesity and its related alterations, but a different nutritional status seems to contribute to differences in these associations. In our study, we examined the association of several polymorphisms at the *PLIN* locus with obesity and lipid profile in children, and then analyzed the mediation of plasma leptin levels on these associations. The single-nucleotide polymorphisms (SNPs) rs894160, rs1052700, and rs2304795 in *PLIN1*, and rs35568725 in *PLIN2*, were analyzed by RT-PCR in 1264 children aged 6–8 years. Our results showed a contrasting association of *PLIN1* rs1052700 with apolipoprotein (Apo) A-I levels in boys and girls, with genotype TT carriers showing significantly higher Apo A-I levels in boys and significantly lower Apo A-I levels in girls. Significant associations of the SNP *PLIN2* rs35568725 with high-density lipoprotein cholesterol (HDL-cholesterol), Apo A-I, and non-esterified fatty acids (NEFA) were observed in boys but not in girls. The associations of the SNPs studied with body mass index (BMI), NEFA, and Apo A-I in boys and girls were different depending on leptin concentration. In conclusion, we describe the mediation of plasma leptin levels in the association of SNPs in *PLIN1* and *PLIN2* with BMI, Apo A-I, and NEFA. Different leptin levels by sex may contribute to explain the sex-dependent association of the *PLIN* SNPs with these variables.

Keywords: PLIN polymorphisms; leptin; BMI; NEFA; HDL-cholesterol; Apo A-I

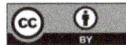

1. Introduction

Perilipins are proteins that coat intracellular lipid droplets [1,2] and play a central role in lipid storage and mobilization. Non-phosphorylated perilipin protects the lipid core from the activity of lipases, such as hormone-sensitive lipase (HSL), which hydrolyze triglycerides into glycerol and fatty acids, preventing basal lipolysis and promoting cellular triglyceride storage by limiting lipase access to triglyceride stores [3–5]. Once phosphorylated, however, perilipin allows lipases to access lipid droplets and, hence, causes active lipolysis. Thus, the activity of perilipin may play a role in body weight and lipid metabolism by regulating adipocyte metabolism, fat storage, and lipolysis [6].

The most widely studied member of the family, perilipin 1 (PLIN1), is the most abundant protein on the surface of adipocyte lipid droplets and the major substrate for the cAMP-dependent protein kinase [7]. The human *PLIN1* gene is found at chromosomal location 15q26.1 [8]. It has been shown to be a susceptibility locus for obesity and hypertriglyceridemia [9]. In fact, some studies have shown that common polymorphisms in the *PLIN1* gene are associated with obesity risk and obesity-related phenotypes [10–12].

Furthermore, *PLIN1* single-nucleotide polymorphisms (SNPs) have also been related to variability in weight loss [12–15]. However, several analyses of the associations between these polymorphisms and body weight and BMI have reported divergent results [16]. A polymorphism in *PLIN2*, another member of the family involved in the formation of lipid droplets, has also been shown to affect the structure and function of the protein. A substitution of serine by proline at the 251 position results in an altered protein structure and a reduction in lipolysis and plasma triglycerides [17,18].

To our knowledge, no studies have investigated the association of the *PLIN* SNPs in a general population of children. A couple of studies in children have focused on specific populations, such as obese children or children in a weight loss intervention [19,20]. Thus, limited evidence is available for Caucasian pre-pubertal children regarding the possible association of these SNPs with obesity-related alterations.

Significant gene–diet interactions involving these *PLIN* SNPs have been reported [21–24], suggesting that nutritional status may modify the association of *PLIN* polymorphisms with these traits. Leptin levels can be considered a good indicator of nutritional status [25].

Leptin, a hormone consistently related to obesity and obesity-related alterations [26], has been shown to exert direct and indirect effects on adipocyte metabolism [27]. As adipocytes express leptin receptors, leptin may influence adipocyte metabolism directly, triggering lipolysis via a lipolytic pathway mediated by cAMP, protein kinase A, perilipin, and HSL. Indeed, cAMP activates the protein kinase A, which is then able to phosphorylate cellular proteins, such as perilipin and HSL. Phosphorylated perilipin may activate HSL function, hydrolyzing triglycerides into glycerol and fatty acids [28,29].

In our study, we aimed to investigate, the association of body mass index (BMI) and plasma lipid levels with several *PLIN1* SNPs (11482G > A (rs894160), 13041A > G (rs2304795), and 14995A > T (rs1052700)) and with the *PLIN2* SNP Ser251Pro (rs35568725) in a large, population-based cohort of Spanish prepubertal children aged between 6 and 8 years. The SNPs selected have been associated with obesity-related phenotypes in adults, but they have not been previously studied in a cohort of children. In addition, we aimed to explore whether leptin modulates the effect of these polymorphisms.

2. Materials and Methods

2.1. Subjects

Our study comprised a population of 1264 children, aged 6–8 years (633 boys and 631 girls), who participated of the Four Provinces Study (4P Study), a cross-sectional study aiming to examine cardiovascular risk factors in Spanish children [30]. All children with a parent-reported chronic disease were excluded. Parents or legal guardians were required to provide written informed consent for their children to participate in the study. The study protocol complied with the Helsinki Declaration guidelines and was approved by the Clinical Research Ethics Committee of the IIS-Fundación Jiménez Díaz (PIC016-2019 FJD).

2.2. Anthropometric Data

Measurements were taken with the children lightly dressed and barefoot as previously described [30]. Height was measured to the nearest millimeter using a portable stadiometer, weight was recorded to the nearest 0.1 kg using a standardized electronic digital scale, and body mass index (BMI, weight in kilograms divided by height in meters squared, kg/m^2) was calculated from these parameters.

2.3. Biochemical Data

Fasting (12 h) blood samples were obtained by venipuncture and centrifuge. Serum and plasma samples were separated and stored at −70 °C. Biochemical determinations were performed as previously described [30]. Cholesterol and triglyceride (TG) concentrations were measured enzymatically (Menarini Diagnostics, Florence, Italy) in a RA-1000 Autoanalyzer (Technicon Ltd., Dublin, Ireland). High-density lipoprotein cholesterol (HDL-cholesterol) was measured after precipitation of apolipoprotein B-containing lipoproteins with phosphotungstic acid and Mg (Roche Diagnostics, Madrid, Spain). Plasma apolipoprotein A-I (Apo A-I) and apolipoprotein B (Apo B) concentrations were measured by immunonephelometry (Dade Berhing, Frankfurt, Germany). Low-density lipoprotein cholesterol (LDL-cholesterol) was calculated according to the Friedewald formula. Non-esterified fatty acids (NEFA) were measured by using the Wako NEFA-C kit (Wako Industries, Osaka, Japan). Leptin concentrations were determined by ELISA using a commercial kit (Leptin EIA-2395, DRG, Marburg, Germany), as described elsewhere [30].

2.4. Genotyping Assays of SNPs in PLIN1 and PLIN2

All DNA was isolated from 10-mL EDTA-blood samples according to standard procedures. To determine the polymorphism in the perilipin genes, the following predesigned TaqMan SNP Genotyping Assays from Applied Biosystems (Waltham, MA, USA) were used: C_8722593_10, C_8722587_10, and C_9304320_20 for the SNPs in *PLIN1* rs894160, rs1052700, and rs2304795, respectively, and C_25764255_10 for the SNPrs35568725 in *PLIN2*. A StepOnePlus™ Real-Time PCR System (Applied Biosystems) was used for allelic discrimination. Additionally, PCR was performed with a mixture of 10 ng of genomic DNA, TaqMan® SNP Genotyping Assay (20X), and TaqPath™ ProAmp™ Master Mix (Applied Biosystems). Samples were cycled under the following recommended conditions: 95 °C for 10 min, 95 °C for 15 sec, and 60 °C for 1 min, repeated over 40 cycles.

2.5. Statistical Analysis

Statistical analyses were performed using the SPSS software package, version 26.0 (IBM, New York, NY, USA) and the GraphPad Prism statistical software (San Diego, CA, USA, Version 8). The normality of quantitative variables was analyzed by the Kolmogorov–Smirnov test, revealing a non-parametric distribution. The Mann–Whitney U test was used to perform sex-based comparisons of median BMI values, lipid profile variables (TC, TG, LDL-cholesterol, Apo B, HDL-cholesterol, Apo A-I, NEFA), and leptin. Differences in median values for the variables under study according to the different genotypes of the SNPs studied were tested using the Mann–Whitney or Kruskal–Wallis tests in our population, divided by sex and grouped according to median plasma leptin levels in each sex (2.26 ng/mL in boys and 5.25 ng/mL in girls).

3. Results

Table 1 shows the anthropometric and biochemical data of the children according to sex. The mean age was similar in boys and girls. Plasma concentrations of HDL-cholesterol and Apo A-I were significantly higher, and concentrations of TG, LDL-cholesterol, and Apo B were significantly lower, in boys compared to girls. Leptin levels were significantly ($p < 0.001$) higher in girls.

When analyzing the relationship of the *PLIN1* SNPs rs894160, rs2304795, and rs1052700 with the variables under study by sex (Table 3), a significant and opposite association was discovered between *PLIN1* rs1052700 and Apo A-I levels between boys and girls. The TT carriers showed significantly higher Apo A-I levels as compared with CC and CT carriers in boys, while significantly lower Apo A-I levels were observed in girls. When analyzing the SNP of *PLIN2* rs35568725 (Table 3), carriers of the AG and GG genotypes were grouped together due to the small number of children who were homozygous for the less common allele (G). Significant differences between AA carriers and carriers of the G allele were observed for HDL-cholesterol ($p = 0.005$), Apo A-I ($p = 0.009$), and NEFA ($p = 0.002$) concentrations in boys, though no such differences were observed in girls. No significant associations were detected between the PLIN polymorphisms and LDL-cholesterol, Apo B, or leptin levels (data not shown).

The frequencies of the genotypes and alleles for the SNPs studied are shown in Table 2. The genotype distributions were within the Hardy–Weinberg equilibrium. These frequencies were similar to those described in other Caucasian populations.

Table 1. Characteristics (means ± SD) of the population studied.

	Overall (n = 1264)	Boys (n = 633)	Girls (n = 631)	p-Value [1]
Age (years)	7.2 ± 0.6	7.2 ± 0.6	7.2 ± 0.6	0.531
BMI (kg/m^2)	17.0 ± 2.4	16.9 ± 2.4	17.0 ± 2.5	0.637
TC (mg/dL)	183.0 ± 28.6	182.6 ± 28.5	183.4 ± 28.7	0.238
TG (mg/dL)	72.9 ± 26.3	71.4 ± 25.4	74.4 ± 27.2	0.014
LDL-C (mg/dL)	109.1 ± 27.3	108.1 ± 27.7	110.0 ± 27.0	0.029
Apo B (mg/dL)	70.3 ± 15.0	69.2 ± 15.0	71.3 ± 15.0	0.001
HDL-C (mg/dL)	59.4 ± 13.3	60.2 ± 13.2	58.7 ± 13.4	0.021
Apo A-I (mg/dL)	137.0 ± 19.1	138.4 ± 19.1	135.5 ± 19.1	0.007
NEFA (mEq/L)	0.70 ± 0.28	0.68 ± 0.27	0.72 ± 0.30	0.074
Leptin (ng/mL)	6.58 ± 8.00	4.65 ± 6.43	8.60 ± 8.97	0.000

[1] p-value: Mann–Whitney U test. Abbreviations are as follows: BMI, body mass index; TC, total cholesterol; TG, triglycerides; LDL-C, low-density lipoprotein cholesterol; Apo B, apolipoprotein B; HDL-C, high-density lipoprotein cholesterol; Apo A-I, apolipoprotein A-I; NEFA, non-esterified fatty acids.

Table 2. Genotypic and allelic distribution of the SNPs studied in PLIN1 and PLIN2.

Gene	SNP	Genotype	% (n)	Allele	%
PLIN1	rs894160	CC	49.4 (625)	C	70.5
		CT	42.1 (532)	T	29.5
		TT	8.5 (107)		
	rs1052700	AA	44.7 (557)	A	66.7
		AT	43.6 (544)	T	33.5
		TT	11.7 (146)		
	rs2304795	AA	34.1 (455)	A	61.0
		AG	47.4 (632)	G	39.0
		GG	13.2 (176)		
PLIN2	rs35568725	AA	88.1 (1110)	A	93.8
		AG	11.5 (145)	G	6.2
		GG	0.4 (5)		

To analyze whether the effect of the polymorphisms studied on BMI and lipid levels was mediated by leptin levels, the relationship of the SNPs (rs894160, rs2304795, and rs1052700 in PLIN1, and rs35568725 in PLIN2) with these parameters was investigated in children classified into two groups according to their plasma leptin levels, i.e., boys and girls with plasma leptin levels above or below their respective median value of leptin. As shown in Figure 1, we observed that the associations of PLIN1 rs894160 and PLIN2 rs35568725 with BMI (Figure 1a) and of PLIN1 rs2304795 and PLIN2 rs35568725 with NEFA (Figure 1b) were different in boys and girls with lower leptin levels compared to subjects with higher leptin concentrations. Significant associations were observed in boys with leptin levels above the median values, as well as in girls with leptin levels below the median leptin value. Additionally, a different association in boys and girls depending on leptin levels was observed concerning the influence of PLIN1 rs1052700 on Apo-I levels (Figure 1c). The association of the PLIN1 rs1052700 SNP with HDL-cholesterol levels (Figure 1d) was evident in girls with high leptin concentrations. Furthermore, the PLIN1 rs894160 and PLIN2 rs35568725 SNPs were also associated with HDL-cholesterol levels depending on leptin concentration and sex (Supplementary Figure S1). No significant results were found when analyzing the association of the SNPs studied with triglyceride concentrations depending on leptin concentration.

Table 3. BMI and lipid profile values (means ± SD) by genotype for *PLIN1* and *PLIN2* SNPs in boys and girls.

Boys			BMI (kg/m^2)	TG (mg/dL)	HDL-C (mg/dL)	APO A-I (mg/dL)	NEFA (mEq/L)
PLIN1	rs894160	CC (n = 306)	17.0 ± 2.4	69.1 ± 28.5	60.6 ± 12.7	137.9 ± 19.3	0.67 ± 0.25
		CT (n = 278)	16.9 −2.5	74.2 ± 28.8	59.8 ± 13.7	138.1 ± 18.7	0.69 ± 0.29
		TT (n = 49)	16.6 ± 1.9	66.5 ± 22.3	60.2 ± 13.1	143.2 ± 17.6	0.70 ± 0.27
		p-value	ns	ns	ns	ns	ns
	rs1052700	AA (n = 270)	17.0 ± 2.4	70.2 ± 23.5	60.2 ± 13.5	137.7 ± 18.9	0.66 ± 0.28
		AT (n = 282)	16.9 ± 2.3	72.4 ± 28.3	59.8 ± 12.8	137.6 ± 19.4	0.69 ± 0.27
		TT (n = 71)	16.9 ± 2.3	70.9 ± 21.0	62.1 ± 13.7	143.6 ± 17.6	0.69 ± 0.21
		p-value	ns	ns	ns	0.013 [a]	ns
	rs2304795	AA (n = 228)	16.8 ± 2.4	69.6 ± 23.4	59.6 ± 14.0	136.8 ± 19.2	0.68 ± 0.28
		AG (n = 317)	17.0 ± 2.4	71.0 ± 27.4	60.9 ± 12.4	139.7 ± 18.9	0.67 ± 0.25
		GG (n = 88)	17.3 ± 2.3	75.7 ± 21.7	59.5 ± 13.1	137.8 ± 18.2	0.71 ± 0.32
		p-value	ns	0.008 [b]	ns	ns	ns
PLIN2	rs35568725	AA (n = 549)	17.0 ± 2.4	71.0 ± 25.2	60.9 ± 13.2	139.3 ± 18.9	0.69 ± 0.28
		AG + GG (n = 80)	16.9 ± 2.7	72.1 ± 26.5	56.1 ± 12.0	133.2 ± 18.6	0.57 ± 0.19
		p-value	ns	0.767	**0.005** [c]	**0.009** [c]	**0.002** [c]
Girls							
PLIN1	rs894160	CC (n = 312)	16.8 ± 2.6	73.2 ± 29.6	58.7 ± 13.1	135.8 ± 19.1	0.73 ± 0.29
		CT (n = 250)	17.1 ± 2.5	75.0 ± 24.1	59.3 ± 13.8	135.8 ± 18.5	0.69 ± 0.31
		TT (n = 57)	17.3 ± 2.3	73.8 ± 19.8	58.5 ± 10.8	136.4 ± 20.1	0.79 ± 0.30
		p-value	ns	ns	ns	ns	ns
	rs1052700	AA (n = 281)	16.8 ± 2.5	75.9 ± 31.6	59.5 ± 14.0	137.9 ± 19.3	0.74 ± 0.31
		AT (n = 257)	17.1 ± 2.6	72.5 ± 21.3	58.6 ± 12.6	135.3 ± 18.3	0.70 ± 0.30
		TT (n = 75)	17.4 ± 2.1	73.1 ± 24.0	57.2 ± 12.5	130.2 ± 19.0	0.69 ± 0.26
		p-value	ns	ns	ns	0.006 [a]	ns
	rs2304795	AA (n = 221)	17.0 ± 2.6	74.8 ± 25.4	58.9 ± 13.8	137.7 ± 17.3	0.73 ± 0.27
		AG (n = 310)	16.9 ± 2.5	74.1 ± 28.7	58.9 ± 13.0	135.0 ± 20.0	0.72 ± 0.30
		GG (n = 87)	17.0 ± 2.4	71.6 ± 22.3	58.9 ± 12.5	134.1 ± 18.9	0.69 ± 0.34
		p-value	0.881	0.551	0.813	0.304	0.175
PLIN2	rs35568725	AA (n = 550)	17.0 ± 2.5	74.4 ± 27.1	58.9 ± 13.0	135.8 ± 18.9	0.72 ± 0.30
		AG + GG (n = 68)	16.6 ± 2.7	70.2 ± 21.9	58.7 ± 14.5	136.4 ± 19.3	0.72 ± 0.30
		p-value	ns	ns	ns	ns	ns

p-value: Mann–Whitney U test; [a] AA + AT vs. TT; [b] AA + AG vs. GG; [c] AA vs. AG + GG. Abbreviations are as follows: ns, not significant; BMI, body mass index; TG, triglycerides; HDL-C, high-density lipoprotein cholesterol; Apo A-I, apolipoprotein A-I; NEFA, non-esterified fatty acids.

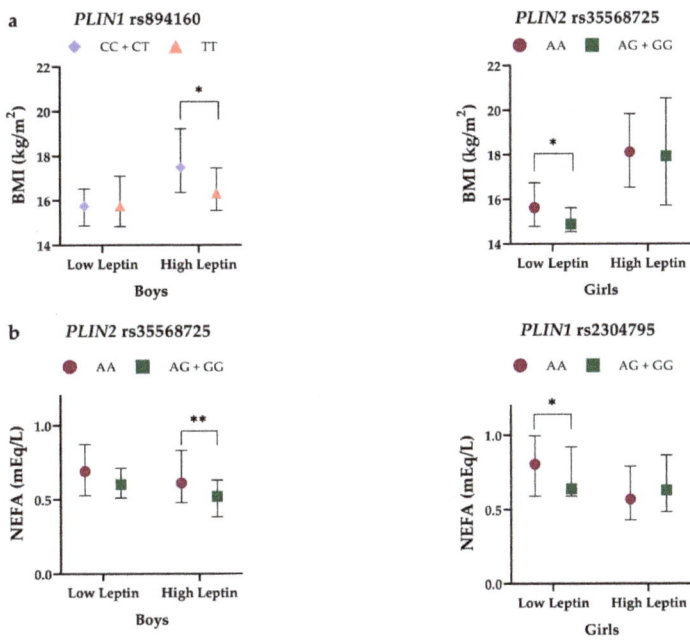

Figure 1. *Cont.*

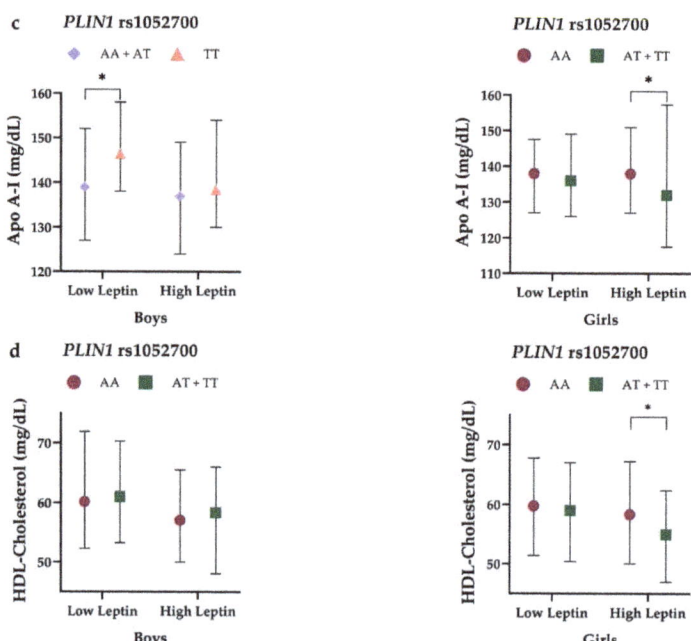

Figure 1. (**a**) BMI values of *PLIN1* rs894160 and *PLIN2* rs35568725 genotypes in boys and girls according to levels of leptin; (**b**) NEFA levels of *PLIN1* rs2304795 and *PLIN2* rs35568725 genotypes in boys and girls by leptin levels; (**c**) Apo A-I levels of *PLIN1* rs1052700 genotypes in boys and girls by levels of leptin. (**d**) HDL-cholesterol levels of *PLIN1* rs1052700 genotypes in boys and girls by levels of leptin. Values are expressed as median and interquartile range. *p*-value: Mann–Whitney U test: * *p*-value < 0.05; ** *p*-value < 0.01.

4. Discussion

Aiming to further clarify the reasons behind reported differences in the association of perilipin polymorphisms with obesity and obesity-related parameters, we analyzed the most commonly studied SNPs in *PLIN1* (11482G > A (rs894160), 14995A > T (rs1052700), and 13041A > G (rs2304795)) and the SNP in *PLIN2* Ser251Pro (rs35568725), causing a missense mutation in exon 6, in a cohort of prepubertal children showing significant differences in plasma leptin concentration between boys and girls [30]. In this population, potential confounding factors are fewer than in the pubertal and adult population. In our analysis, sex-dependent differences were observed in the association of the SNP rs1052700 of *PLIN1* with Apo A-I concentrations. Furthermore, an association of the SNP rs35568725 of *PLIN2* was found with NEFA, HDL-cholesterol, and Apo A-I concentrations in boys, which was not observed in girls. No significant associations of the polymorphisms in *PLIN1* and *PLIN2* were observed with body weight, BMI, LDL-cholesterol, or Apo B.

The association of *PLIN* SNPs with anthropometric traits and obesity has been described in studies in adults, including populations of different ethnic groups [10,11,31–33]. Although studies analyzing the association of *PLIN* SNPs with plasma lipid concentrations are scarce, some studies have also reported an association of these SNPs with triglycerides and HDL-cholesterol levels [10,15]. However, other studies have failed to detect association between these SNPs and obesity or obesity-related parameters [34–39]. Interaction of *PLIN* SNPs with nutritional factors may represent a plausible explanation for discrepancies among studies [16]. Another important issue is the sex-dependent association between SNPs at the *PLIN* locus and the obesity risk reported in adult populations [31,40] which may contribute to explaining divergent findings.

Few studies have analyzed the relationship of *PLIN* SNPs with obesity or obesity-related alterations in children [19,20]. The design of these studies differs from ours, as Deram et al. [19] analyzed the effect of *PLIN* gene variation on weight loss in children with obesity aged 7–14 year, while the study of Tokgöz analyzed their association with obesity in a case-control study including 206 children with obesity and 102 healthy controls [20], which complicates efforts to compare our findings, as we analyzed a general child population and the analysis is not performed in overweight/obese children.

Here, we described a different sex-based association, particularly concerning the SNP rs1052700 of *PLIN1* and the SNP rs35568725 of *PLIN2* in a cohort of children in which a different nutritional status by sex, as reflected by plasma leptin levels, had been previously described [30].

Differences in diet have been associated with variations in the effect of the PLIN polymorphisms on obesity and obesity-related parameters [21–24]. Diet-induced changes in body fat and energy metabolism may be responsible for a different nutritional metabolism status, and these changes affect leptin levels. We hypothesized that the differences found in the effect of the polymorphism between boys and girls would be associated with the fact that the boys and girls in our population had significantly different leptin levels, and that plasma leptin levels could modulate the association of the polymorphisms with NEFA concentrations, which conditions its association with BMI and lipid metabolism. The *PLIN1* rs894160 and *PLIN1* rs1052700 have been associated with changes in abdominal fat and blood NEFA levels that occur in weight loss [41], which may also suggest an influence on these associations exerted by changes in leptin levels associated with changes in body weight.

In our study, when analyzing the effect of the SNPs studied in children grouped according to plasma leptin levels, we observed that the relationship of the polymorphisms with BMI, Apo A-I, and NEFA varied depending on leptin concentrations. The effect of leptin on adipocyte metabolism has been demonstrated, and both direct and indirect effects of leptin on adipocyte metabolism have been suggested [27]. As adipocytes express leptin receptors, leptin may influence adipocyte metabolism directly and, as adipocytes are insulin-responsive, leptin can also modify adipocyte metabolism indirectly [27].

As described previously, perilipin is a protein that coats lipid droplets (LDs) in adipocytes [42] and plays an important role in lipolysis as, upon activation by protein kinase A, phosphorylated perilipin translocates from the lipid droplet and allows HSL to hydrolyze the TG and release NEFA. An important triggering role of leptin has been suggested for this intracellular lipolytic pathway. Indeed, PLIN1, the most abundant protein associated with LDs [43], is highly expressed in white adipocytes [44], and lower PLIN1 expression is related to higher rates of lipolysis [43]. Additionally, *PLIN* genetic variants may affect the protein content and lipolytic rates of adipocytes. Mottagui-Tabar et al. linked the rs894160 polymorphism of *PLIN1* to perilipin content in the adipocyte and basal and noradrenaline-induced lipolysis, with the 11482A allele being associated with a decreased perilipin content and with an increase in lipolysis [4]. The rs35568725 polymorphism of *PLIN2* has also been associated with an alteration of the gene that affects lipolysis and which is related to lower concentrations of TG [17]. Thus, based on the hypothesis that leptin triggers the lipolytic pathway that leads to phosphorylated perilipin and stimulates lipolysis, we assume a different effect of the genetic variants of *PLIN*, which determine the perilipin content in the adipocyte and PLIN functionality, and on BMI and lipid metabolism depending on leptin levels.

We should mention the lack of information regarding body composition as the main limitation of our study, as information on body fat might help us to understand differences on plasma leptin levels between boys and girls. An inherent limitation of all cross-sectional studies is the inability to demonstrate causality. Therefore, further studies are needed to confirm the causal nature of these associations.

5. Conclusions

Based on our results, we may conclude that the association of the *PLIN1* and *PLIN2* polymorphisms with BMI, NEFA, and Apo A-I concentrations seems to be modulated by plasma leptin levels in prepubertal children. Our data may contribute to elucidate the discrepancies observed in previous studies analyzing these associations in adult populations. Our data allow us to speculate that different plasma leptin concentration by sex through life, affecting the relationship of the *PLIN* SNPs with cardiovascular risk factors, such as BMI and lipid profile, may contribute to explaining the different predisposition to cardiovascular disease depending on sex across life. Further studies analyzing these aspects in other groups of age should be performed.

Supplementary Materials: The following supporting information can be downloaded at: https://www.mdpi.com/article/10.3390/nu14153072/s1, Figure S1: (**a**) HDL-cholesterol levels of *PLIN1*rs894160 genotypes in boys and girls according to levels of leptin; (**b**) HDL-cholesterol levels of *PLIN2*rs35568725 genotypes in boys and girls by leptin levels. Values are expressed as median and interquartile range. p-value: Mann–Whitney U test: * p-value < 0.05; ** p-value < 0.01.

Author Contributions: Conceptualization, C.G.; methodology, C.V.-V., I.P.-N. and O.d.D.; software, C.V.-V. and J.L.-C.; formal analysis, C.V.-V., J.L.-C. and C.G.; investigation, C.V.-V., I.P.-N. and O.d.D.; resources, T.G.-P., L.S.-G. and C.G.; data curation, T.G.-P. and C.G; writing—original draft preparation, C.G.; writing—review and editing, C.V.-V., J.L.-C., T.G.-P. and L.S.-G.; visualization, C.V.-V. and J.L.-C.; supervision, C.G.; project administration, C.G.; funding acquisition, L.S.-G. and C.G. All authors have read and agreed to the published version of the manuscript.

Funding: This research was supported by a grant from the Fondo de Investigación Sanitaria (FIS 18/01016) and Biobank grant FEDER RD09/0076/00101. Claudia Vales-Villamarín is recipient of a research contract from Carlos III Institute of Health (pFIS). Jairo Lumpuy-Castillo received grant support in the form of an FPI contract from Universidad Autónoma, Madrid.

Institutional Review Board Statement: The study was conducted in accordance with the Declaration of Helsinki, and approved by the Clinical Research Ethics Committee of the IIS-Fundación Jiménez Díaz (PIC016-2019 FJD).

Informed Consent Statement: Informed consent was obtained from all subjects involved in the study.

Data Availability Statement: Not applicable.

Acknowledgments: The article is dedicated to the late Manuel de Oya as the warmest homage to his memory. We thank Oliver Shaw for his assistance with language editing.

Conflicts of Interest: The authors declare no conflict of interest.

References

1. Londos, C.; Brasaemle, D.L.; Gruia-Gray, J.; Servetnick, D.A.; Schultz, C.J.; Levin, D.M.; Kimmel, A.R. Perilipin: Unique proteins associated with intracellular neutral lipid droplets in adipocytes and steroidogenic cells. *Biochem. Soc. Trans.* **1995**, *23*, 611–615. [CrossRef] [PubMed]
2. Blanchette-Mackie, E.J.; Dwyer, N.K.; Barber, T.; Coxey, R.A.; Takeda, T.; Rondinone, C.M.; Theodorakis, J.L.; Greenberg, A.S.; Londos, C. Perilipin is located on the surface layer of intracellular lipid droplets in adipocytes. *J. Lipid Res.* **1995**, *36*, 1211–1226. [CrossRef]
3. Brasaemle, D.L.; Rubin, B.; Harten, I.A.; Gruia-Gray, J.; Kimmel, A.R.; Londos, C. Perilipin A increases triacylglycerol storage by decreasing the rate of triacylglycerol hydrolysis. *J. Biol. Chem.* **2000**, *275*, 38486–38493. [CrossRef] [PubMed]
4. Mottagui-Tabar, S.; Rydén, M.; Löfgren, P.; Faulds, G.; Hoffstedt, J.; Brookes, A.J.; Andersson, I.; Arner, P. Evidence for an important role of perilipin in the regulation of human adipocyte lipolysis. *Diabetologia* **2003**, *46*, 789–797. [CrossRef] [PubMed]
5. Marcinkiewicz, A.; Gauthier, D.; Garcia, A.; Brasaemle, D.L. The phosphorylation of serine 492 of perilipin A directs lipid droplet fragmentation and dispersion. *J. Biol. Chem.* **2006**, *281*, 11901–11909. [CrossRef]
6. Tai, E.S.; Ordovas, J.M. The role of perilipin in human obesity and insulin resistance. *Curr. Opin. Lipidol.* **2007**, *18*, 152–156. [CrossRef]
7. Sztalryd, C.; Brasaemle, D.L. The perilipin family of lipid droplet proteins: Gatekeepers of intracellular lipolysis. *Biochim. Biophys. Acta BBA Mol. Cell Biol. Lipids* **2017**, *1862*, 1221–1232. [CrossRef]
8. Nishiu, J.; Tanaka, T.; Nakamura, Y. Isolation and chromosomal mapping of the human homolog of perilipin (PLIN), a rat adipose tissue-specific gene, by differential display method. *Genomics* **1998**, *48*, 254–257. [CrossRef]

9. Mori, Y.; Otabe, S.; Dina, C.; Yasuda, K.; Populaire, C.; Lecoeur, C.; Vatin, V.; Durand, E.; Hara, K.; Okada, T.; et al. Genome-wide search for type 2 diabetes in Japanese affected sib-pairs confirms susceptibility genes on 3q, 15q, and 20q and identifies two new candidate Loci on 7p and 11p. *Diabetes* **2002**, *51*, 1247–1255. [CrossRef]
10. Qi, L.; Corella, D.; Sorlí, J.V.; Portolés, O.; Shen, H.; Coltell, O.; Godoy, D.; Greenberg, A.S.; Ordovas, J.M. Genetic variation at the perilipin (PLIN) locus is associated with obesity-related phenotypes in White women. *Clin. Genet.* **2004**, *66*, 299–310. [CrossRef]
11. Qi, L.; Tai, E.S.; Tan, C.E.; Shen, H.; Chew, S.K.; Greenberg, A.S.; Corella, D.; Ordovas, J.M. Intragenic linkage disequilibrium structure of the human perilipin gene (PLIN) and haplotype association with increased obesity risk in a multiethnic Asian population. *J. Mol. Med.* **2005**, *83*, 448–456. [CrossRef] [PubMed]
12. Corella, D.; Qi, L.; Sorlí, J.V.; Godoy, D.; Portolés, O.; Coltell, O.; Greenberg, A.S.; Ordovas, J.M. Obese subjects carrying the 11482G>A polymorphism at the perilipin locus are resistant to weight loss after dietary energy restriction. *J. Clin. Endocrinol. Metab.* **2005**, *90*, 5121–5126. [CrossRef] [PubMed]
13. Garaulet, M.; Vera, B.; Bonnet-Rubio, G.; Gómez-Abellán, P.; Lee, Y.-C.; Ordovás, J.M. Lunch eating predicts weight-loss effectiveness in carriers of the common allele at *PERILIPIN1*: The ONTIME (Obesity, Nutrigenetics, Timing, Mediterranean) study. *Am. J. Clin. Nutr.* **2016**, *104*, 1160–1166. [CrossRef]
14. Luglio, H.F.; Sulistyoningrum, D.C.; Susilowati, R. The role of genes involved in lipolysis on weight loss program in overweight and obese individuals. *J. Clin. Biochem. Nutr.* **2015**, *57*, 91–97. [CrossRef] [PubMed]
15. Soenen, S.; Mariman, E.C.M.; Vogels, N.; Bouwman, F.G.; den Hoed, M.; Brown, L.; Westerterp-Plantenga, M.S. Relationship between perilipin gene polymorphisms and body weight and body composition during weight loss and weight maintenance. *Physiol. Behav.* **2009**, *96*, 723–728. [CrossRef]
16. Smith, C.E.; Ordovás, J.M. Update on perilipin polymorphisms and obesity. *Nutr. Rev.* **2012**, *70*, 611–621. [CrossRef]
17. Magné, J.; Aminoff, A.; Perman Sundelin, J.; Mannila, M.N.; Gustafsson, P.; Hultenby, K.; Wernerson, A.; Bauer, G.; Listenberger, L.; Neville, M.J.; et al. The minor allele of the missense polymorphism Ser251Pro in perilipin 2 (*PLIN2*) disrupts an α-helix, affects lipolysis, and is associated with reduced plasma triglyceride concentration in humans. *FASEB J.* **2013**, *27*, 3090–3099. [CrossRef]
18. Sentinelli, F.; Capoccia, D.; Incani, M.; Bertoccini, L.; Severino, A.; Pani, M.G.; Manconi, E.; Cossu, E.; Leonetti, F.; Baroni, M.G. The perilipin 2 (*PLIN2*) gene Ser251Pro missense mutation is associated with reduced insulin secretion and increased insulin sensitivity in Italian obese subjects. *Diabetes Metab. Res. Rev.* **2016**, *32*, 550–556. [CrossRef]
19. Deram, S.; Nicolau, C.Y.; Perez-Martinez, P.; Guazzelli, I.; Halpern, A.; Wajchenberg, B.L.; Ordovas, J.M.; Villares, S.M. Effects of perilipin (PLIN) gene variation on metabolic syndrome risk and weight loss in obese children and adolescents. *J. Clin. Endocrinol. Metab.* **2008**, *93*, 4933–4940. [CrossRef]
20. Tokgöz, Y.; Işık, I.A.; Akbari, S.; Kume, T.; Sayın, O.; Erdal, E.; Arslan, N. Perilipin polymorphisms are risk factors for the development of obesity in adolescents? A case-control study. *Lipids Health Dis.* **2017**, *16*, 52. [CrossRef]
21. Corella, D.; Qi, L.; Tai, E.S.; Deurenberg-Yap, M.; Tan, C.E.; Chew, S.K.; Ordovas, J.M. Perilipin gene variation determines higher susceptibility to insulin resistance in Asian women when consuming a high-saturated fat, low-carbohydrate diet. *Diabetes Care* **2006**, *29*, 1313–1319. [CrossRef] [PubMed]
22. Smith, C.E.; Tucker, K.L.; Yiannakouris, N.; Garcia-Bailo, B.; Mattei, J.; Lai, C.-Q.; Parnell, L.D.; Ordovás, J.M. Perilipin polymorphism interacts with dietary carbohydrates to modulate anthropometric traits in hispanics of Caribbean origin. *J. Nutr.* **2008**, *138*, 1852–1858. [CrossRef] [PubMed]
23. Smith, C.E.; Arnett, D.K.; Corella, D.; Tsai, M.Y.; Lai, C.Q.; Parnell, L.D.; Lee, Y.C.; Ordovás, J.M. Perilipin polymorphism interacts with saturated fat and carbohydrates to modulate insulin resistance. *Nutr. Metab. Cardiovasc. Dis.* **2012**, *22*, 449–455. [CrossRef]
24. Holzbach, L.C.; Silveira, A.G.Z.; Franco, L.P.; Horst, M.A.; Cominetti, C. Polymorphism *PLIN1* 11482 G>A interacts with dietary intake to modulate anthropometric measures and lipid profile in adults with normal-weight obesity syndrome. *Br. J. Nutr.* **2021**, 1–9. [CrossRef]
25. Keisler, D.H.; Daniel, J.A.; Morrison, C.D. The role of leptin in nutritional status and reproductive function. *J. Reprod. Fertil. Suppl.* **1999**, *54*, 425–435. [CrossRef] [PubMed]
26. Landecho, M.F.; Tuero, C.; Valentí, V.; Bilbao, I.; de la Higuera, M.; Frühbeck, G. Relevance of Leptin and Other Adipokines in Obesity-Associated Cardiovascular Risk. *Nutrients* **2019**, *11*, 2664. [CrossRef] [PubMed]
27. Harris, R.B.S. Direct and indirect effects of leptin on adipocyte metabolism. *Biochim. Biophys. Acta BBA Mol. Basis Dis.* **2014**, *1842*, 414–423. [CrossRef]
28. Zhang, H.H.; Souza, S.C.; Muliro, K.V.; Kraemer, F.B.; Obin, M.S.; Greenberg, A.S. Lipase-selective functional domains of perilipin A differentially regulate constitutive and protein kinase A-stimulated lipolysis. *J. Biol. Chem.* **2003**, *278*, 51535–51542. [CrossRef]
29. Clifford, G.M.; Londos, C.; Kraemer, F.B.; Vernon, R.G.; Yeaman, S.J. Translocation of hormone-sensitive lipase and perilipin upon lipolytic stimulation of rat adipocytes. *J. Biol. Chem.* **2000**, *275*, 5011–5015. [CrossRef]
30. Jois, A.; Navarro, P.; Ortega-Senovilla, H.; Gavela-Pérez, T.; Soriano-Guillén, L.; Garcés, C. Relationship of high leptin levels with an adverse lipid and insulin profile in 6–8 year-old children in Spain. *Nutr. Metab. Cardiovasc. Dis.* **2015**, *25*, 1111–1116. [CrossRef]
31. Qi, L.; Shen, H.; Larson, I.; Schaefer, E.J.; Greenberg, A.S.; Tregouet, D.A.; Corella, D.; Ordovas, J.M. Gender-specific association of a perilipin gene haplotype with obesity risk in a white population. *Obes. Res.* **2004**, *12*, 1758–1765. [CrossRef] [PubMed]
32. Sone, Y.; Yamaguchi, K.; Fujiwara, A.; Kido, T.; Kawahara, K.; Ishiwaki, A.; Kondo, K.; Morita, Y.; Tominaga, N.; Otsuka, Y. Association of lifestyle factors, polymorphisms in adiponectin, perilipin and hormone sensitive lipase, and clinical markers in Japanese males. *J. Nutr. Sci. Vitaminol.* **2010**, *56*, 123–131. [CrossRef] [PubMed]

33. Richardson, K.; Louie-Gao, Q.; Arnett, D.K.; Parnell, L.D.; Lai, C.-Q.; Davalos, A.; Fox, C.S.; Demissie, S.; Cupples, L.A.; Fernandez-Hernando, C.; et al. The *PLIN4* variant rs8887 modulates obesity related phenotypes in humans through creation of a novel miR-522 seed site. *PLoS ONE* **2011**, *6*, e17944. [CrossRef]
34. Yan, W.; Chen, S.; Huang, J.; Shen, Y.; Qiang, B.; Gu, D. Polymorphisms in *PLIN* and hypertension combined with obesity and lipid profiles in Han Chinese. *Obes. Res.* **2004**, *12*, 1733–1737. [CrossRef] [PubMed]
35. Meirhaeghe, A.; Thomas, S.; Ancot, F.; Cottel, D.; Arveiler, D.; Ferrières, J.; Amouyel, P. Study of the impact of perilipin polymorphisms in a French population. *J. Negat. Results Biomed.* **2006**, *5*, 10. [CrossRef] [PubMed]
36. Bergmann, A.; Li, J.; Reimann, M.; Hentrich, T.; Hanefeld, M.; Bornstein, S.R.; Schwarz, P.E.H. Polymorphisms in perilipin gene (*PLIN*) are not associated with obesity and weight variation in people with high risk of type 2 diabetes. *Exp. Clin. Endocrinol. Diabetes* **2008**, *116*, S56–S58. [CrossRef] [PubMed]
37. Hu, D.-S.; Xie, J.; Yu, D.-H.; Xu, G.-H.; Lu, J.; Yang, J.-X.; Li, C.-Y.; Li, Y.-Y. Perilipin gene 1237 T > C polymorphism is not associated with obesity risk in northern Chinese Han adults. *Biomed. Environ. Sci.* **2009**, *22*, 442–447. [CrossRef]
38. Peeters, A.; Beckers, S.; Verrijken, A.; Mertens, I.; Van Gaal, L.; Van Hul, W. Possible role for *ENPP1* polymorphism in obesity but not for *INSIG2* and *PLIN* variants. *Endocrine* **2009**, *36*, 103–109. [CrossRef]
39. Angeli, C.B.; Kimura, L.; Auricchio, M.T.; Vicente, J.P.; Mattevi, V.S.; Zembrzuski, V.M.; Hutz, M.H.; Pereira, A.C.; Pereira, T.V.; Mingroni-Netto, R.C. Multilocus analyses of seven candidate genes suggest interacting pathways for obesity-related traits in Brazilian populations. *Obesity* **2011**, *19*, 1244–1251. [CrossRef]
40. Ordovas, J.M. Gender, a significant factor in the cross talk between genes, environment, and health. *Gend. Med.* **2007**, *4* (Suppl. S2), S111–S122. [CrossRef]
41. Jang, Y.; Kim, O.Y.; Lee, J.H.; Koh, S.J.; Chae, J.S.; Kim, J.Y.; Park, S.; Cho, H.; Lee, J.E.; Ordovas, J.M. Genetic variation at the perilipin locus is associated with changes in serum free fatty acids and abdominal fat following mild weight loss. *Int. J. Obes.* **2006**, *30*, 1601–1608. [CrossRef] [PubMed]
42. Greenberg, A.S.; Egan, J.J.; Wek, S.A.; Garty, N.B.; Blanchette-Mackie, E.J.; Londos, C. Perilipin, a major hormonally regulated adipocyte-specific phosphoprotein associated with the periphery of lipid storage droplets. *J. Biol. Chem.* **1991**, *266*, 11341–11346. [CrossRef]
43. Grahn, T.H.M.; Zhang, Y.; Lee, M.-J.; Sommer, A.G.; Mostoslavsky, G.; Fried, S.K.; Greenberg, A.S.; Puri, V. FSP27 and PLIN1 interaction promotes the formation of large lipid droplets in human adipocytes. *Biochem. Biophys. Res. Commun.* **2013**, *432*, 296–301. [CrossRef]
44. Shijun, L.; Khan, R.; Raza, S.H.A.; Jieyun, H.; Chugang, M.; Kaster, N.; Gong, C.; Chunping, Z.; Schreurs, N.M.; Linsen, Z. Function and characterization of the promoter region of perilipin 1 (PLIN1): Roles of E2F1, PLAG1, C/EBPβ, and SMAD3 in bovine adipocytes. *Genomics* **2020**, *112*, 2400–2409. [CrossRef] [PubMed]

MDPI
St. Alban-Anlage 66
4052 Basel
Switzerland
Tel. +41 61 683 77 34
Fax +41 61 302 89 18
www.mdpi.com

Nutrients Editorial Office
E-mail: nutrients@mdpi.com
www.mdpi.com/journal/nutrients

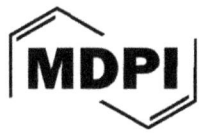

www.ingramcontent.com/pod-product-compliance
Lightning Source LLC
LaVergne TN
LVHW070045120526
838202LV00101B/632